Advanced Structured Materials

Volume 53

More information about this series at http://www.springer.com/series/8611

Juliana Marchi
Editor

Biocompatible Glasses

From Bone Regeneration to Cancer Treatment

Springer

Editor
Juliana Marchi
Centro de Ciências Naturais e Humanas
Universidade Federal do ABC
Santo André
Brazil

ISSN 1869-8433 ISSN 1869-8441 (electronic)
Advanced Structured Materials
ISBN 978-3-319-44247-1 ISBN 978-3-319-44249-5 (eBook)
DOI 10.1007/978-3-319-44249-5

Library of Congress Control Number: 2016950409

Printed on acid-free paper

This Springer imprint is published by Springer Nature
The registered company is Springer International Publishing AG
The registered company address is: Gewerbestrasse 11, 6330 Cham, Switzerland

To my parents, Flavia and Alvaro (in memoriam) for being my life example; to my husband Cleidson due to his complicity; to my brother Sergio due to our conversations that always enrich my scientific productions; and to my sons Beatriz and Gabriel.

Foreword

Bioglasses are an intriguing and challenging class of biomaterials, which present important technological application, involving health and life.

The results of the elaboration of this book, which involve historic concepts, evolution and knowledge consolidation, and directions for the future of the developed glass materials and its application as a biomaterial, are a precious contribution not only for researchers, but for students that intent to start or are developing their studies as well as for professionals from correlated areas.

The contribution of authors from different places of the world, allowed the covering of current issues presented in 13 consistent chapters, which allow the general comprehension of each explained subject and encourage the continuing to learn more about the development and application of these always innovative materials.

At the end of this book, we are certain that this is an important work and a great gift to all material science community.

Frank Ferrer Sene
José Roberto Martinelli (in memorian)
Materials Science and Technology Center,
Energy and Nuclear Research Institute,
São Paulo, Brazil

Acknowledgments

To my editor Mayra Castro, by encouraging me and believing in this work.

To the authors and their staff who made the 13 chapters of this book, by accepting this challenge, and trusting in the final result of this work.

To Dr. José Roberto Martinelli (in memoriam) for sharing an incredible desire of working with biocompatible glasses, and appreciating distinct applications of these materials that will make difference in life quality of many people in a near future. I hope to give you some flavors of these huge knowledges along these chapters.

To my research group (counting those who do not work direct with biocompatible glasses) including undergraduate and graduate students, as well as all my professional colleagues; In special, Roger Borges for the operational support and for being always available to help me when required.

Contents

Editor's Notes

The aim of this book is to provide an in-depth understanding about the main technological breakthroughs in biocompatible glasses and their applications. Recently, thanks to the scientific progress in biology, materials science, and computational simulation, it has been observed significant evolution in the knowledge concerning glass structure, mechanism of reactions, and biological response of biocompatible glasses.

This book was didactically organized; therefore, even a layperson will easily be introduced to the fascinating biocompatible glasses world, since the basic concepts are shown over the initial chapters, being followed by more advanced topics.

The first two chapters refer to the history of biomaterials focused on bioactive glasses. Concepts regarding tissue engineering, tissue regeneration, and bioactivity are explored as from the advent of bioactive glasses. The history of these materials is presented taking into consideration not only the most common compositions, but also those recently developed. These two chapters offer the basic concepts needed to understand very specific and advanced issues in the field of biocompatible glasses. On third, fourth, and fifth chapters, it is established a relationship between concepts of chemical composition and structure of bioactive glasses and their bioactivity properties, including both experimental and theoretical approach. In addition, on the sixth chapter, it is given a deep description about preparation and properties of the different forms of bioactive glasses, in which suggestive applications related to microstructure are addressed. From Chapters "45S5 Bioglass Based Scaffolds for Skeletal Repair" to "Glasses for Treatment of Liver Cancer by Radioembolization", these applications are discussed from bone regeneration (Chapter "45S5 Bioglass Based Scaffolds for Skeletal Repair") to cancer treatment (Chapter "Biocompatible Glasses for Cancer Treatment"). Chapter "Glasses for Treatment of Liver Cancer by Radioembolization" highlights the usage of biocompatible glasses for cancer treatment by radioembolization due to the importance of this issue in the field of glasses. Many of these applications have used glasses as biomaterial, however, these glasses have compositions that exceed the usual ones of bioactive glasses. These specific glasses are reviewed on Chapters "Vitreous Materials for Dental Restoration and Reconstruction" and "Glasses for Treatment of

Liver Cancer by Radioembolization." Chapter "Biocompatible Glasses for Controlled Release Technology" shows how bioactive glasses can be used as technologies for controlled release such as drug delivery systems. This chapter also shows how these glasses can be used to improve the aforementioned applications. Finally, on Chapter "Future Applications of Bioglass" future perspectives and applications of biocompatible glasses are addressed.

The usage of glass materials for biomedical applications goes beyond the use of common bioactive glasses, such as the Bioglass 45S5®. Other glasses like borate and phosphate have been explored, as well as those doped with therapeutic ions. Then, this book have authors who use the term bioglass, bioactive glass and biocompatible glasses as synonym. Particularly, in Chapters "45S5 Bioglass Based Scaffolds for Skeletal Repair" and "Vitreous Materials for Dental Restoration and Reconstruction," bioglass is generically used for glasses made of quaternary, ternary or binary systems similar to Bioglass 45S5®. On Chapters "Biocompatible Glasses for Cancer Treatment" and "Biocompatible Glasses for Controlled Release Technology," the authors used the term biocompatible glasses, which is a more comprehensive term including not only silicate glasses like bioactive glasses, but phosphate and borate glasses which also show bioactivity and biocompatibility properties. On Chapters "Bioactive Materials: Definitions and Application in Tissue Engineering and Regeneration Therapy," "Structure and Percolation of Bioglasses," "Bioactive Glasses: Advancing From Micro to Nano and Its Potential Application" and "Future Applications of Bioglass" the term bioactive glass is used as synonym of bioglass. On the other hand, on Chapters "An Introduction and History of the Bioactive Glasses," "The Evolution, Control, and Effects of the Compositions of Bioactive Glasses on their Properties and Applications," "What Can We Learn From Atomistic Simulations of Bioactive Glasses?" and "Special Applications of Bioactive Glasses in Otology and Ophthalmology," the term bioactive glass is used as synonym of biocompatible glass. These terms are exchangeable because bioactivity is synonym of biocompatibility, and both terms are strongly related one to each other along bioactive materials history.

In conclusion, it is expected that the reader can have the knowledge needed to understand biocompatible glasses under a critical point of view, and be able to use this expertise to conduct its own scientific research in this field, contributing to the scientific community by developing materials for new applications not yet covered in this book.

Enjoy it!

Santo André, Brazil Juliana Marchi

Bioactive Materials: Definitions and Application in Tissue Engineering and Regeneration Therapy

Jon Whitlow, Arghya Paul and Alessandro Polini

Abstract The field of biomaterials has been evolving at an astonished rate in the last decades, leading to the design of *bioactive materials*, materials able to elicit specific and predictable cells and tissues responses. This chapter will go through the key milestones achieved during this exciting development with special emphasis on the meaning of material-driven bioactivity and its importance in the optimization of highly performing tissue regeneration and regeneration therapy methodologies. An overview on the history of bioactive glasses (bioglasses) (please consult the Editor's note in order to clarify the usage of the terms bioglass, bioactive glass and biocompatible glass) and their biological properties will describe the huge potential of these materials in regenerative medicine applications. Finally, an introduction on stem cells and their role in the physiological development of tissues and organs will be given, shedding light on therapeutic synergistic approaches based on the use of bioactive materials and stem cells.

1 Biomaterials History

According to the American National Institute of Health "any substance or combination of substances, other than drugs, synthetic or natural in origin, which can be used for any period of time, which augments or replaces partially or totally any tissue, organ or function of the body, in order to maintain or improve the quality of

J. Whitlow · A. Paul
BioIntel Research Laboratory, Department of Chemical and Petroleum Engineering, Bioengineering Graduate Program, School of Engineering, University of Kansas, Lawrence, KS, USA

A. Polini
Radboud Excellence Initiative, Radboud University, Nijmegen, The Netherlands

A. Polini (✉)
Department of Biomaterials, Radboud University Medical Center, Nijmegen, The Netherlands
e-mail: alessandro.polini@radboudumc.nl; apolini00@gmail.com

J. Marchi (ed.), *Biocompatible Glasses*, Advanced Structured Materials 53,
DOI 10.1007/978-3-319-44249-5_1

life of the individual" can be intended as biomaterial. This definition is largely accepted but it is far from being fully comprehensive (e.g., orthodontic brackets and surgical instruments are not included). The last decades have shown how the idea of biomaterials can be differently interpreted and giving a sharp definition is extremely difficult [1]. The main reason relies on the huge dynamicity of the biomaterials research, developed rapidly in the last fifty years.

Although the above mentioned concept of biomaterials has been developed in the modern age, their use dates to more than 2000 years ago when Egyptians, Romans, Chinese, and Aztecs used to employ largely available materials, such as wood, gold and ivory, for repairing craniofacial defects. Poly (methyl methacrylate) (PMMA), a non-degradable polyacrylate, can be considered the first biomaterial of the modern age. Its excellent tissue biocompatibility was accidentally studied in World War II military pilots that experienced intraocular implantation of PMMA fragments during aircraft crushes, opening the way to the use as biomaterial for contact lenses, orthopedic fillers and medical devices. Since then, the field has matured swiftly with increasing focus on how biomaterials interact with the body (Fig. 1).

At the beginning of the modern biomedical research (during the 1960s and 1970s), biomaterials were chosen among (bio)inert, often synthetic, materials able to evoke (nearly) no tissue response, similarly to the case of PMMA. Their main function was largely structural: they needed to provide mechanical integrity in a reproducible way and avoid a massive immune response, which could potentially

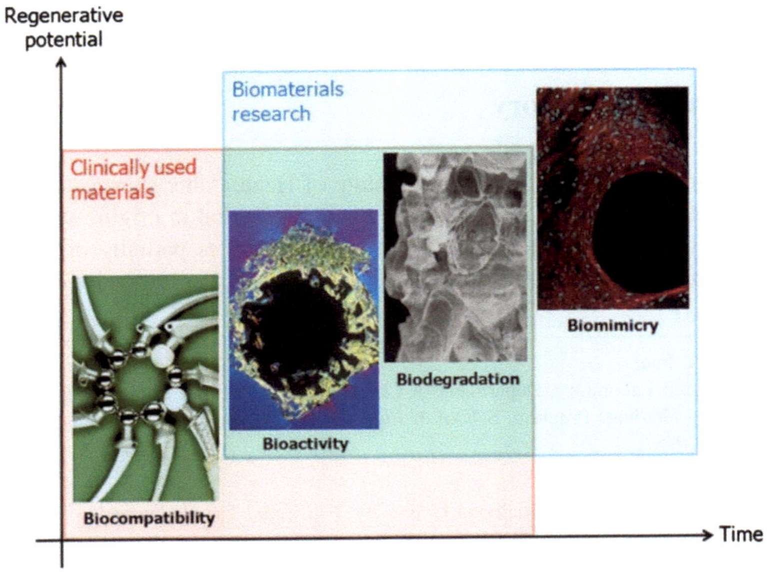

Fig. 1 Summary of the development of biomaterials field in the modern age: different generation of biomaterials focused on different fundamental aspects. Figure reprinted with permission from the publisher [2]

affect the device performance and patient health [3]. During the development of this first-generation biomaterials, the typical approach was based more on a trial and error basis rather than a scientific hypothesis driven method, mostly due to a very limited knowledge regarding how materials and biological components (cells, tissues, body) could interact. The aim was to obtain a material with the right combination of chemical and physical properties in order to match the body target [4]. A plethora of different materials were studied as part of medical implants and devices, such as hip replacements, dental restoratives, contact lenses and vascular stents. For example, metals such as stainless steel and, later, passivated cobalt-chromium alloys replaced carbon and vanadium, often suffering by corrosion, while as polymers we witnessed a switch from nylons and polyesters to not-degradable polymers, such as polytetrafluorethylene (PTFE), PMMA, polyethylene and silicones. Overall, *inert* materials, i.e., having very limited biological activity, were chosen in order to minimize the immune response and prevent body rejection: they caused the formation of a thin, acellular fibrous capsule, with no or limited adhesion with the surrounding tissues [5]. Due to their robust use in routine surgical procedures and vast knowledge of their interaction with body tissues, some of these materials are still applied today.

The molecular biology revolution of the 1970s brought new tools and information to better understand the foreign body response and, therefore, the field of biomaterials was positively affected. Second-generation biomaterials were mostly designed to be bioactive, showing ability to trigger specific biological responses at the biomaterial-tissue interface in a controlled way [5]. Mainly orthopedic and dental fields exploited the use of bioactive materials, such as bioactive glasses, ceramics, glass–ceramics and composites, to guarantee a bioactive implant fixation and bone tissue regeneration (larger description of the bioactivity concept will be provided in the following paragraph). In addition, this phase mainly focused on resorbable biomaterials: the chemical degradation of the foreign biomaterial at the biomaterial-host tissue interface was replaced by neo-tissue with, ultimately, no distinct differences between the implant site and host tissue [4]. However, survival analysis regarding some of these biomaterials used in skeletal prosthetic devices and synthetic heart valves reported that a third to half of them failed within 10 to 25 years, leading to the need of a revision surgery [4]. This drawback is related to the main difference between the highly dynamic living tissue and the relatively static synthetic biomaterials, which fail to respond actively to changes of the microenvironment. This consideration stimulated the development of more biology-based biomaterials.

The advancements in genomics and proteomics in the 1990s and 2000s considerably modified the concept of biomaterials leading to a new (third) generation where the concept of bioactivity and resorbability were merged [4]. Scientists focused on modification of resorbable materials at the molecular level, by adding distinct moieties able to modify specific cell functions. Cell proliferation, differentiation and production/organization of extracellular matrix (ECM) components were affected towards the final goal of tissue regeneration. Specific molecules fundamental for the development of functional tissues started to be incorporated in commercial products, like in the case of bone morphogenetic proteins for osteogenic implants.

Aimed at meeting increasingly high clinical and patient expectations, scientists developed the current (fourth) generation of biomaterials that includes the so often called smart or biomimetic biomaterials [2]. The idea underneath this new class comes from the hypothesis that only by mimicking nature's hierarchical structures and mechanisms, optimized in millions of years, we can obtain a functional and physiological recovery of body tissues. The design of new materials is therefore continuously re-shaped following the latest advancements in the understanding of tissue development and regeneration. From a clinical point of view, smart materials are engineered to actively respond to internal or external stimuli (e.g., changes in pH, ionic strength, magnetism, temperature) and participate to the regeneration of tissue damages. Materials such as ceramics, glasses and polymers, proposed in older generations of biomaterials, can be further modified with tissue engineering approaches, e.g., by partially altering their components or being processed with different procedures, to confer smart capabilities. Aspects such as chemistry, nano/micro architecture, and porosity as well as degradation rate assume new importance for directing the cell behavior [6–8].

2 Bioactivity Concept and Bioactive Materials

According to the pioneering definition of Larry L. Hench et al., "a bioactive material is one that elicits a specific biological response at the interface of the material which results in the formation of a bond between the tissues and the material" [9]. It is well-known that the biomaterial-host tissue interface plays a crucial role in the fate of any implant. Different materials can elicit different responses at the implant site, e.g., generating the formation of non-adherent fibrous capsule as in the case of inert biomaterials. The thickness of such fibrous capsule can vary in accordance to the implant material and the stress at the implant microenvironment, and progressively increases due to the micromotion at the capsule-host tissue interface [10]. The micromotion can be minimized by morphological and biological fixation processes: in the first case, a dense (non-porous) material fits the defect, while in the second case the material presents pores larger than 100–150 μm for allowing tissue ingrowth. In the case of bioactive materials, they generate several biophysical and biochemical reactions at the biomaterial-host tissue interface, with the formation of mechanically strong chemical interfacial bonding as final result (bioactive fixation). This phenomenon is largely due to the biochemical and biomechanical compatibility of the bioactive material with the target tissue: the bioactive material generates an environment favorable for bone growth and its mineralized interface (a layer of biologically active hydroxyl carbonate apatite, HCA, formed on the implant) represents the connection between living and non-living material [10]. Several ceramics based on calcium phosphate, bioactive glass, and their composites have shown such bioactivity, although mechanism, time dependence, strength and thickness of the bonding are different.

The most common bioactive calcium phosphates are hydroxyapatite (HA) and tricalcium phosphate (TCP), due to their osteoconductivity properties and chemical/crystallographic similarity to the mineral phase of skeletal tissue. They differ mostly in the degradability in vivo: synthetic HA is considered non-resorbable, while TCP is resorbable and able to react with body fluids to form HA [11]. The main differences between synthetic and natural HA from mineralized tissues are the following [10]: (a) Natural HA is a Ca-deficient HA (CDHA) where 3.2–5.8 % is carbonate (therefore it is often referred as HCA) and few other elements (Mg, Na, K as well as trace elements Sr, Pb, Ba) are present, marginally affecting the HA lattice structure; (b) The natural HA shows a slightly anisotropic microstructure while synthetic HA is more isotropic and has larger grain size; (c) Natural HA contains an organic component (1 and 25 % in weight for enamel and bone, respectively). Despite these differences, synthetic HA is able to bond to living tissue with a mechanism that can be described by two models. Following the dissolution/precipitation model, the acidic environment, created by cellular and enzymatic activity at the implant site [12], favors the partial dissolution of HA (with release of Ca^{2+}, HPO_4^{2-} and PO_4^{3-}). This creates a supersaturation of calcium phosphates ions in the surroundings generating a precipitation of a HCA natural-like layer on the synthetic HA crystals that bonds pristine HA from the host. This mechanism results to be slow and strongly affected by the crystallinity and dissolution characters of the synthetic HA. When this shows high crystallinity and poor dissolution, the bone tissue constituents can directly bond to synthetic HA as described by the epitaxial growth model [13]. Globular deposits (0.1–1.1 μm in thickness) and an organized network of collagen fibers are deposited on the implant surface creating a fused cement-like matrix that directs the uniaxial ordered formation of HA crystallites [14].

Most of bioactive glasses compositions processed by the traditional way (high temperature melting, casting and sintering) contains SiO_2, Na_2O, CaO and P_2O_5. As described in the chapter "An introduction and history of the bioactive glasses", the first and most studied bioactive glass is 45S5 Bioglass®, which is composed by 45 % SiO_2, 24.5 % Na_2O, 24.5 % CaO and 6 % P_2O_5 (in weight percent). The bonding of bioactive glasses to bone tissues involves the formation of a HCA, able to create a stable bond with the collagen fibers of damaged tissue [15]. Similarly to bioactive calcium phosphates, the mechanism of HCA layer formation is well defined but the specific steps of the HCA layer-bone tissue integration are less described: protein adsorption from the bone microenvironment, deposition of collagen fibers and other ECM proteins, adhesion and differentiation of bone cells, mineralization processes are probably part of the implant integration process [16]. The formation of the HCA layer is favored by the dissolution of ions from the glass surface that creates surface sites for the growth of HCA from one side and a change in pH able to facilitate the nucleation from the other side [11]. The glass composition is the most important parameter affecting the HCA layer formation and bonding to bone tissue capability. A lower silica content is often correlated with a

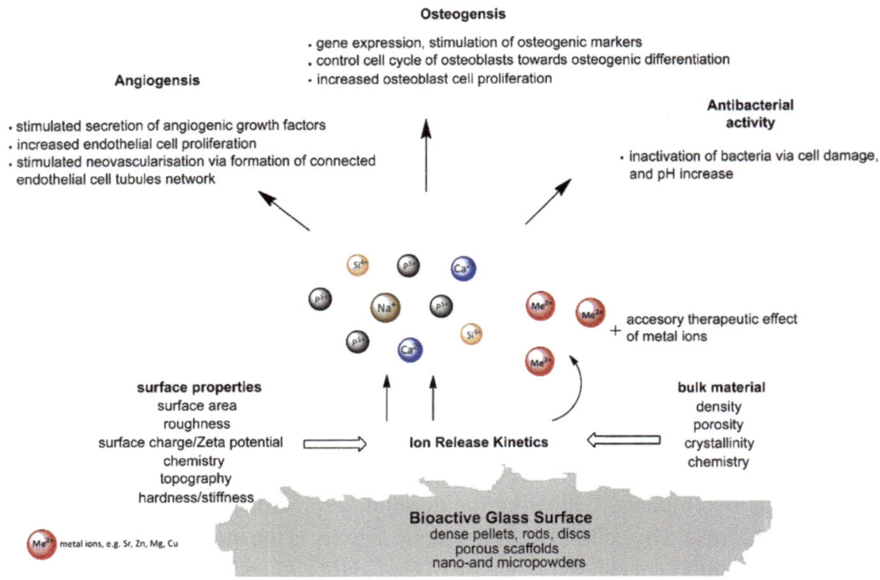

Fig. 2 Summary of biological effects triggered by dissolution products of bioactive glasses. Figure reprinted with permission from the publisher [25]

looser glass network that is more prone to dissolution and leads to faster HCA layer formation. The complexity of the glass network is also modified by the type of other cations present in the composition: for example, when sodium partially replaces silicon, the dissolution rate is increased, while the presence of multivalent ions (e.g., Al^{3+}, Ti^{4+} or Ta^{5+}) decrease this rate and, therefore, the bioactivity [17]. Generally, 60 % represents the maximum amount of SiO_2 that a traditional glass composition can support without losing bioactivity, while sol-gel derived glasses can show bioactivity even at 90 mol% SiO_2 content [18].

More recently, it was observed that dissolution products from bioactive glasses possess further unique properties (Fig. 2) [16]. As mentioned, the HCA layer itself, responsible for the strong bond to bone tissue, is a perfect place for bone cells to adhere, differentiate and form new collagenous matrix that leads to bone nodules, as showed by in vitro experiments where no conventional stimulating factors such as dexamethasone and β-glycerophosphate were employed [19]. In recent years, it was reported that ionic products derived by dissolution of bioactive glass materials are able to affect the gene expression in osteoblastic cells triggering the osteogenic differentiation [20]. Beside the most studied osteogenic pathway, ionic dissolution products can positively interfere with other pathways involving angiogenesis [21], antibacterial and inflammatory responses [22, 23]. These effects are not fully unforeseen considering the effects on bone metabolism belonging to elements such as Sr, Cu, Zn or Co, present as trace in our body [24]. The current challenge in bioactive glass design is to enrich the therapeutic effects of these materials by adding specific ions to their composition: in this way new materials can act as ions depot, making therapeutic ions available upon dissolution. To have a better understanding of the plethora of effects due to the release of these ions from glass materials, more information can be found on the next chapters.

Although calcium phosphate ceramics and bioactive glasses interact with pristine bone tissue in a very effective way, creating a mechanically strong interfacial bond with bone, they show important differences with natural bone: they equal, or even exceed, the strength of the host bone but they do not generally reach its flexural strength, strain-to-failure, and fracture toughness and possess higher elastic moduli. This biomechanical mismatch has limited the use of bioactive materials in load bearing applications, but bioactive composites have been proposed to expand the applicability of these materials. Bioactive glasses can be reinforced with a high fracture tough phase (e.g., metal fibers or ceramic particles) for obtaining bioactive composites with improved bending strength and fracture toughness [26]. These composites are still bioactive as they create a layer of HCA on the surface, although the rate is often lower, and their elastic modulus is generally still higher than bone, leading to stress shielding of bone. Bioactive glass (fibers or particles) can also be used to reinforce a biocompatible polymer phase (polyethylene, poly methyl methacrylate, polysulfone, or collagen), as introduced by Bonfield in the early 1980s [27]. These materials match the elastic modulus of cortical bone (10–20 GPa) and avoid any stress shielding, but no long term (20–40 years) lifetime reports are available and their durability is still to be proven. Another strategy for broadening the use of bioactive glasses in load-bearing applications involves their use as coating material on mechanically suitable materials, such as metals, by enamelling, electrophoretic deposition, laser cladding, thermal spray, sol-gel coating and thin film technologies [28]. Traditionally, bioactive coatings offer a great advantage for fixation of orthopedic implants in the short-term, while their long-term stability and reliability can show limitations.

3 Introduction to Stem Cells for Regeneration Therapy

Stem cells are defined as cells that have the ability to self-renew and differentiate into various lineages upon cell division. The term dates back as early as the 1860s, when German scientist Ernst Haeckel reported his observations on the development of different germ layers from a zygote. Just as the definition of biomaterials has changed over time, as mentioned previously in this chapter, the interpretation and classification of stem cells have also evolved as new discoveries are made. The term was ambiguously defined until the 1960s when McCulloch and Till isolated multipotent hematopoietic stem cells from bone marrow [29]. This discovery spurred extensive research into utilizing stem cells to regenerate or replace damaged tissues. Stem cells are classified by their origin and also by their potency. Embryonic stem cells (ESCs), derived from the inner mass of the blastocyst of an embryo, are pluripotent stem cells, which means that they have the plasticity to differentiate into any type of cell of an organism. ESCs are able to form cells of all three germ layers (the ectoderm, endoderm, and mesoderm) of the body, and they express this pluripotency naturally during gastrulation of embryonic development. When human ESCs were first isolated from blastocysts in 1998, the distinct property of unlimited self-renewal was demonstrated as ESCs that had been cultured in vitro for nearly five months without differentiation were still capable of forming cells of all three germ layers. ESCs inherently express heightened telomerase activity, which accounts for their nearly unlimited self-renewal ability [30]. Adult stem cells (ASCs), first discovered in bone marrow, are multipotent stem cells, which means that they possess a more restricted ability to differentiate and are typically limited to the lineages of the tissue from which the cells are derived. In addition to bone marrow, ASCs are found in adipose, neonatal, muscle, neural, and other tissues of mature organs.

The plasticity of stem cells has been an area of active research by cell biologists for decades. This ability to form cells of an entirely new lineage is in part due to the overlapping expression of many transcription factors. Recent discoveries have found that adult cells can be genetically reprogrammed to attain pluripotency. Induced pluripotent stem cells (iPSCs) were first developed in 2006 by Shinya Yamanaka, by the genetic reprogramming of adult murine fibroblasts. Pluripotency was synthetically induced by retrovirally transducing the fibroblast cells with Oct4, Sox2, cMyc, and Klf4 genes, which are four of the main transcription factors that regulate and maintain pluripotency [31]. Shortly after the discovery of hematopoietic stem cells, bone marrow transplants became the very first clinical procedure to utilize stem cells. The first successful bone marrow transplant in 1968 cured a patient with genetic thymic alymphoplasia and aplastic anemia from graft-verse-host-disease (GVHD) [32]. With over 50,000 transplants per year, bone marrow transplants have become the most prevalent clinical stem cell therapies and are used to treat patients with leukemia and autoimmune disorders [33]. The ease of sourcing ASCs coupled with their relative lack of immunogenicity in transplant procedures has popularized ASCs for use in other clinical treatments such as skin grafting. ESCs have very few clinical applications due to ethical controversies, limited sources, and difficulty in controlling their differentiation. iPSCs, on the other hand, are not implicated with ethical controversy and have a virtually unlimited cell source—however, the formation of iPSCs is a costly process with current technologies. As with ESCs, iPSCs are difficult to control in vivo and can be problematic since they are formed by genetic reprogramming with oncogenes.

4 Bioactive Ceramics and Stem Cells: A Synergistic Approach for Regeneration Therapy

One of the challenges impeding stem cell research is the inability to control the differentiation and quiescence in vivo. This presents a barrier between the lab and the clinic for many potential stem cell treatments. The microenvironment that a stem cell is subjected to modulates the cell's capacity to regenerate and form cells of new lineages. For instance, if ESCs were implanted into an injured organ without any control over the differentiation, the ESCs would generate cells from a variety of lineages and form a teratoma rather than replacement tissue for the damaged organ. Thus, the study of controlled (tissue-specific) stem cell differentiation is of utmost importance for the field of regenerative medicine.

Biomaterials serve as excellent tools for modulating the behavior of stem cells. Bioactive constructs are utilized as platforms for mimicking stem cell niche to induce differentiation towards a desired lineage and enhancing cell engraftment. Stem cell differentiation and proliferation is governed by paracrine and autocrine signaling, i.e., the induction of cell-soluble factors by cell-cell interactions. However, the mechanical properties of the surrounding 3D microenvironment are also vital factors in regulating the physiological environment that is the stem cell niche. Mesenchymal stem cells, for example, develop lineage specificity based on the elasticity of the microenvironment matrix (despite addition of cell-soluble factors). MSCs cultured in soft matrices follow neurogenic pathways while rigid matrices similar to bone invoke a distinct osteogenic pathway [34]. The extracellular matrix (ECM) of cells is a complex 3D network of proteins that provides the microenvironmental structure and the integrin-mediated cell-ECM interactions in naturally occurring tissues. The ECM is a cornerstone for the design of smart biomaterials that direct stem cell differentiation for regenerative therapies. A wide variety of bioactive materials, such as hydroxyapatite (HA), tricalcium phosphate (TCP), chitosan, collagen, and silk fibroin, have been characterized by their interactions with stem cells and abilities to form ECM-mimetic constructs.

4.1 Hydroxyapatite

Given its structural similarity with bone, hydroxylapatite, has been highly praised as a bioactive ceramic among the scientific and medical community for its osteoinductivity and osteoconductivity. Though HA is naturally derived from ECM and is bioactive as a standalone material, applying this material in a tissue scaffold in vivo requires introduction of synthetic composites to match the native biomechanics of bone. Polymers such as polyamide (which shares similarities with collagen) in conjunction with HA can promote the adhesion, proliferation, and differentiation of MSCs to osteoblasts by heightened alkaline phosphatase (ALP) activity and collagen type I expression [35]. The use of specific osteogenic peptide sequences, able to bind selectively HA surfaces, can be another potential way to improve HA materials [36]. A multitude of other composite scaffolds, such as HA in chitosan-gelatin networks, have shown similar osteoconductive interactions with BMSCs in porous 3D scaffolds [37]. Osteoconductivity of HA is the attributed to paracrine/autocrine signaling that is activated by the dissolution of calcium phosphate ions and formation of the interfacial HCA layer described previously in this chapter. The presence of these ions in the extracellular microenvironment causes a cascade of signaling pathways in stem and progenitor cells including upregulation of BMP, Wnt, TGF-β, and MAPK pathways and activation of soluble factor Il1α [38]. Recent efforts in developing osteogenic scaffolds have emphasized the benefits of nanoparticle hydroxyapatite. Nano-HA is a more reactive material than its micro-sized counterpart due to the large surface area to volume ratio. Rod, fiber, and spherical shaped nano-HA impart an enhanced osteogenic effect on BMSCs and favorable mechanical properties in tissue scaffolds [39–41]. Nano-HA has also shown success as a non-viral gene delivery vector for promoting osteogenesis and angiogenesis upon transfection of human BMSCs [42].

4.2 TCP and Biphasic Calcium Phosphates

Tricalcium phosphate is another calcium salt that has a profound osteogenic effect on BMSCs. Through the same mechanisms of osteoinduction as HA, TCP stimulates the formation of the HCA layer and stem cell adhesion, proliferation, and differentiation. TCP ceramics have even been utilized with great success in clinical studies for spinal fusion therapies [43]. TCP is regarded as a more soluble (resorbable) source of CaP ions, while HA is slower to degrade in the human body. Biphasic calcium phosphates (BCPs) such as HA-TCP have been developed to harness the benefits of this solubility difference. The resorption rate of a BCP ceramic scaffold can be tuned by altering the ratio of the soluble phase to the more stable phase. Soluble ceramics (high TCP/low HA concentration) can stimulate BMSC osteogenesis and bone remodeling in vivo [44, 45]. BCPs are also capable of inducing osteogenic differentiation of ESCs [46].

4.3 Silicate Nanoclay

For several decades, silicon has been well documented for its vital role in bone development. Silicate ions, the products of dissolution or degradation of silicon-based scaffolds, activate various cell signaling pathways in BMSCs including the Shh and Wnt pathways [47]. Silica nanoparticles and nanoclays are common bioactive materials that enable stem cell differentiation. Silica nanoplatelets, at a therapeutic threshold, induce osteogenic differentiation of BMSCs and ASCs by increased Col I expression, collagen fibril assembly, and ECM deposition [48, 49]. These bioactive materials can guide stem cells to an osteoblastic phenotype in the absence of dexamethasone or osteogenic cytokines. Mesoporous silica nanoparticles (MSNs) are a promising class of biomaterials that, due to their tunable surface properties and pore sizes, facilitate drug delivery. Though silicates have an inherent ability to stimulate osteogenesis, MSNs can be conjugated with specific drugs to promote specificity to a different stem cell lineages, such as the MSN-induced differentiation of ESCs to cardiomyocytes [50]. Layered silicates known as nanoclays are another form of Si nanoparticle that are gaining attention as bioactive osteogenic materials. Nanoclays in conjunction with calcium phosphates or polymers are viable candidates for stem cell bone regeneration [51, 52].

4.4 Bioactive Glass

As elucidated previously, the dissolution of different types of ions from resorbable bioactive scaffolds has a therapeutic effect towards bone regeneration. The HCA layer, which forms as a result of the signaling pathways triggered by presence of ions, is the bioactive interface that recruits osteoprogenitor cells responsible for bone remodeling and regeneration. Bioglass (BG) is an especially attractive material for osteogenic stem cell treatments due to the therapeutic value of auto/paracrine signal-inducing ions released as the BG degrades. BGs supersede the bioactivity of HA since these materials not only serve as a source of CaP ions but also ions of Si, B, Zn, Mg, Sr, Cu, and Mn. The array of ion species that BG presents on the HCA interface elicits a primary set of cell signaling pathways which combinatorially activates further cellular signals; therefore it is difficult to pinpoint the effects of individual ion species among the mixture. In general, HCA formation and ionic dissolution by BGs promotes osteogenic differentiation of stem cells, such as the controlled differentiation of BMSCs to osteoblasts by culture on BG surfaces [53]. 45S5 Bioglass® (and BGs of other compositions) is also well known to endogenously induce angiogenesis in various cell lines by autocrine upregulation of vascular endothelial growth factor (VEGF) [54]. The ability to promote both bone remodeling as well as vascularization among multipotent, autologous/allogeneic stem cells, simply by ion-mediated cell signaling, renders bioactive glass a novel material for stem cell therapies.

The interactions between stem cells and various ion-doped BG scaffolds have shed light on the functions of specific ion species in the regulation of osteogenesis and angiogenesis. Some examples of ion-doped BG will be given in this section, relating them to stem cell regulation, but, as aforementioned, we suggest you to read the chapters "An introduction and history of the bioactive glasses" and "Structure and percolation of bioglasses", so that you would appreciate further information in which go beyond the stem cells-related examples.

Zinc plays a significant role in osteostimulation by activating transcription factors that regulate stem cell differentiation (osteopontin, osteocalcin, ALP, collagen type I) and helps stimulate HCA formation to drive BMSCs toward an osteogenic lineage [58]. Silicon modulates cell signaling pathways, and initiates collagen I formation as well as bone remodeling (osteoblast differentiation). The therapeutic effects of the dissolution of Si ions from bioglass are illustrated by the histological analysis of fetal osteoblasts in Fig. 3a–c. As the Si concentration is increased in 45S5 Bioglass® scaffolds seeded with fetal osteoblasts, the extent of mineralization of the matured osteoblasts is increased. The highest Si concentration correlates to the greatest extent of calcium nodule formation (Fig. 3c). It has been proposed that Si ions lead to OCN and Col I upregulation in a dose-dependent

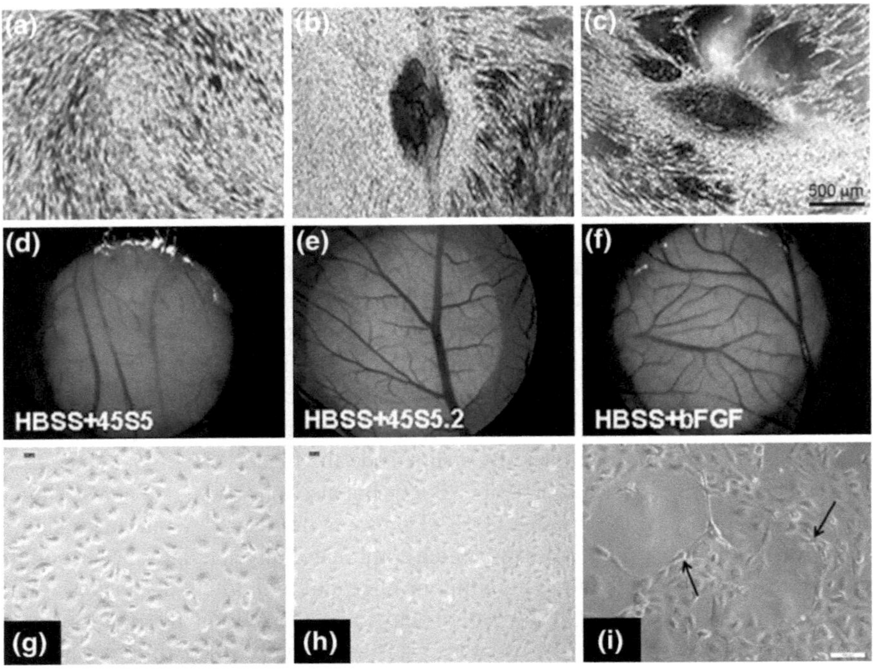

Fig. 3 Osteogenic and angiogenic effects of ion-doped bioglass on stem and progenitor cells: **a–c** Silicon-doped bioglass promotes bone mineralization in fetal osteoblasts. As revealed by red alizarin stains for calcium nodules, an increase in Si concentration in bioglass correlates to increased mineralization, evidenced by **a** 0 μg/mL Si, **b** 15 μg/mL Si and **c** 20 μg/mL Si [55]. **d–f** Boron-doping of bioglass stimulates neovascularization in embryonic quail chorioallantoic membranes. Microscopic imaging reveals that (**d**) bioglass alone induces negligible angiogenic response while (**e**) boron-doped bioglass promotes vascularization to the same extent as **f**, the response to a therapeutic dosage of basic fibroblast growth factor [56]. **g–i** Dissolution of copper ions from BG in conjunction with BMSCs induces a similar angiogenic effect in endothelial cells. **g** BG alone does not promote significant vascularization, nor does (**h**) BG delivered in co-culture with BMSCs. However, **i** copper-doped bioglass administered in co-culture with BMSCs results in significant angiogenic remodeling. Cu ions trigger BMSC-mediated growth of tube-like vasculature, which is denoted by the *arrows* [57]. Figures reprinted with permission from the publishers

manner [55] which explicates the mechanism through which Si ions induce osteogenesis of BMSCs [59]. Regarding strontium, its ions promote differentiation but not proliferation of BMSCs [58]. Other ions, such as manganese ions, when incorporated with bioglass, promote osteogenesis by upregulation of ALP and BMP in progenitor cells [60], while magnesium ions inhibit osteogenesis of multipotent stem cells [59].

Fewer studies underly mechanisms through which bioactive glass stimulates angiogenesis. Though 45S5 Bioglass® has an inherent angiogenic property, ion-doping can further augment this property. For instance, boron-doped 45S5 Bioglass® stimulates neovascularization in the embryonic model of chorioallantoic membrane (Fig. 3d–f). Therapeutic quantities of angiogenic growth factors can be generated in vivo by the release of B ions (by the activation of the $\alpha_v\beta_3$ integrin) [56]. Figure 3e provides evidences that the B ions from bioglass can stimulate vascularization to the same extent as controlled delivery of bFGF. Angiogenic effects are similarly noted for copper-doped bioglass. Dissolution of Cu ions from BG can stimulate both osteogenesis and angiogenesis [57, 61]. Figure 3i represents the angiogenic response to Cu ions in co-culture with endothelial cells and BMSCs and, in contrast to Fig. 3g, h, it is the only group with tube-like vascular networks clearly visible.

4.5 *Polymers and Biomaterials*

Calcium phosphates and ceramic biomaterials have great osteogenic potential in vitro, but to utilize these interactions in a potential stem cell therapy, the material must be arranged in a construct that mimics the structure and biomechanics of natural bone. As established previously in this chapter, the elasticity of the stem cell microenvironment dictates the cells' preference of lineage. A bioactive bone scaffold must be a three-dimensional porous structure that not only enables cell adhesion and proliferation but also promotes vascularization. Synthetic, biocompatible polymers enriched with osteogenic biomaterials can be constructed under these parameters, while allowing for precise tuning of the mechanical properties to match that of bone. Among the most common polymers utilized for this effect are polyethylene glycol (PEG), polylactic acid (PLLA), polycaprolactone (PCL), polyvinyl alcohol (PVA), and polyglycolic acid (PGA). Composites based on these polymers with bioactive materials such as HA, TCP, and bioglass are formed to further construct porous 3D scaffolds that mimic the complex environment required for bone regeneration. Bioactive polymer composites, such as PVA/PLLA/PCL-bioglass/TCP, have synergistic osteogenic effects when combined with multipotent stem cells [7, 62, 63].

4.6 *Emerging Carbon Based Nanomaterials*

Carbon nanomaterials are another class of materials that hold stake in the future of stem cell therapies. Carbon nanotubes (CNTs), nanodiamonds (NDs), and graphene have rich surface chemistries that promote adhesion and proliferation of stem and progenitor cells. CNTs are cylindrical fullerenes that, in conjunction with polymers such as PEG or polyacrylic acid, have shown capabilities as a substrate conducive of not only osteogenic differentiation from BMSCs [64] but also neuronal differentiation of ESCs [65]. Diamond nanoparticles, though more biologically inert that CNTs, can be functionalized with polymers, drugs, peptides, nucleic acids, and other molecules for targeted delivery within the cytoplasm of cells. NDs loaded with cytokines such as BMP-2 can direct BMSCs towards an osteogenic lineage

[66]. Furthermore, defects within the carbon core of NDs enable them to fluoresce in the far red spectrum rendering them useful for long term in vivo fluorescent stem cell labeling [67]. Graphene is a novel fullerene with a two-dimensional honeycomb structure that exhibits an array of exciting mechanical, electrical, and biological properties. Graphene and graphene oxide have proven to be useful substrates for stem cell culture with the ability to stimulate osteogenic differentiation of mesenchymal stem cells [68] as well as a viable substrate for adhesion and proliferation of neural stem cells [69] and iPSCs [70].

Acknowledgments Arghya Paul would like to acknowledge the Institutional Development Award (IDeA) from the National Institute of General Medical Sciences of National Institutes of Health (NIH), under Award Number P20GM103638-04 and University of Kansas New Faculty General Research Fund. Alessandro Polini would like to acknowledge the Radboud Excellence Initiative from Radboud University for funding.

References

1. Williams, D.F.: On the nature of biomaterials. Biomaterials **30**(30), 5897–5909 (2009)
2. Holzapfel, B.M., et al.: How smart do biomaterials need to be? A translational science and clinical point of view. Adv. Drug Deliv. Rev. **65**(4), 581–603 (2013)
3. Ratner, B.D., Bryant, S.J.: Biomaterials: where we have been and where we are going. Annu. Rev. Biomed. Eng. **6**, 41–75 (2004)
4. Hench, L.: Biomaterials. Science **208**(4446), 826–831 (1980)
5. Hench, L.L., Thompson, I.: Twenty-first century challenges for biomaterials. J. R. Soc. Interface **7**(Suppl 4), S379–S391 (2010)
6. Shin, H., Jo, S., Mikos, A.G.: Biomimetic materials for tissue engineering. Biomaterials **24** (24), 4353–4364 (2003)
7. Polini, A., et al.: Osteoinduction of human mesenchymal stem cells by bioactive composite scaffolds without supplemental osteogenic growth factors. PLoS ONE **6**(10), e26211 (2011)
8. Polini, A., Bai, H., Tomsia, A.P.: Dental applications of nanostructured bioactive glass and its composites. Wiley Interdiscip. Rev. Nanomed. Nanobiotechnol. **5**(4), 399–410 (2013)
9. Hench, L.L., et al.: Bonding mechanisms at the interface of ceramic prosthetic materials. J. Biomed. Mater. Res. **5**(6), 117–141 (1971)
10. Cao, W., Hench, L.L.: Bioactive materials. Ceram. Int. **22**(6), 493–507 (1996)
11. Hench, L.L.: Bioceramics: from concept to clinic. J. Am. Ceram. Soc. **74**(7), 1487–1510 (1991)
12. Baron, R.: Cell-mediated extracellular acidification and bone resorption: evidence for a low pH in resorbing lacunae and localization of a 100-kD lysosomal membrane protein at the osteoclast ruffled border. J. Cell Biol. **101**(6), 2210–2222 (1985)
13. Bagambisa, F.B., Joos, U., Schilli, W.: Mechanisms and structure of the bond between bone and hydroxyapatite ceramics. J. Biomed. Mater. Res. **27**(8), 1047–1055 (1993)
14. de Bruijn, J.D., van Blitterswijk, C.A., Davies, J.E.: Initial bone matrix formation at the hydroxyapatite interface in vivo. J. Biomed. Mater. Res. **29**(1), 89–99 (1995)
15. Hench, L.L., Paschall, H.A.: Direct chemical bond of bioactive glass-ceramic materials to bone and muscle. J. Biomed. Mater. Res. **7**(3), 25–42 (1973)
16. Hench, L.L., Polak, J.M.: Third-generation biomedical materials. Science **295**(5557), 1014–1017 (2002)
17. Jones, J.R.: Review of bioactive glass: from Hench to hybrids. Acta Biomater. **9**(1), 4457–4486 (2013)

18. Vallet-Regí, M., Ragel, C.V., Antonio, J.: Salinas, glasses with medical applications. Eur. J. Inorg. Chem. **2003**(6), 1029–1042 (2003)
19. Bosetti, M., Cannas, M.: The effect of bioactive glasses on bone marrow stromal cells differentiation. Biomaterials **26**(18), 3873–3879 (2005)
20. Xynos, I.D., et al.: Gene-expression profiling of human osteoblasts following treatment with the ionic products of Bioglass® 45S5 dissolution. J. Biomed. Mater. Res. **55**(2), 151–157 (2001)
21. Gorustovich, A.A., Roether, J.A., Boccaccini, A.R.: Effect of bioactive glasses on angiogenesis: a review of in vitro and in vivo evidences. Tissue Eng. Part B Rev. **16**(2), 199–207 (2010)
22. Zhang, D., et al.: Antibacterial effects and dissolution behavior of six bioactive glasses. J. Biomed. Mater. Res. A **93**(2), 475–483 (2010)
23. Day, R.M., Boccaccini, A.R.: Effect of particulate bioactive glasses on human macrophages and monocytes in vitro. J. Biomed. Mater. Res. A **73**(1), 73–79 (2005)
24. Beattie, J.H., Avenell, A.: Trace element nutrition and bone metabolism. Nutr. Res. Rev. **5**(1), 167–188 (1992)
25. Hoppe, A., Guldal, N.S., Boccaccini, A.R.: A review of the biological response to ionic dissolution products from bioactive glasses and glass-ceramics. Biomaterials **32**(11), 2757–2774 (2011)
26. Wang, M.: Developing bioactive composite materials for tissue replacement. Biomaterials **24** (13), 2133–2151 (2003)
27. Bonfield, W., et al.: Hydroxyapatite reinforced polyethylene—a mechanically compatible implant material for bone replacement. Biomaterials **2**(3), 185–186 (1981)
28. Sola, A., et al.: Bioactive glass coatings: a review. Surf. Eng. **27**(8), 560–572 (2011)
29. Ramalho-Santos, M., Willenbring, H.: On the origin of the term "stem cell". Cell Stem Cell **1** (1), 35–38 (2007)
30. Thomson, J.A., et al.: Embryonic stem cell lines derived from human blastocysts. Science **282** (5391), 1145–1147 (1998)
31. Takahashi, K., Yamanaka, S.: Induction of pluripotent stem cells from mouse embryonic and adult fibroblast cultures by defined factors. Cell **126**(4), 663–676 (2006)
32. Gatti, R., et al.: Immunological reconstitution of sex-linked lymphopenic immunological deficiency. Lancet **292**(7583), 1366–1369 (1968)
33. Gratwohl, A., et al.: Hematopoietic stem cell transplantation: a global perspective. JAMA **303** (16), 1617–1624 (2010)
34. Engler, A.J., et al.: Matrix elasticity directs stem cell lineage specification. Cell **126**(4), 677–689 (2006)
35. Wang, H., et al.: Biocompatibility and osteogenesis of biomimetic nano-hydroxyapatite/polyamide composite scaffolds for bone tissue engineering. Biomaterials **28**(22), 3338–3348 (2007)
36. Polini, A., et al.: Stable biofunctionalization of hydroxyapatite (HA) surfaces by HA-binding/osteogenic modular peptides for inducing osteogenic differentiation of mesenchymal stem cells. Biomater. Sci. **2**, 1779–1786 (2014)
37. Zhao, F., et al.: Effects of hydroxyapatite in 3-D chitosan-gelatin polymer network on human mesenchymal stem cell construct development. Biomaterials **27**(9), 1859–1867 (2006)
38. Liu, H., et al.: Composite scaffolds of nano-hydroxyapatite and silk fibroin enhance mesenchymal stem cell-based bone regeneration via the interleukin 1 alpha autocrine/paracrine signaling loop. Biomaterials **49**, 103–112 (2015)
39. Zandi, M., et al.: Biocompatibility evaluation of nano-rod hydroxyapatite/gelatin coated with nano-HAp as a novel scaffold using mesenchymal stem cells. J. Biomed. Mater. Res. A **92**(4), 1244–1255 (2010)
40. Zhou, D.S., et al.: Repair of segmental defects with nano-hydroxyapatite/collagen/PLA composite combined with mesenchymal stem cells. J. Bioact. Compat. Polym. **21**(5), 373–384 (2006)

41. Huang, Y., et al.: Micro-/nano- sized hydroxyapatite directs differentiation of rat bone marrow derived mesenchymal stem cells towards an osteoblast lineage. Nanoscale **4**(7), 2484–2490 (2012)
42. Curtin, C.M., et al.: Combinatorial gene therapy accelerates bone regeneration: non-viral dual delivery of VEGF and BMP2 in a collagen-nanohydroxyapatite scaffold. Adv. Healthcare Mater. **4**(2), 223–227 (2015)
43. Gan, Y., et al.: The clinical use of enriched bone marrow stem cells combined with porous beta-tricalcium phosphate in posterior spinal fusion. Biomaterials **29**(29), 3973–3982 (2008)
44. Arinzeh, T.L., et al.: A comparative study of biphasic calcium phosphate ceramics for human mesenchymal stem-cell-induced bone formation. Biomaterials **26**(17), 3631–3638 (2005)
45. Sun, H., et al.: The upregulation of osteoblast marker genes in mesenchymal stem cells prove the osteoinductivity of hydroxyapatite/tricalcium phosphate biomaterial. Transpl. Proc. **40**(8), 2645–2648 (2008)
46. Tang, M., et al.: Human embryonic stem cell encapsulation in alginate microbeads in macroporous calcium phosphate cement for bone tissue engineering. Acta Biomater. **8**(9), 3436–3445 (2012)
47. Han, P., Wu, C., Xiao, Y.: The effect of silicate ions on proliferation, osteogenic differentiation and cell signalling pathways (WNT and SHH) of bone marrow stromal cells. Biomater. Sci. **1**(4), 379–392 (2013)
48. Mihaila, S.M., et al.: The osteogenic differentiation of SSEA-4 sub-population of human adipose derived stem cells using silicate nanoplatelets. Biomaterials **35**(33), 9087–9099 (2014)
49. Mieszawska, A.J., et al.: Osteoinductive silk-silica composite biomaterials for bone regeneration. Biomaterials **31**(34), 8902–8910 (2010)
50. Ren, M., et al.: Ascorbic acid delivered by mesoporous silica nanoparticles induces the differentiation of human embryonic stem cells into cardiomyocytes. Mater. Sci. Eng. C **56**, 348–355 (2015)
51. Ambre, A.H., Katti, D.R., Katti, K.S.: Nanoclays mediate stem cell differentiation and mineralized ECM formation on biopolymer scaffolds. J. Biomed. Mater. Res. A **101**(9), 2644–2660 (2013)
52. Gaharwar, A.K., et al.: Nanoclay-enriched poly(ε-caprolactone) electrospun scaffolds for osteogenic differentiation of human mesenchymal stem cells. Tissue Eng. Part A **20**(15–16), 2088–2101 (2014)
53. Ohgushi, H., et al.: Osteogenic differentiation of cultured marrow stromal stem cells on the surface of bioactive glass ceramics. J. Biomed. Mater. Res. **32**(3), 341–348 (1996)
54. Day, R.M.: Bioactive glass stimulates the secretion of angiogenic growth factors and angiogenesis in vitro. Tissue Eng. **11**(5–6), 768–777 (2005)
55. Tsigkou, O., et al.: Differentiation of fetal osteoblasts and formation of mineralized bone nodules by 45S5 Bioglass conditioned medium in the absence of osteogenic supplements. Biomaterials **30**(21), 3542–3550 (2009)
56. Haro Durand, L.A., et al.: Angiogenic effects of ionic dissolution products released from a boron-doped 45S5 bioactive glass. J. Mater. Chem. B **3**(6), 1142–1148 (2015)
57. Rath, S.N., et al.: Bioactive copper-doped glass scaffolds can stimulate endothelial cells in co-culture in combination with mesenchymal stem cells. PLoS ONE **9**(12), e113319 (2014)
58. Wu, X., et al.: Zn and Sr incorporated 64S bioglasses: material characterization, in-vitro bioactivity and mesenchymal stem cell responses. Mater. Sci. Eng. C **52**, 242–250 (2015)
59. Ojansivu, M., et al.: Bioactive glass ions as strong enhancers of osteogenic differentiation in human adipose stem cells. Acta Biomater. **21**, 190–203 (2015)
60. Miola, M., et al.: In vitro study of manganese-doped bioactive glasses for bone regeneration. Mater. Sci. Eng. C **38**, 107–118 (2014)
61. Wu, C., et al.: Copper-containing mesoporous bioactive glass scaffolds with multifunctional properties of angiogenesis capacity, osteostimulation and antibacterial activity. Biomaterials **34**(2), 422–433 (2013)

62. Larrañaga, A., et al.: Effect of bioactive glass particles on osteogenic differentiation of adipose-derived mesenchymal stem cells seeded on lactide and caprolactone based scaffolds. J. Biomed. Mater. Res. A **103**, 3815–3824 (2015)
63. Handel, M., et al.: 45S5-Bioglass((R))-based 3D-scaffolds seeded with human adipose tissue-derived stem cells induce in vivo vascularization in the CAM angiogenesis assay. Tissue Eng. Part A **19**(23–24), 2703–2712 (2013)
64. Nayak, T.R., et al.: Thin films of functionalized multiwalled carbon nanotubes as suitable scaffold materials for stem cells proliferation and bone formation. ACS Nano **4**(12), 7717–7725 (2010)
65. Chao, T.-I., et al.: Carbon nanotubes promote neuron differentiation from human embryonic stem cells. Biochem. Biophys. Res. Commun. **384**(4), 426–430 (2009)
66. Suliman, S., et al.: Release and bioactivity of bone morphogenetic protein-2 are affected by scaffold binding techniques in vitro and in vivo. J. Controlled Release **197**, 148–157 (2015)
67. Wu, T.-J., et al.: Tracking the engraftment and regenerative capabilities of transplanted lung stem cells using fluorescent nanodiamonds. Nat. Nano **8**(9), 682–689 (2013)
68. Nayak, T.R., et al.: Graphene for controlled and accelerated osteogenic differentiation of human mesenchymal stem cells. ACS Nano **5**(6), 4670–4678 (2011)
69. Akhavan, O., Ghaderi, E.: Differentiation of human neural stem cells into neural networks on graphene nanogrids. J. Mater. Chem. B **1**(45), 6291–6301 (2013)
70. Chen, G.Y., et al.: A graphene-based platform for induced pluripotent stem cells culture and differentiation. Biomaterials **33**(2), 418–427 (2012)

An Introduction and History of the Bioactive Glasses

Gurbinder Kaur, Steven Grant Waldrop, Vishal Kumar, Om Prakash Pandey and Nammalwar Sriranganathan

Abstract When the hierarchy turns towards higher level, the molecular events become more complex and convoluted. The human embryo development is quite complex as it originates from a 32-celled stage and metamorphoses by a series of metabolic and physical processes. The process of fetus formation is full of breathtaking complexity as it involves the development of lungs, heart, gut, nerves, limbs, bones, blood vessels, cartilages, circulatory system, nervous system and excretory system. The constant wear and tear of muscles, joints and other vital body tissues takes place during the lifetime of human body. Due to the advancement of medical science, artificial limbs and transplantation have helped the human body to resume the day-to-day chores, but the biomaterials have revolutionized the world due to their capability to repair the damaged tissues by self-healing mechanism. These days, the bioactive materials have become an imperative and indispensable tool for the medical science due to their numerous advantages. Hence, the current focus is given on the history, categories and requirements of the biomaterials especially bioactive glasses (please consult the Editor's note in order to clarify the usage of the terms bioglass, bioactive glass and biocompatible glasses).

1 Bioactive Glasses as Biomaterials

The naturally occurring or man-made non-natural materials, which are used to supplement, replenish or enhance the living tissue functionality, are regarded as biomaterials [1]. Biomaterials can be classified as (a) metals (b) synthetic or natural polymers (c) ceramics/bioactive glasses and (d) composites, which are shown in

S.G. Waldrop · N. Sriranganathan
Blacksburg, VA, USA

G. Kaur (✉) · O.P. Pandey
SPMS, Thapar University, Patiala 147004, India
e-mail: gkaur82@vt.edu

V. Kumar
SGGSWU, Fatehgarh Sahib, India

J. Marchi (ed.), *Biocompatible Glasses*, Advanced Structured Materials 53,
DOI 10.1007/978-3-319-44249-5_2

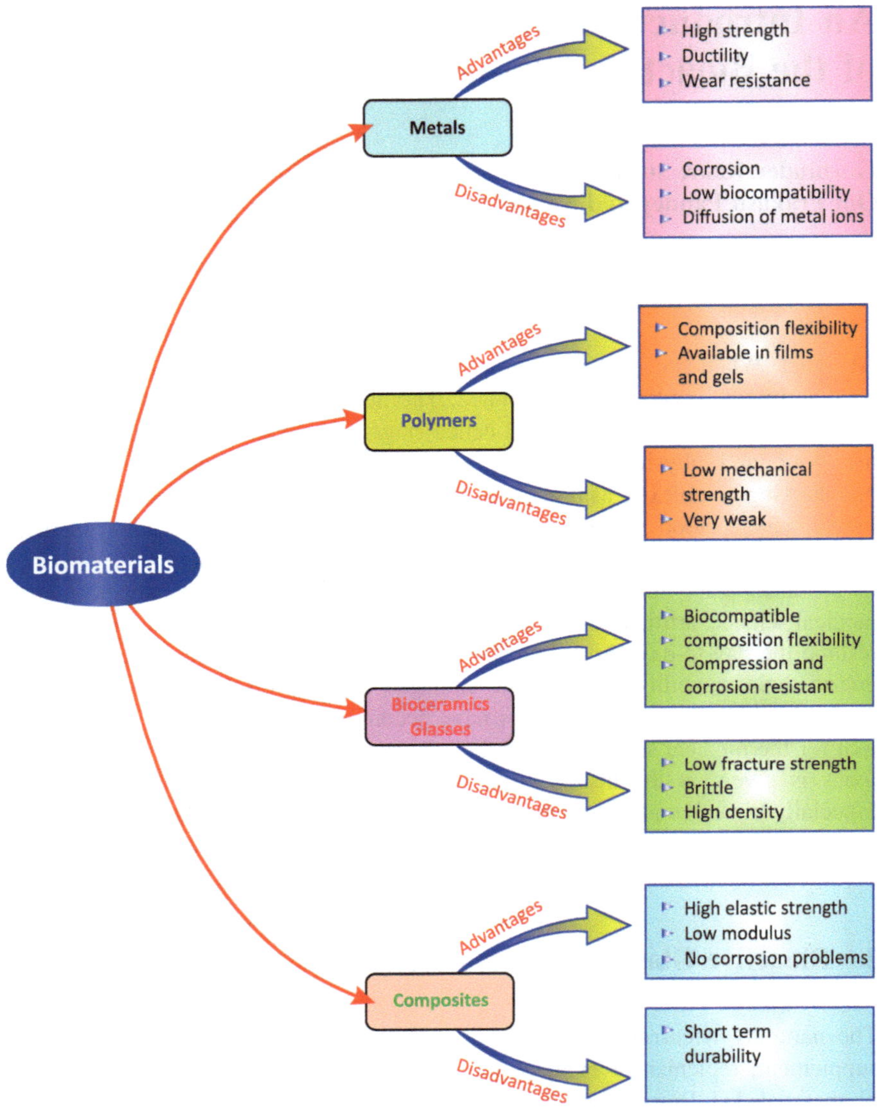

Fig. 1 Categorization of bioactive materials

Fig. 1. Metals possess high strength, wear resistance and ductility. Anyhow, their low biocompatibility and high corrosion rate are detrimental for living tissues. Furthermore, allergic reactions may be caused due to the high diffusion of metal ions, which result in irreparable loss to the human tissues [2]. Polymers are endowed with the composition flexibility, which endows them with their distinctive features. However, polymers cannot withstand the stresses required in various orthopedic and load bearing applications due to their low mechanical strength. In contrast to this, the composites compose of cross-linked elastomer units, which endow them with high elastic moduli and is beneficial for the biocompatibility. Ceramics is a superior category of materials, which generally posses resistance to corrosion and compression along with good biocompatibility. The brittle nature, high density, low fracture strength and small resilience of ceramics can cause problems in their bioactive properties. Individually, these materials may pose different problems, but when combined together to form a composite, the synergistic effect of all the components can enhance their mechanical and bioactive properties. For instance, biodegradable polymer scaffolds do not posses hydroxyapatite (HA) inorganic phase, which is mechanically biocompatible and hence its use is challenging. In contrast to this, the scaffolds fabricated from the bioceramics such as bioactive glass or calcium phosphate-based inorganic materials usually provide enhanced bioactive properties as well as higher mechanical strength [3, 4]. All these biomaterials find potential applications inside the human body as shown in Fig. 2. Almost every joint and body part needs biomaterial in direct or indirect way.

The eminence of human lives has been influenced to a large extent by a special class of materials regarded as bioceramics. Bioceramics exist as composites (polyethylene-hydroxyapatite), monocrystals (sapphire) or polycrystalline materials (hydroxyapatite) [5]. When the bioceramic material/bioactive glasses are implanted inside the host tissue, then time-dependent kinetic modification takes place on their surface due to interface formation biological hydroxyapatite layer [6, 7]. More specifically, when we define the word "bioactive glasses", it refers the glass endowed with an ability of hydroxyapatite (HA) layer formation on the surface via a chain of certain specific reactions and possesses compatibility with the surrounding living tissues. Broadly, a bioactive material yields target specific biological activity after incorporation of metal ions in their composition. Since 1969, many research groups have been working tirelessly in developing novel bioactive glasses as the potential breakthrough in the hot field of regenerative medicines and tissue engineering. Biomaterials are foci of attraction due to their ability to yield wide change in bioactive/thermal/physical properties even after minor tailoring of constituents in their chemical composition [5–9]. Resorbability is one of the indispensable requirements for any biomaterial (including bioactive glasses) i.e. the biomaterials should degrade over period of time after implantation, so that its functionality can be replaced by the natural host tissue [5, 9]. During the degradation period, resorbable biomaterials require stable interface as well as the matching of resorption rates, which makes tissues repairing easy. The bioactive glasses should also be non-carcinogenic, non-antigenic, non-toxic and non-mutagenic, in order to avoid any detrimental effect on the host cells [6–8]. A bioactive material undergoes a two-step process when implanted inside the body i.e. it comes in contact with the simulated body fluid (SBF) and undergoes a set of specific surface reactions thereby forming a HA-like biological layer, responsible for the hard and soft tissues interactions [10].

These days, for the bone repair applications, the attention has shifted towards materials possessing crystallographic and chemical similarity to the biphasic calcium phosphate (BCP), calcium phosphate-based bioceramics such as natural bone mineral HA ($Ca_{10}(PO_4)_6(OH)_2$), fluorapatite, β-tricalcium phosphate (β-TCP, $Ca_3(PO_4)_2$), and other calcium phosphates [11]. HA is a carbonated phosphate and

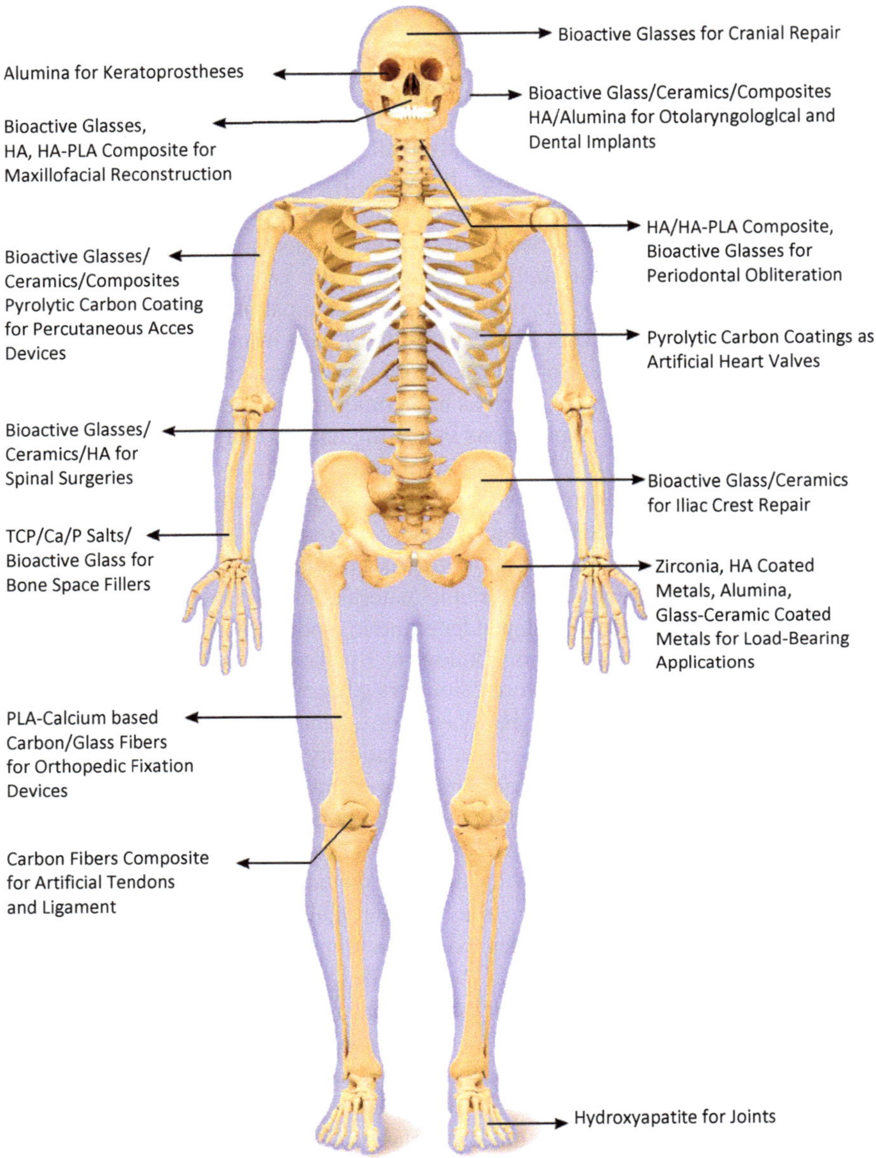

Fig. 2 Use of biomaterials/bioactive glasses inside the human body for various applications

calcium-deficient bone mineral and regarded as one of most stable phase among other reported calcium phosphates. HA is osteoconductive because it supports bone regeneration by showing excellent bonding at the bone–implant interface. Though, amorphous HA possess high degradation rates, but it does not exhibit enough mechanical strength to build and sustain a 3-dimensional porous network. In spite

Table 1 Calcium phosphates along with their Ca/P ratios [17]

Calcium phosphate	Chemical formula	Ca/P
Calcium metaphosphate	$Ca(PO_3)_2$	0.5
Calcium phosphate monohydrate	$Ca(H_2PO_4)_2 \cdot H_2O$	0.5
Tetracalcium phosphate diacid	$Ca_4H_2P_6O_{20}$	0.67
Heptacalcium phosphate	$Ca_7(P_5O_{16})_2$	0.7
Calcium pyrophosphate dehydrate	$Ca_7P_2O_7 \cdot 2H_2O$	1
Calcium phosphate	$Ca_7P_2O_7$	1
Dicalcium phosphate	$CaHPO_4$	1
Dicalcium phosphate dihydrate	$CaHPO_4 \cdot 2H_2O$	1
Octacalcium phosphate	$Ca_8H_2(PO_4)_6 \cdot 5H_2O$	1.33
Tricalcium phosphate	$Ca_3(PO_4)_2$	1.5
Calcium phosphate	$Ca_{10-x}H_{2x}(PO_4)_6(OH)_2$	–
Hydroxyapatite	$Ca_{10}(PO_4)_6(OH)_2$	1.67
Tetracalcium phosphate	$Ca_{10}O(PO_4)_2$	2.0

of the fact that in vitro formation of an HA-like biological surface layer takes place upon immersion in a SBF for some materials like dicalcium phosphate dehydrate, no evidence of direct in vivo bone bonding could be reported [12, 13]. Contrary to this, β- TCP shows extensive bonding to bone, inspite of the fact that it necessarily does not lead to the formation of a biological HA-layer upon its contact with the SBF [14]. HA possess relatively slower resorption rates and undergoes slight conversion to a bone-like material upon implantation. As compared to other calcium phosphates, HA yields higher mechanical strength [11, 12]. A better control over biological behavior and degradation rates could be obtained using DCP with different HA to β-TCP ratios [15].

Ca/P ratio is the fundamental criteria, used to determine the stoichiometry, acidity and solubility of apatites. Ca/P ratios for some prominent calcium phosphates is listed in Table 1. Higher Ca/P ratio yields lower acidity and solubility and vice versa. The Ca/P ratio of the converted material usually varies from the surface to the interior of the reacted glass. The carbon presence in apatite results in lattice distortion causing micro-stresses and crystalline defects in the network, which play an imperative role in the apatite solubility. Clinical investigations confirmed that the implanted calcium phosphates and hydroxyapatites remain within the body for 6 to 7 years post-implantation and hence regarded as virtually inert [16].

2 Implantation and Transplantation

Bone structure consists of the encased cells in composite matrix composed of collagen fibers and apatite phase [18, 19]. Bone possesses excellent mechanical properties such as flexural strength and hardness. Anyhow, due to age related problems like osteoarthritis, osteoporosis, the bone requires regeneration, which can

Table 2 The first transplants of heart, lung and kidney [20–25]

Transplant	USA	Europe	Asia
First heart transplant	Dr. Denton A. Cooley and his team, in Texas (1968)	Dr. Maurice on 66 year old man, in Paris (1968)	Dr. Wada at Sapporo Medical University, in Japan (1968)
First lung transplant	Dr. James Hardy at the University of Mississippi, in Missisippi (1963)	John Wallwork at Papworth Hospital (UK), in UK (1984)	Dr. Tan and team in Singapore, in Singapore (2009)
First kidney transplant	Dr. J.E. Murray at the Peter Bent Brigham Hospital, in Boston (1954)	Dr. D. Alfani and group at Clinica Chirurgica, in Italy (1982)	Dr. Kusunoki in University of Tokyo, in Tokyo (1956)

be achieved via transplantation or implantation. Organ transplantation involves the transfer of an organ from a donor site to another location on the person's own body (autografts) or from one body to another to replace the damaged/absent organ of recipient. Transplants are composed of nonliving or living tissues and may include the harvesting of patient's own tissue from a donor region, thereby followed by the transplantation on the damaged region. Organs like heart, kidneys, lungs, liver, pancreas, and intestine can be transplanted. Globally, the most common transplant is the kidney transplant followed by the heart and liver. Dr Christiaan Barnard, a South African doctor at Groote Schuur Hospital (Cape Town, South Africa) performed world's first human to human heart transplant on 3 December 1967 [20]. Table 2 lists some of the vital human organs transplants [20–25]. Tissue transplants have outnumbered the organ transplant because bones, heart valves, muscoskeletal grafts, cornea transplants, skin, nerves, and veins have been widely practiced with higher success rates over decades.

In contrast to this, during the implantation process, some man-made biocompatible materials like bioceramics/glasses especially scaffolds are used for the regeneration purpose. The organ transplantation requires matching of tissue type, blood type, body statistics and potential recipient availability etc. whereas for the bioactive glass implantation process, the important parameters to be considered are resorbability, dissolution and biocompatibility. During the glass network dissolution, a silica-rich layer is formed on the glass surface, which is further followed by the calcium phosphate apatite layer formation. Apatite layer formation depends upon the glass composition, surface, pore size, along with the preparation conditions. Bioactive glasses fall under the category of class A bioactive materials, which reveals their ability to bond well with the bone and the soft tissue via HA layer formation [26].

3 Elements Required by Human Body

Certain elements are required by human body for regulating the body fluids and maintaining the acid–base balance because they are the vital constituents of human organs or body parts. Almost 90 % of human tissues consist of water whereas hydrogen, carbon, nitrogen and oxygen, are the major constituents of proteins, amino acids, ribonucleic acids (RNA) and deoxyribonucleic acids (DNA) [27]. Hence, all these elements are deemed as the basic building blocks of human body, which makes it necessary to obtain an insight of their relative abundance in the biological tissues/cells. Broadly, the elements required for the vital functioning of human body are classified as microelements and macroelements. The elements required by human tissues are summed up in Table 3 along with their importance. Macroelements are required >100 mg/dl whereas microelements are required up to <100 mg/dl. Calcium, phosphorus, sodium, chlorine, potassium etc. fall into the category of macroelements whereas magnesium, copper, strontium, zinc, iron, sulphur, chromium, etc. are the microelements [2, 28–30]. Both the deficiencies and excess of these elements can result in major public health problems. Hence, the intake of all these elements shall be balanced in order to sustain healthy functioning of organs. The bioactive glasses composition may consist of these elements and for the non-hindered working of these bioactive glasses, the in vivo glass degradation is relevant such that the trace elements release from the scaffolds must be less than the toxic level.

The basic building block of bioactive glasses is silicon, which contributes to the structure and resilience of the connective tissues due to its cross-linking properties [31, 32]. Silicic acid is the physiological form of silica and it interacts with the aqueous aluminum to yield less harmful/toxic hydroxyl aluminosilicates [33]. Chlorine (Cl), Sodium (Na), and potassium (K) are the principal constituents of the extracellular fluids and regulate osmotic pressure. Their deficiency can cause decreased motor response and slow neural activity. Calcium is required for the membrane permeability, muscle contraction, as well as neuromuscular excitability. For the synthesis of phospholipids and phosphoproteins, phosphorus is required.

The excess of phosphorus can cause chronic nephritis and hypoparathyroidism whereas its deficiency leads to osteomalacia or De-Toni Fanconi syndrome. Both calcium and phosphorus are important constituents of bones and teeth, and low Ca/P ratio is included in hypothyroidism [34]. Magnesium is also present in bones and is an essential activator for the diphosphopyridinenucleotide kinase, phosphate-transferring enzymes myokinase and creatine kinase whereas strontium helps in bone resorption and calcification. Strontium has yielded promising results during the osteoporosis treatment [35, 36]. The tendon reflexes get deeply depressed due to the deficiency of magnesium. Barium oxides increase the surface adherence by reducing surface tension and barium crystals are used in radio-opaque bioactive glasses and bone cements as an opacifier [37, 38]. Barium oxide provides non-bridging oxygen (NBO's) to the glass structure because it is a very strong modifier, thereby enhancing the apatite layer formation [39]. Chromium is an effective cross-linking agent for collagen and plays a role in maintaining the RNA molecule configuration. "Glucose tolerance factor" (GTF), which activates/binds/potentiates insulin action composes of trivalent chromium.

Other elements like cobalt, iron, copper, manganese, zinc, and iodine etc. also play an imperative role to sustain the normal functioning of the human body/organs. Cobalt is required as a cofactor of enzymes involved in amino acid metabolism and DNA biosynthesis and constituent of vitamin B12. Copper is considered to be

Table 3 Role of elements in human body

Name of the element	Role
Silicon	Mucopolysaccharides component, bone calcification, connective tissue component, biological cross linking agent, to maintain connective tissues resiliency
Sodium	Plasma volume regulation, Principal constituent cation of extracellular fluid, osmotic pressure maintenance, nerve impulses transmission, amino acids and bile salts absorptive processes
Potassium	Principal constituent cation in the extracellular fluid, osmotic pressure maintenance, glycogenesis, helps in cardiac muscle contraction
Chlorine	Electrolyte and fluid balance, principal constituent anion in gastric juice and extracellular fluid
Calcium	Bones and teeth constituent, nerve regulation, activation of enzymes, neuromuscular excitability
Phosphorous	Teeth and bones constituent, constituent of nucleic acids and adenosine triphosphate
Magnesium	Constituent of enzyme system containing thymine pyrophosphate cofactor, bones and teeth component, activator for phosphate transferring enzymes
Strontium	Promote bones and teeth calcification along with bone healing and bone resorption
Barium	Bone opacifier
Chromium	RNA molecule configuration maintenance, primary ingredient in glucose tolerant factor
Cobalt	Component of vitamin B_{12}, cofactor of enzymes involved in DNA biosynthesis
Copper	Required for neurologic and hematologic systems, myelin sheath formation in nervous systems, enzyme constituent, promotes iron absorption
Iodine	Constituent of thyroid hormones
Iron	Vital component of hemoglobin, cellular respiration enzymes, required in spinal cord myelination, neurotransmitters synthesis and packaging
Manganese	Hydrolase and decarboxylase cofactor, required in glycoprotein, constituent of enzymes required for pyruvate metabolism and urea formation
Molybdenum	Metalloenzymes constituent, regulates cellular metabolism
Selenium	Component of glutathione peroxidase, involved in defense system protecting organisms from oxidant with vitamin E and harmful free radicals
Zinc	Enzyme cofactor, cell replication, vitamin A and E metabolism, wound healing and tissue repair
Fluorine	Increases bone hardness and enamel remineralization, dental caries prevention
Sulfur	Required for connective tissue, nails, skin, hair and amino acid
Nickel	Membrane structure maintenance, prolactin control
Boron	Promotes bone formation

essential micro-nutrient required for the haematologic and neurologic systems. The proteins containing copper are regarded as erythrocuprein in red blood cells, hepatocuperin in liver and cerebrocuperin in brain [34]. Copper is also reported to promote bone formation but 10^{-6} M concentration of Cu^{2+} is found to inhibit the osteoclast activity [40, 41]. Copper is and angiogenic agent and triggers endothelial cells towards angiogenesis. Cu enhances the mesenchymal stem cells differentiation towards the osteogenic lineage [29]. Cu is required for the myelin sheaths formation in the nervous systems and helps in iron incorporation in haemoglobin as well as supports iron absorption from the gastrointestinal tract (GIT) long with the iron transfer from tissues to the plasma [29]. The excess of copper causes Wilson disease and liver poisoning, though its deficiency is associated with cardiac hypertrophy and cardiac failure and anaemia due to reduced ferroxidase function. Iodine is stored in thyroid as thyroglobulin and one of the essential component of the thyroxine, thyroid hormones, and mono-, di-, and tri-iodothyronine. Many enzymes such as phosphohydrolases and phosphotransferases, which are involved in the proteoglycans synthesis in cartilage have manganese as cofactor. Mn is also an essential part of the enzymes involved in urea formation, pyruvate metabolism and the galactotransferase of connective tissue biosynthesis. The enzymes involved for the metabolism of nitrogen-containing compounds present in DNA and RNA production and sulphur-containing amino acid and production of uric acid contain molybdenum as a cofactor. Selenium acts as a synergistic antioxidant with vitamin E and its activities are closely related to the antioxidative properties of coenzyme Q (ubiquinone) and tocopherol (vitamin E) [29, 30]. Connective tissue, Coenzyme A, skin, hair and nails and amino acids like cystine, cysteine and methionine are sulfur rich. Biotin and thiamine are the members of vitamin B complex and also contain sulfur in their respective molecules.

Zinc plays a vital role in insulin and plasma component and also acts as a cofactor for many dehydrogenase enzymes, regarded necessary for the cell replication as well as macronutrient metabolism [30]. It also helps in healing wounds and tissue repair, developing taste buds and anti-inflammation [42]. Zinc binds specific DNA regions to monitor genetic control of cell proliferation and helps in vitamin A and E metabolism. Iron is essential for the white matter myelination of cerebellar folds in brain and it is also a cofactor for many neurotransmitter system enzymes. Basically, Fe is transferred as transferrin, accumulated as ferritin/hemosiderin and vanishes in sloughed cells. Iron (Fe) is an important component of heme of hemoglobin (Hb), succinate dehydrogenase, cytochrome and myoglobin [29, 30]. Anemia is caused by iron deficiency whereas its excessive accumulation can cause hemosiderosis, neurologic disorders like Alzheimer, Parkinson disease and neuro-degeneration [43]. Conclusively, for the healthy uninterrupted functioning of human body, all these elements shall be optimized through the intake of balanced diet. Boron is a trace element, required for the bone health.

4 Design Criteria for Biomaterials/Bioactive Glasses

Biomaterials should be designed in such a manner to provide required essential structural compatibility without posing any adverse effects on the living tissues [15–18]. The most outstanding property of bioactive glasses, is their ability to enhance revascularization, osteoblast adhesion, enzyme activity, and mesenchymal stem cell differentiation. In addition to this, bioactive glasses act as promising filler materials/coatings for polymer structures empowering them to work bone tissue engineering applications [16–18, 26]. The indispensable criteria, which shall be considered while designing the bioactive biomaterials is the cytotoxicity in order to ensure that the elemental release is lower than their biologically safe levels. Figure 3 lists all the essential features that must be kept in consideration while designing suitable bioactive glass. To obtain bioactive glass ceramics, glass is heated at a fixed temperature for fixed duration in controlled atmosphere leading to the formation of crystalline phases embedded in the amorphous glassy matrix. The flexural/mechanical strength and viscous behavior of the glass gets enhanced during crystallization process. Crystallization process in bioactive glass causes decrease in bioactivity, indicating that the glass ceramic compromises for the bioactivity though it is mechanically stronger than the counterpart amorphous glass [44, 45]. The bioactive glass cells of potential biomedical interest are harvested into the scaffold, such that a scaffold symbolizes a macroporous 3-dimensional structural device retaining the geometry and environmental conditions as that of the host-replacement

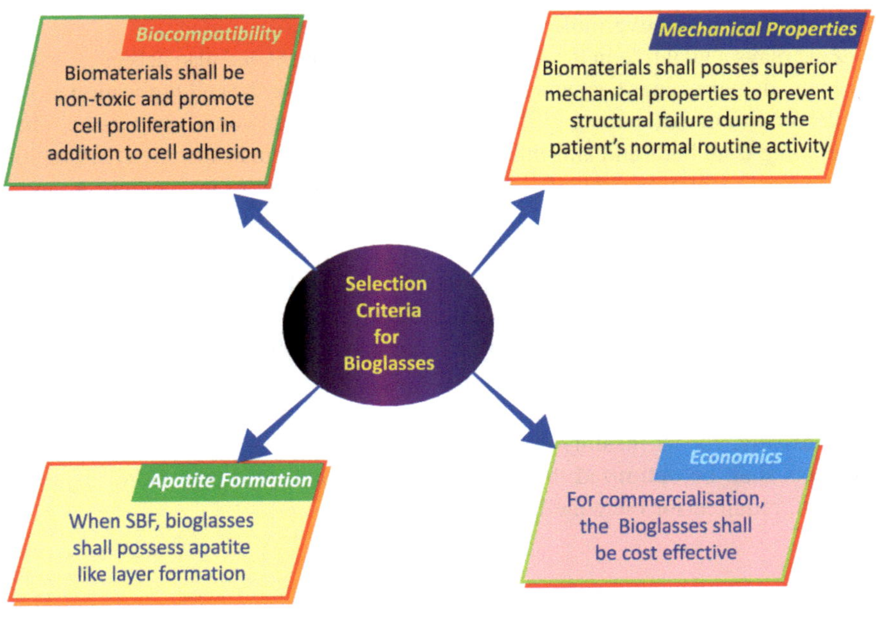

Fig. 3 Design consideration of bioactive glass

tissues required for stimulating tissue regeneration [46]. The properties of bioactive glasses due to their particle size and shape/size of granules shall be considered while using bioactive glasses for producing filler materials, porous scaffolds and dental materials. Some of essential parameters required for the bioactive glass scaffolds to retain its functionality as a suitable biomaterial are listed as follows [2, 16–18, 47]:

1. The bioactive glass is heat treated at a suitable temperature for particular time duration to obtain scaffolds. During the heat treatment, nucleation and growth of the crystalline phases may occur in the glassy matrix. The formed crystalline phases must not hamper interrupt the bioactive processes inside the cell/tissue induced due to the cytotoxic effect.
2. Bioactive glass scaffolds shall not demonstrate immunogenicity/cytotoxicity or posses any inflammatory response.
3. Tissue scaffolds must exhibit neogenesis as they shall deliver a temporary structure required for new tissue synthesis. Moreover, they should degrade into easily resorbable nontoxic products, which can be excreted by the body.
4. The mechanical properties of bioactive glass scaffolds must possess superior mechanical properties as that of the host tissue for better biocompatibility. Also, both the bulk materials and surface shall be sterile.
5. For bone engineering, bioactive glass should exhibit a typical porosity of almost 90 % with a minimum pore diameter of almost 100 μm to enhance tissue vascularization. The controllable interconnected porosity supports vascularization and also direct cells to proliferate into the required physical structure.
6. The glass scaffolds must have porous 3-D architecture for cell vascularization, proliferation and nutrient diffusion, thereby providing an optimized microenvironment for new tissue synthesis.

Therefore, all the above-mentioned criteria are required for obtaining suitable bioactive glasses/scaffolds for the technological and biomedical applications.

5 Different Types of Bioactive Glasses

Due to the versatile applications of the bioactive glasses (Fig. 2), the research interest has been in the field of biomedical application of bioactive glasses since last four decades. The importance of this fuming field of bioactive glasses is clearly depicted from the constantly increasing number of publications. Many research groups are actively engaged to fabricate borate/borosilicate, silicate, and phosphate bioactive glasses. Some mesoporous glasses have also been investigated for the targeted drug delivery applications. Many trace elements have also been incorporated into the glass network for obtaining the desired properties for bone remodeling and/or associated angiogenesis. This section describes different bioactive glasses and their bioactive properties.

5.1 *Silicate Glasses*

Most silica structures consist of basic tetrahedra $(SiO_4)^{4-}$ and the connectivity can be in 1-, 2-, and 3-dimensional arrangements. Each oxygen anion is coordinated by two Si cations corresponding to corner sharing of the oxide tetrahedral, thereby resulting in relatively open structures and prevention of the close-packing of anion layers [48, 49]. Silicon plays a vital role in bone mineralization and gene activation. The deciding factor for the intracellular and extracellular response of bioactive glasses is the release of soluble ionic forms of Si, Na, P and Ca from the glass surface, 45S5 Bioglass W, a silica-based composition has shown enhanced secretion of vascular endothelial growth factor in vitro [50]. Silicate bioactive glasses (13-93 or 45S5) support the proliferation and differentiation of MLO-A5 and MC3T3-E1 osteoblastic cells, in vitro cell culture [51]. Silica spheres and organic ligands find desirable applications in immuno arrays and biological molecule detection. Hence, silica based bioactive glasses are attracting attention of researchers especially in the field of drug delivery and nanomedicine [52].

5.2 *Borate/Borosilicate Glasses*

Though, 45S5 silicate compositions have been the main theme of investigation for many years but borosilicate and borate compositions have also been investigated extensively [47, 51, 53–55]. The first borosilicate glasses for biomedical applications was proposed in 1990 by Brink et al. [53]. The content of B_2O_3 was tailored to achieve desirable properties. Borate glasses have lower chemical durability and are very reactive, hence they degrade rapidly and get converted to HA as compared to their silica counterparts [54]. Borate glasses lead to high level of local boron content near the vicinity of the glass as they quickly release high concentrations of boron. Therefore, the degradation and sintering behavior of borate/borosilicate glass is more controlled compared to silicate glasses. Tissue infiltration in vivo, cell proliferation and differentiation in vitro is enhanced by borate glasses. However, some reports indicate that toxicity is associated with the $(BO_3)^{3-}$ ions and certain borate glasses compositions exhibited cytotoxic effects under static conditions, in vitro [55]. The toxic effects of borate bioactive glasses can be reduced by dilution of the phosphate solution, dynamic cell culture, or partial conversion of borate-based glass to hydroxyapatite (prior to tissue culture).

5.3 *Phosphate Glasses*

Phosphate based glasses were first proposed in 1980 and P_2O_5 acts as a network former oxide in them. Phosphate glasses contain a highly asymmetric phosphate

$[PO_4]$ tetrahedron structural unit [48, 49]. This asymmetry is the origin of low durability of these glasses and hence eases P–O–P bonds hydration [56]. The special feature of phosphate glasses, which endows them for soft-tissue engineering as guides for muscle/nerve repair is that they can be spun into glass fibers. Phosphate glasses have been regarded as "smart materials" for soft-tissue engineering applications as they yielded positive results for in vivo tests performed on phosphate glass nerve guides, such as tubes or meshes [57]. The phosphate glasses are regarded as bone tissue regenerative materials for hard tissue engineering. Phosphate glasses are strongly dependent on composition and possess great potential as regenerative medicine. The dissolution rate of phosphate glasses can be monitored by doping appropriate metal oxides to their composition, such as TiO_2, MnO, NiO, SrO, CuO, and Fe_2O_3 [2]. Phosphate glasses have also been widely investigated for 3D construction of muscular tissues and as drug carriers of antibacterial ions such as silver, zinc, copper and gallium.

5.4 Doped Glasses

Glass properties like bioactivity, bioresorbability and/or biodegradability can be modified to a large extent using "dopants" or additional additives such as La, In, Y, Fe, Cu, Zn, Cr, Sr and Ba in their composition to make it [58, 59]. To endow particular properties to the glass, different oxides can be incorporated in the glass network in addition to SiO_2, B_2O_3, and P_2O_5. Bioactive glass compositions doped with silver have yielded antibacterial properties while retaining their bioactive function whereas K_2O, Na_2O, CaO, and MgO are helpful in adjusting the pH of surroundings [60]. Apart from AgO, other oxides like ZnO, TiO_2 and CuO also allow the ion release imparting antibacterial properties to the material. Zinc and magnesium have exerted a stimulatory effect on proliferation/differentiation of osteoblasts and bone mineralization. To strengthen the mechanical properties of glasses, Al_2O_3 is used due to its high hardness, abrasion resistance and bioinertness making it suitable material for dental and bone implants [61]. The incorporation of strontium in the bioactive glass can accelerate bone-healing processes and osteogenesis along with reduced bone resorption [35]. The drug strontium ranelate has increased the fracture-healing ability of rat bones in terms of callus resistance. A significant increase in callus resistance compared to the untreated control group could be seen in the group of rats treated with strontium ranelate.

5.5 Metallic Glasses

The bulk metallic glasses [BMG] possess outstanding properties of superior strength, high fracture toughness, high elastic strain limit, and low young's modulus [62, 63]. In addition to this, these glasses are biodegradable without hydrogen evolution, in vivo. Zirconium based metallic glasses has found potential applications in biomedical engineering as Zirconium has high mechanical strength and fracture toughness. The presence of trace radio elements in zirconium may affect the cytotoxicity of BMG.

5.6 *Mesoporous Glasses*

Conventional bioactive glasses are without mesopore structures (thereby reducing drug delivery) whereas pure mesopore SiO_2 like Mobil Composition of Matters (MCM)-4 1exhibit low bioactivity. A new class of biomaterials known as mesoporous glasses is developed to overcome these demerits of materials (in 2004 for $CaO–SiO_2–P_2O_5$ composition), which is endowed with enhanced drug delivery and excellent bioactivity [47, 64, 65]. The mesoporous glasses are fabricated by the sol-gel method and then involve incorporation of structure directing agents like P123 (EO20-PO70-EO20), F127 (EO106-PO70-EO106) and cetyltrimethyl ammonium bromide (CTAB) into the glass network structure [64, 65]. The mesoporous bioactive glasses belong to third generation bioactive glasses, and hence act as controlled delivery systems attributed to the entrapment and subsequent release of different drug molecules in the mesopore cavities. Mesoporous bioactive glasses (MBG) exhibit better cytocompatibilty, enhanced in vitro/in vivo bioactivity, along with excellent drug-delivery capability due to their highly ordered pore wall and mesoporous structure with a pore diameter ranging from 5 to 20 nm [64–66]. MBG is a solution to the problem of osteomyelitis (due to bacterial infection) in bone reconstruction as the drugs can be released through a local drug system on the implant site.

6 History and State of Art of Bioglasses

Bioactive materials have revolutionized the field of biomedical engineering due to their versatile characteristics. These days the time span of human organs like knees, joints, hips and degenerated tissues can be increased by incorporated suitable biomaterials. The first revolution of biomaterials came into existence during the 1960–1970 decade and it was an era of implantation of prosthetic devices inside human body with maximum compatibility. These biomaterials were bio-inert, non-toxic and corrosion resistant metals/polymers. Inspite of these superior features, biomaterials are subject to wear and tear causing mismatch of elastic moduli between bone and implanted biomaterial, tissue breakdown and loosening with passage of time duration. The second major breakthrough in the field of medical science occurred with the development of second generation biomaterials i.e. when a special category of "bioactive glasses" was discovered by L.L. Hench (1967–1969), while working at University of Florida, Gainesville, USA [67]. The idea of developing the special Bioglass was seeded into his brain by Colonel Klinker, who returned to US after a duty tour in Vietnam. Both of them were sharing a bus ride and colonel Klinker

Table 4 Composition of the glasses developed by Hench and co-workers from SiO_2–Na_2O–CaO–P_2O_5 system

Glass	Na_2O	CaO	SiO_2	P_2O_5	Additives
45S5 (Novabone)	24.5	24.5	45	6	
A-W glass ceramic (Cerabone)	0	44.7	34	16.2	0.5 CaF_2 + 4.6 MgO
S53P4 (AbminDent1)	23	20	53	4	

asked a life changing question to Dr. Hench "If you can make a material that will survive exposure to high energy radiation, can you make a material that will survive exposure to the human body". Colonel also expressed the need of materials that shall be accepted by the body. In 1968, Hench and his coworkers (Ray Splinter, Bill Allen, Ted Greenlee) submitted a proposal to the US Army Medical R&D command. Three compositions were designed from the SiO_2–Na_2O–CaO–P_2O_5 phase diagram (listed in Table 4). All these compositions exhibited strong bonding ability with the bone. The bioactivity of this glass system can vary from bulk degradable to surface bioactive i.e., resorbed within 10–30 days in tissue.

45S5 Bioglass displayed rapid osteostimulation and osteoconduction mechanism as evident from the swift regeneration of trabecular bone with matching strength and architecture as that of the original bone. In addition to this, the in vitro experiments revealed the superior ability of 45S5 Bioglass to form HA layer.

Different groups were actively engaged to determine the bonding ability of Bioglass. Professor Peter Griss confirmed the bond bonding ability of Bioglass while testing load bearing prostheses in sheep (1976), whereas Professor Gross found that upon adding K_2O and MgO in Bioglass [CeraVital], the mechanical strong interface of glass-ceramic/bone could be obtained. The apatite-Wollastonite (A/W) bioactive glasses developed by Professor Yamamuro and coworkers has been approved in orthopaedic applications in Japan with success in 3000 vertebral prostheses, 20,000 iliac crest prostheses and 12,000 laminoplasty cases. In 1985, MEP named device (based on Bioglass) used for treating conductive hear loss by replacing bones of middle ear was commercialized [67]. Another Bioglass based device ERMI came into market in 1988, which was designed for application in denture construction by supporting lingual and tibial plates in natural tooth. In 1993, the first particulate 45S5 product was used as a synthetic bone graft for jaw defects and treating periodontal diseases. In 1999, Novabone particulate was released in the market for the orthopaedic load bearing applications. NovaBone particulate is mixed with the defect site blood to form a putty like material and then push it into the defect site before it clots. Since 2004, Bioglass 45S5 have been of commercial success as an active repair agent in the toothpaste under the name NovaMin (Glaxosmithkline, UK). BIOMET3i is another Bioglass composition with narrower particle size in the range of 300–360 μm, which is used to treat the jawbone defects. In 2006, the particulates of S53P4 compositions known as BonAlive have been approved as orthopaedic bone graft substitute [68]. Infact, BonAlive enhanced bone growth as compared to the 13-93 glass, which can be due to the higher magnesium content of 13-93. Among 45S5 and BonAlive, the HA thickness is observed more for the 45S5 indicating its high reactivity.

The invention of Bioglass revolutionized biomaterial development and doped bioglass system for the human body. Thus many scientists and research groups engaged themselves in the study of silicate, borate, phosphate, doped, metallic and mesoporous system of glasses for tissue regeneration, orthopedic and biomedical applications. To reconstruct the defective parts of the body, ancient civilizations like Chinese, Egyptians, Indian used biomaterials but Bioglass in the fine particulate form has been in clinical practice since 1985 to the present for dental application (Perioglas, NovaBone, USA).

Currently, the current area of investigation for many researchers is the substitution of silicon for calcium into synthetic hydroxyapatite. Fu and coworkers proposed 13-93 glass, which exhibits facile viscous flow behavior than bioglass [51]. Considerably smaller weight loss in comparison to 45S5 and high bioactivity during the 12 h of immersion in SBF was observed for the diopside system synthesised by Goel and coworkers [69]. Huang and coworkers replaced SiO_2 with B_2O_3 in steps and found increase in the HA layer formation (borate-rich layer formations) [54]. Borate based 13-93B2 glass is attracting attention these days as it exhibits promising characteristics to be a scaffold material. 13-93B2 scaffolds possessed microstructure similar to the human trabecular bone making them very favourable candidates for the clinical applications especially as bone grafts [70, 71]. Liu and coworkers studied the mechanism of conversion of 13-93B2 scaffolds in HA after soaking them in dilute phosphate solutions [70, 71]. After 15 days soaking in phosphate solution, significant drop in the 13-93B2 scaffold strength is observed i.e. from 6.2 to 2.8 MPa attributed to the progressive material degradation, In contrast to this, silica free 13-93B3 borate glass scaffolds were regarded as toxic for murine MLO-A5 osteogenic cells in vitro [72]. Anyhow, the same scaffolds were non toxic to the cells in vivo and enhanced new tissue infiltration upon subcutaneous implantation in rats. Vitale-Brovarone et al. developed phosphate glass-ceramic scaffolds [73] using ICEL2 powders as glassy inorganic phase and observed these scaffolds to be resorbable and bioactive. Abou Neel and coworkers studied Na_2O–CaO–SrO–P_2O_5 system and [74] obtained that the substitution of Na_2O with SrO from 0 to 5 mol% produced a significant increase in the degradation rate of these glasses. Superior mechanical properties (up to 6 MPa) with respect to pure b-TCP scaffolds (up to 2.3 MPa) could be obtained upon reinforcing the phosphate glass phase in b-TCP-based composite scaffolds (b-TCP/PG1), as during the sintering process, glass must have acted as a viscous binder causing strengthening of the final scaffold structure [75].

On adding dopants, the glasses may possess superior bioactive properties. For treatment of cancer, Luderer [76], incorporated Fe_2O_3 in aluminoborosilicate glasses whereas Singh and coworkers [77] obtained a iron doped a borosilicate glass composition and found that the samples with 10–15 % Fe_2O_3 revealed apatite layer formation on the glass. The effect on La, Al, Y and Cr on the bioactive behavior of calcium borosilicate glasses is also studied where chromium and yttria based glasses revealed apatite formation after soaking in SBF solution [78]. The formation of brushite and whitlockite could be seen, though no hydroxyapatite formation could be observed on the barium zinc alumino-borosilicate glass surface for $Al_2O_3 > 5$ %

[38]. According to the results of Branda et al. [58], the dopants like In, Ga and La etc. show less bioactive behavior of glasses as compared to the indium doped glasses. The sintered 6P53B glass scaffolds show a compressive strength of (136 ± 22 MPa) is obtained, comparable with human cortical bone whereas porosity of (60 %) is obtained in the range of trabecular bone. Titania doped glass compositions based on the P_2O_5–CaO–Na_2O–TiO_2 system have shown controlled solubility and the chemical composition is close to the bone mineral phase [80].

Metallic glasses have also geared up in the glass revolution and the studies yielded superior properties for BMG than the conventional biomaterials. Hiromoto [81] found lower metal dissolution during the re-passivation process of $Zr_{65}Cu_{17.5}Ni_{10}A_{17.5}$ amorphous alloy in the Hank's solution. Morrison compared the corrosion resistance of $Zr_{41.2}Ti_{13.8}Ni_{10}Cu_{12.5}Be_{22.5}$ with conventional biomaterials like 316L steel and Ti–6Al–4V alloy [82]. The biocompatibility of Zr–10Al–5Ti–17.9Cu–14.6Ni is confirmed by viability of cells on the cell surface [83]. Anyhow, BMG possess a major drawback due to the nickel inclusion in its composition and Ni is possibly carcinogenic and can cause an allergic response [84]. Hence the current efforts are focussed to develop Ni free metallic glasses. $(Zr_xCu_{100-x})_{80}(Fe_{40}Al_{60})_{20}$(x = 62–81) glasses, have yielded excellent biocompatibility with the cell. Zirconium oxide formed on the surface of the glass helps in controlling the toxic ion dissolution. A series of MgZnCa glasses with high tensile strength [85] have been developed by Loffler SWISS group.

Another fascinating field of bioactive glasses endowed with the drug delivery applications known as mesoporous glass is among the hottest research field these days. In 2004, the highly ordered mesoporous glass CaO–SiO_2–P_2O_5 composition with channels of 5 nm was produced using the sol-gel method and the incorporation of structure directing agents like F127 (EO106-PO70-EO106), P123 (EO20-PO70-EO20) and cetyltrimethyl ammonium bromide (CTAB) into the glass network structure [64, 66, 86]. Different structure-directing agents influence the properties of bioactive glasses i.e. F127 gives a wormlike mesopore structure whereas P123 is produces a two-dimensional hexagonal (p6mm) mesopore structure of pore size 4–10 nm [87]. Generally, CTAB-induced bioactive glasses posses small pore size of 2–3 nm and low orderings of the mesopores.

Mesoporous bioglass powders of high specific surface area were synthesised by acetic acid as a structure-assisting agent [88]. Li and co-workers fabricated Mg-, Zn- or Cu-containing multicomponent mesoporous bioglass particles using P123 and hydrothermal treatment [89]. Ultrathin mesoprous bioglass fibres ($70SiO_2$–$25CaO$–$5P_2O_5$ in mol%) with high matrix homogeneities were synthesized using phase-seperation-induced agent P123–PEO co-templates and the electrospinning technique [90, 91]. Wu et al. [92] prepared millimetre-sized mesoporous bioglass sphere using alginate cross-linking with Ca^{2+} ions. The same group developed porous mesoporous nanospheres using hydrothermal method and also synthesised mesoporous particles for haemostatic applications [93]. Using sol-gel method, mesoporous–macroporous bioglass spheres in the micrometers range were prepared and the triblock copolymer templating [94]. By sol-gel technique using polyethylene glycol template, mesoporous shell of diameter 500 nm was prepared [88].

Hong et al. [91] developed mesoporous bioactive glass hollow fibers (MBGHFs) of the fiber length: (A) 5–10 mm, (B) 2–2.5 mm, (C) 0.2–0.3 mm and (D) <20 μm. Kang et al. [95] developed luminescent calcium silicate mesoporous bioglass microspheres of mesopore size 6 nm. Zhao and co-workers fabricated mesoporous bioglass microspheres of 4–5 μm using structure directing agents P123 and CTAB, is prepared [96]. Due to the excellent mineralization ability of these nanospheres, it was desired for the infected canal treatment.

7 Techniques for Bioactive Glass Fabrication

Major portion of economy for USA and European countries is dominated by the glass industry because glass is an indispensable material for sophisticated applications in biomedical engineering, optoelectronics, photonics and biotechnologies. From centuries, the glass making has followed different techniques. The fabrication method has a huge impact on determining the structural properties of the biomaterial. Conventionally, the bioactive glasses are prepared using sol-gel techniques or melt-quenching techniques (Table 5).

In the melt-quenching technique, glass is obtained by fusing a mixture of raw materials and subsequent solidification by quenching into glass frits. The batch of glasses is prepared by uniformly mixing an appropriate mole/weight fraction of well-desired initial ingredients. Subsequently, the ground powder is melted in a high temperature furnace such as automatized molybdenum disilicide ($MoSi_2$) furnace. For certain aluminosilicate compositions, the temperature of the furnace can go up to 1500 °C, whereas borate and phosphate compositions melt at lower temperatures of 1200–1300 °C. The molten glass is poured in a preheated graphite mold and hence glasses can be made of desirable sizes and shapes by pouring them into moulds of particular shapes. Hench [67] casted 45 % SiO_2–24.5 % Na_2O–24.5 % CaO–6 % P_2O_5 bioactive glass composition, which was easy to melt as it was near to the ternary eutectic.

In the sol-gel methodology, the organic precursors are used for gelation and drying to prepare the amorphous glass. Sol less viscous liquid whereas an abrupt increase in the viscosity is observed for the gel. The hydrolysis and polycondensation of an organometallic precursor leads to the formation of an interconnected 3-D network to form a gel. Then syneresis/aging of a gel is done to decrease the porosity, which increase the strength due to the continued process of polycondensation and reprecipitation of the gel network [5, 6]. The aged gel must be dried by removing the pore liquid from the interconnected rigid 3-D network. When the resulting gel is heated at high temperatures, then the elimination of pores result in the densification of network.

Both the processes result in different mechanical properties, porosity, uniformity and especially bioactive properties. Sol-gel glasses are attributed with mesoporous character, which is attributed to their pore diameter in the range of 2–50 nm [18, 47]. Moreover, the sol-gel method provides high purity glasses with more

Table 5 The bioactive glasses with their composition and synthesis techniques [38, 45, 47, 69, 70, 74, 97–119]

Glass label	SiO_2	CaO	P_2O_5	B_2O_3	MgO	Na_2O	Dopants TiO_2/K_2O/SrO/BaO/CaF_2/Al_2O_3	wt%/mol %	Technique used
13-93	53	20	4		5	6	12 K_2O	wt%	Melt-quench
13-93B1	34.4	19.5	3.8	19.9	4.9	5.8	11.7 K_2O	wt%	Melt-quench
13-93B3		18.5	3.7	56.6	4.6	5.5	11.1 K_2O	wt%	Melt-quench
1	64	26	5				5 ZnO	mol%	Sol-gel
ICSW 1	51.06	22.84				26.10		mol%	Sol-gel
ICSW 2	47.84	23.33	2.16			26.67		mol%	Sol-gel
ICSW 3	44.47	23.85	4.42			27.26		mol%	Sol-gel
ICSW 4	37.28	24.95	9.25			28.52		mol%	Sol-gel
ICSW 5	40.96	24.39	6.78			27.87		mol%	Sol-gel
ICSW 6	48.98	23.33	1.02			26.67		mol%	Sol-gel
ICSW 7	47.07	23.78	1.95			27.19		mol%	Sol-gel
ICSW 8	43.66	24.60	3.62			28.12		mol%	Sol-gel
ICSW 9	38.14	25.91	6.33			29.62		mol%	Sol-gel
ICSW 10	40.71	25.31	5.07			28.91		mol%	Sol-gel
Undoped	74.7	25.3					0 ZnO	wt%	Sol-gel
Zn1	73.7	25.3					1.0 ZnO	wt%	Sol-gel
Zn2	74.0	21.2					4.8 ZnO	wt%	Sol-gel
BG-B_0	60.68	35.83	3.49	0				mol%	Sol-gel
BG-B_{10}	49.02	39.46	1.54	9.98				mol%	Sol-gel
BG-B_{20}	29.87	48.43	1.70	20.00				mol%	Sol-gel
45S5	46.1	26.9	2.6			24.4		mol%	Sol-gel
45S5F	46.1	20.9	2.6			24.4	6 CaF_2 + 6 TiO_2	mol%	Sol-gel
63S	63	28	9					mol%	Sol-gel
BGNP	80.7	16.8	2.5					mol%	Sol-gel

(continued)

Table 5 (continued)

Glass label	SiO_2	CaO	P_2O_5	B_2O_3	MgO	Na_2O	Dopants $TiO_2/K_2O/SrO/BaO/CaF_2/Al_2O_3$	wt%/mol %	Technique used
BGMP	55.5	35.8	8.7					mol%	Sol-gel
58S	58	33	9				0 ZnO	mol%	Sol-gel
58S0.5Z	58	32.5	9				0.5 ZnO	mol%	Sol-gel
58S4Z	58	29	9				4 ZnO	mol%	Sol-gel
70S30C	70	30							Sol-gel
1	40.36	31.4	1.35	4.48	13.45	4.48	4.48 CaF_2	mol%	Melt-quench
1a	40.10	31.18	2.00	4.45	13.37	4.45	4.45 CaF_2	mol%	Melt-quench
1b	39.82	30.97	2.65	4.43	13.27	4.43	4.43 CaF_2	mol%	Melt-quench
2	41.15	32.92	1.23	4.12	12.34	4.12	4.12 CaF_2	mol%	Melt-quench
3	41.82	34.22	1.15	3.80	11.41	3.80	3.80 CaF_2	mol%	Melt-quench
A-3	54.5	15.0	6.0		8.5	12	4 K_2O	wt%	Melt-quench
A-5	56.5	15.0	6.0		8.5	11	3 K_2O	wt%	Melt-quench
A-6	54.8	14.6	5.8		8.2	10.7	3 TiO_2 + 2.9 K_2O	wt%	Melt-quench
6P57	56.5	15.0	6.0		8.5	11.0	3 K_2O	wt%	Melt-quench
6P61	61.1	12.6	6.0		7.2	10.3	2.8 K_2O	wt%	Melt-quench
6P68	67.7	10.1	6.0		5.7	8.3	2.2 K_2O	wt%	Melt-quench
A	42	5					53 ZnO	mol%	Melt-quench
B	57	14					29 ZnO	mol%	Melt-quench
46S6	46	24	6			24	0.00 ZnO	wt%	Melt-quench
46S6Zn10	46	23.94	6			23.94	0.12 ZnO + 0.1 Zn	wt%	Melt-quench
D-Alk-B (13-93B2	18	22	2	36	8	6	8 K_2O	mol%	Melt-quench
10C50P		18.2	45.4			36.4		mol%	Melt-quench
20C50P		33.3	41.7			25		mol%	Melt-quench
30C50P		46.2	38.4			15.4		mol%	Melt-quench

(continued)

Table 5 (continued)

Glass label	SiO_2	CaO	P_2O_5	B_2O_3	MgO	Na_2O	Dopants $TiO_2/K_2O/SrO/BaO/CaF_2/Al_2O_3$	wt%/mol %	Technique used
40C50P		57.2	35.7			7.1		mol%	Melt-quench
50C50P		66.7	33.3			0		mol%	Melt-quench
HZ5	42.54	23.4	5.64			23.27	4.94 ZnO	wt%	Melt-quench
HZ10	40.44	22.02	5.39			22.08	10.05 ZnO	wt%	Melt-quench
HZ 20	37.14	18.86	4.64			18.75	20.13 ZnO	wt%	Melt-quench
TCP-10	44.39	31.14	8.80		14.89		0.77 CaF_2	wt%	Melt-quench
TCP-20	38.84	33.98	13.37		13.03		0.77 CaF_2	wt%	Melt-quench
TCP-30	33.3	36.81	17.95		11.17		0.77 CaF_2	wt%	Melt-quench
TCP-40	27.75	39.65	22.53		9.31		0.77 CaF_2	wt%	Melt-quench
Zn-0	38.49	36.07	5.61		19.24		0 ZnO + 0.59 CaF_2	mol%	Melt-quench
Zn-2	38.49	36.07	5.61		17.24		2 ZnO + 0.59 CaF_2	mol%	Melt-quench
Zn-4	38.49	36.07	5.61		15.24		4 ZnO + 0.59 CaF_2	mol%	Melt-quench
Zn-6	38.49	36.07	5.61		13.24		6 ZnO + 0.59 CaF_2	mol%	Melt-quench
Zn-8	38.49	36.07	5.61		11.24		8 ZnO + 0.59 CaF_2	mol%	Melt-quench
Zn-10	38.49	36.07	5.61		9.24		10 ZnO + 0.59 CaF_2	mol%	Melt-quench
CNP		30	50			20	0 SrO	mol%	Melt-quench
CNP Sr1		30	50			19	1 SrO	mol%	Melt-quench
CNP Sr3		30	50			17	3 SrO	mol%	Melt-quench
CNP Sr5		30	50			15	5 SrO	mol%	Melt-quench
BT110	40	10				10	20 SrO + 20 ZnO	mol%	Melt-quench
BT111	40	10				20	20 SrO + 10 ZnO	mol%	Melt-quench
BT112	40	10				30	20 SrO	mol%	Melt-quench
BT113	40	0				10	30 SrO + 20 ZnO	mol%	Melt-quench
BT114	40	0				20	30 SrO + 10 ZnO	mol%	Melt-quench

(continued)

Table 5 (continued)

Glass label	SiO_2	CaO	P_2O_5	B_2O_3	MgO	Na_2O	Dopants $TiO_2/K_2O/SrO/BaO/CaF_2/Al_2O_3$	wt%/mol %	Technique used
BT115	40	0				30	30 SrO	mol%	Melt-quench
ICIE1	49.46	23.08	1.07			26.38	0 SrO	mol%	Melt-quench
ICIE1 Sr2.5	49.46	22.5	1.07			1.07	0.58 SrO	mol%	Melt-quench
ICIE1 Sr10	49.46	20.77	1.07			1.07	2.31 SrO	mol%	Melt-quench
ICIE1 Sr50	49.46	11.54	1.07			1.07	11.54 SrO	mol%	Melt-quench
ICIE1 Sr100	49.46	0	1.07			1.07	23.08 SrO	mol%	Melt-quench
CP5	60	20	5	5			10 ZnO	mol%	Sol-gel
CP10	60	15	10	5			10 ZnO	mol%	Sol-gel
CP10	60	10	15	5			10 ZnO	mol%	Sol-gel
CP20	60	5	20	5			10 ZnO	mol%	Sol-gel
BZA (I)	40			10			30 BaO + 20 ZnO	mol%	Melt-quench
BZA (II)	40			7.5			30 BaO + 2.5 Al_2O_3 + 20 ZnO	mol%	Melt-quench
BZA (III)	40			5			30BaO + 5 Al_2O_3 + 20 ZnO	mol%	Melt-quench
BZA (IV)	40			2.5			30 BaO + 7.5 Al_2O_3 + 20 ZnO	mol%	Melt-quench
BZA (V)	40			0			30 BaO + 10 Al_2O_3 + 20 ZnO	mol%	Melt-quench
CaAl	40	30		20			10 Al_2O_3	mol%	Melt-quench

homogeneity. Moreover, a lower processing temperature is required. In contrast to this, the melt-quenched glasses have enhanced mechanical properties like hardness and flexural strength etc. [47]. The sol-gel-derived scaffolds have low strength (2–3 MPa) and consequently they are suitable for substituting defects in low-load sites only. Nano pores present in the glass prepared from a sol-gel-method yield a high surface area, which leads to the degradation and a faster conversion of sol-gel glasses to HA than their counterpart melt-derived glass with the same composition. Some common bioactive glasses along with their composition and their route of synthesis are listed in Table 4 [47, 97–119].

8 Conclusions

While designing the bioactive glass scaffolds, mechanical strength, pore size and pore inter-connectivity hall be kept under consideration. An oriented microstructure is more beneficial compared to the random microstructure because it can provide higher strength in the direction of orientation. Disordered macro-porous structures of polymers and bioceramics can be produced by freezing of aqueous solutions and suspensions [2]. Porous scaffolds with an oriented microstructure can be prepared by optimizing and controlling freezing techniques due to the preferred direction of the ice-growth. By thermally bonding a random packing of loose particles in a mold of the desired geometry, the scaffolds can be obtained but they lack in desired porosity and connectivity. One method for forming a scaffold is by mixing the bioactive glass particles with some organic material and then removing it before the sintering process but does not fully resolve the pore size issues. Silicate, borosilicate and borate bioactive glass have been prepared with porosities in the range 60–90 % using polymer foam replication method. This method usually produces scaffolds similar to human trabecular bones. Sponge replication method is relatively inexpensive, quick and very advantageous processing technique for making scaffolds. Anyhow, this technique yield scaffolds with poor mechanical strength. Scaffolds produced by the polymer burning-out method show higher mechanical strength than that obtained through sponge replication. An electrospinning method is also used to produce nano-fibrous bioactive glass scaffolds and offers the advantage of silica content variation over a larger composition range. These glass scaffolds have higher surface area than sol-gel derived glasses. Many research groups are actively engaged in the fabrication of scaffolds with desirable features.

References

1. Ramakrishna, S., Meyer, J., Wintermantel, E., Leong, K.W.: Biomedical applications of polymer-composite materials: a review. Comput. Sci. Technol. **61**, 1189–1224 (2001)
2. Kaur, G., et al.: A review of bioactive glasses: their structure, properties, fabrication, and apatite formation. J. Biomed. Mater. Res. A **102**, 254–274 (2013)

3. Rehman, M.N., Ray, D.E., Bal, B.S., Fu, Q., Jung, S.B., Bonewald, L.F., Tomsia, A.P.: Bioactive glass in tissue engineering. Acta Biomater. **7**, 2355–2373 (2011)
4. Kim, S.-S., Ahn, K.M., Park, M.S., Lee, J.-H., Choi, C.Y., Kim, B.-S.: A poly(lactide coglycolide)/hydroxyapatite composite scaffold with enhanced osteoconductivity. J. Biomed. Mater. Res. **80A**, 206–215 (2007)
5. Hench, L.L.: Bioceramics: from concept to clinic. J. Am. Ceram. Soc. **74**, 1487–1510 (1991)
6. Hench, L.L.: Bioactive Ceramics, Annals of the New York Academy of Sciences, vol. 523, pp. 54–71. Wiley, New York (1988)
7. Yamamuro, T., Hench, L.L., Wilson, J.: Calcium phosphate and hydroxylapatite ceramics. In: Handbook of Bioactive Ceramics, vol 2. CRC Press, Boca Raton (1990)
8. Hoppe, A., Guldal, N.S., Boccaccini, A.R.: A review of the biological response to ionic dissolution products from bioactive glasses and glass-ceramics. Biomaterials **32**, 2757–2774 (2011)
9. Chen, Q.Z., Rezwan, K., Armitage, D., Nazhat, S.N., Boccaccini, A.R.: The surface functionalization of 45S5 Bioglass (R)-based glass-ceramic scaffolds and its impact on bioactivity. J. Mater. Sci. Mater. Med. **17**(11), 979–987 (2006)
10. Kokubo, T., Takadama, H.: How useful is SBF in predicting in vivo bone bioactivity? Biomaterials **27**, 2907–2915 (2006)
11. Witte, F., Kaese, V., Haferkamp, H., Switzer, E., Meyer-Lindenberg, A., Wirth, C.J., et al.: In vivo corrosion of four magnesium alloys and the associated bone response. Biomaterials **26**, 3557–3563 (2005)
12. Apelt, D., Theiss, F., El-Warrak, A.O., Zlinszky, K., Bettschart-Wolfisberger, R., Bohner, M., et al.: In vivo behavior of three different injectable hydraulic calcium phosphate cements. Biomaterials **25**, 1439–1451 (2004)
13. Theiss, F., Apelt, D., Brand, B., Kutter, A., Zlinszky, K., Bohner, M., et al.: Biocompatibility and resorption of a brushite calcium phosphate cement. Biomaterials **26**, 4383–4394 (2005)
14. LeGeros, R.Z., LeGeros, J.P.: Phosphate minerals in human tissues. In: Nriagu, J.O., Moore, P.B. (eds.) Phosphate Minerals, pp. 351–385. Springer-Verlag, Berlin (1984)
15. Wagoner Johnson AJ: Herschler BA. A review of the mechanical behavior of CaP and CaP/polymer composites for applications in bone replacement and repair. Acta Biomater. **7**, 16–30 (2011)
16. Regi, M.V.: Ceramics for medical applications. J. Chem. Soc., Dalton Trans. **2**, 97–108 (2001)
17. Marcacci, M., Kon, E., Moukhachev, V., Lavroukov, A., Kutepov, S., Quarto, R., Mastrogiacomo, M., Cancedda, R.: Stem cells associated with macroporous bioceramics for long bone repair: 6- to 7-year outcome of apilot clinical study. Tissue Eng. **13**, 947–955 (2007)
18. Baino, F., Brovarone, C.V.: Three-dimensional glass-derived scaffolds for bone tissue engineering: current trends and forecasts for the future. J. Biomed. Mater. Res. A **97A**, 514–535 (2010)
19. Schlickewei, W., Schlickewei, C.: The use of bone substitutes in the treatment of bone defects—The clinical view and history. Macromol. Symp. **253**, 10–23 (2007)
20. Hoffenberg, R.: Christiaan Barnard: his first transplants and their impact on concepts of death. BMJ **323**, 22–29 (2001)
21. Alfani, D., et al.: Kidney transplantation from living unrelated donors. Clin. Transpl. **117**, 205–212 (1998)
22. Vathsala, A.: Immunosuppression use in renal transplantation from Asian transplant centers: a preliminary report from the Asian Transplant Registry. Transpl. Proc. **36**(7), 1868–1870 (2004)
23. Ota, K.: Organ transplantation in Japan present status and problems. Transpl. Int. **2**, 61–67 (1989)

24. Lysaght, M.J., Jaklenec, A., Deweerd, E.: Great expectations: private sector activity in tissue engineering, regenerative medicine, and stem cell therapeutics. Tissue Eng. Part A **14**(2), 305–315 (2008)
25. Bruck, A., et al.: Heart-lung transplantation successful therapy for patients with pulmonary vascular disease. Engl. J. Med. **306**, 557–564 (1982)
26. Hench, L.L., Polak, J.M.: Third generation biomaterials. Science **295**, 1014–1017 (2002)
27. Darby, W.J.: In: Prasad, A.S., Oberleas, D. (eds.) Trace Elements in Human Health and Disease. Academic Press, New York, vol. 1, p. 17 (1976)
28. Seeley, R.R., Stephens, T.D.: Rate P Anatomy and physiology, 8th edn. McGrew Hill, New York (2006)
29. Soetan, K.O., Olaiya, C.O., Oyewole, O.E.: The importance of mineral elements for humans, domestic animals and plants: a review. Afr. J. Food Sci. **4**, 200–222 (2010)
30. Whitney, E.N., Rolfes, S.R.: Understanding Nutrition. Wadsworth Publishing, Belmon (2010)
31. Schwarz, K.: A bound form of silicon in glycosaminoglycans and polyuronides. Proc. Natl. Acad. Sci. USA **70**, 1608–1612 (1973)
32. Barrett, A.J.: In: Florkin, M., Stotz, E.H. (eds.) Comprehensive Biochemistry. Elsevier, New York, vol. 26 B, pp. 438–442 (1968)
33. Birchall, J.D., Bellia, J.P., Roberts, N.B.: On the mechanisms underlying the essentiality of silicon interactions with aluminium and copper. Coord. Chem. Rev. **49**, 231–240 (1996)
34. Murray, R.K., Granner, D.K., Mayer, P.A., Rodwell, V.W.: Harper's Biochemistry, 25th edn. Mc-Graw Hill, Health Profession Division, USA (2000)
35. Meunier, P.J., Slosman, D.O., Delmas, P.D., Sebert, J.L., Brandi, M.L., Albanese, C., Lorenc, R., Pors-Nielsen, S., de Vernejoul, M.C., Roces, A., Reginster, J.Y.: Strontium ranelate: dose-dependent effects in established postmenopausal vertebral osteoporosis—a 2-year randomized placebo controlled trial. J. Clin. Endocrinol. Metab. **87**, 2060–2066 (2002)
36. Marie, P.J., Ammann, P., Boivin, G., Rey, C.: Mechanisms of action and therapeutic potential of strontium in bone. Calcif. Tissue Int. **69**, 121–129 (2001)
37. Kaur, G., Pandey, O.P., Singh, K.: Interfacial study between high temperature SiO_2-B_2O_3-AO-La_2O_3 (A = Sr, Ba) glass seals and Crofer 22 APU for solid oxide fuel cell applications. Int. J. Hydrogen Energy **37**, 6862–6874 (2012)
38. Kaur, G., Sharma, P., Kumar, V., Singh, K.: Assesment of *in-vitro* bioactivity of SiO_2-BaO-ZnO-B_2O_3-Al_2O_3 glasses: an optico-analytical approach. Mater. Sci. Eng. C **32**, 1941–1947 (2012)
39. Madanat, R., Moritz, N., Vedel, E., Svedstro, E., Aro, H.T.: Radio-opaque bioactive glass markers for radiostereometric analysis. Acta Biomater. **5**, 3497–3505 (2009)
40. Zhang, J.C., Huang, J.A., Xu, S.J., Wang, K., Yu, S.F.: Effects of Cu2 + and pH on osteoclastic bone resorption in vitro. Prog. Nat. Sci. **13**, 266 (2003)
41. Smith, B.J., King, J.B., Lucas, E.A., Akhter, M.P., Arjmandi, B.H., Stoecker, B.J.: Skeletal unloading and dietary copper depletion are detrimental to bone quality of mature rats. J. Nutr. **132**, 190–196 (2002)
42. Yamaguchi, M.: Role of zinc in bone formation and bone resorption. J. Trace Elem. Exp. Med. **11**, 119–135 (1998)
43. Sadarzadeh, S.M., Saffari, Y.: Iron and brain disorder. Am. J. Clin. Pathol. **121**, 64–70 (2004)
44. Filho, O.P., Latorre, G.P., Hench, L.L.: Effect of crystallization on apatite-layer formation of bioactive glass 45 S5. J. Biomed. Mater. Res. **30**, 509–514 (1996)
45. Kaur, G., et al.: Synthesis, cytotoxicity, and hydroxypatite formation in 27-Tris-SBF for sol-gel based CaO-P_2O_5-SiO_2-B_2O_3-ZnO bioactive glasses. Sci. Rep. **4**, 1–14 (2014)
46. Place, E.S., Evans, N.D., Stevens, M.M.: Complexity in biomaterials for tissue engineering. Nature **8**, 457–470 (2009)

47. Kaur, G., Pickrell, G., Sriranganathan, N., Kumar, V., Homa, D.: Review and the state of the art: sol-gel and melt quenched bioactive glasses for tissue engineering. J. Biomed. Mater. Res. B Appl. Biomater. (2015). doi:10.1002/jbm.b.33443
48. Kingery, W.D., Bowen, H.K., Uhlmann, D.R.: Introduction to Ceramics, 2nd edn. John Wiley and Sons, New York (1976)
49. Shelby, J.E.: Introduction to Glass Science and Technology, 2nd edn. The Royal Society of Chemistry, Cambridge (2005)
50. Day, R.M., Boccaccini, A.R., Shurey, S., Roether, J.A., Forbes, A., Hench, L.L., Gabe, S.: Assessment of polyglycolic acid mesh and bioactive glass for soft tissue engineering scaffolds. Biomaterials **25**, 5857–5866 (2004)
51. Fu, Q., Rahaman, M.N., Bal, B.S., Brown, R.F., Day, D.E.: Mechanical and in vitro performance of 13–93 bioactive glass scaffolds prepared by a polymer foam replication technique. Acta Biomater. **4**, 1854–1864 (2008)
52. Regi, M.V., Bala, F.: Silica material for biomedical applications. Open Biomed. Eng. J. **2**, 1–9 (2008)
53. Brink, M.: The influence of alkali and alkali earths on the working range for bioactive glasses. J. Biomed. Mater. Res. **36**, 109–117 (1997)
54. Huang, W.H., Day, D.E., Kittiratanapiboon, K., Rahaman, M.N.: Kinetics and mechanisms of the conversion of silicate (45 S5), borate, and borosilicate glasses to hydroxyapatite in dilute phosphate solutions. J. Mater. Sci. Mater. Med. **17**, 583–596 (2015)
55. Zhang, X., Jia, W., Gua, Y., Wei, X., Liu, X., Wang, D., Zhang, C., Huang, W., Rahaman, M.N., Day, D.E., Zhou, N.: Teicoplanin-loaded borate bioactive glass implants for treating chronic bone infection in a rabbit tibia osteomyelitis model. Biomaterials **31**, 5865–5874 (2010)
56. Bunker, B.C., Arnold, G.W., Wilder, J.A.: Phosphate glass dissolution in aqueous solutions. J. Non Cryst. Solids **64**, 291–316 (1984)
57. Shah, R., Sinanan, A.C.M., Knowles, J.C., Hunt, N.P., Lewis, M.P.: Craniofacial muscle engineering using a 3-dimensional phosphate glass fibre construct. Biomaterials **26**, 1497–1505 (2005)
58. Branda, F., Arcobello-Varlese, F., Costantini, A., Luciani, G.: Effect of the substitution of M_2O_3 (M = La, Y, In, Ga, Al) for CaO on the bioactivity of $2.5CaO{\cdot}2SiO_2$ glass. Biomaterials **23**, 711–716 (2002)
59. Hoppe, A., Guldal, N.S., Boccaccini, A.R.: A review of the biological response to ionic dissolution products from bioactive glasses and glass-ceramics. Biomaterials **32**, 2757–2774 (2011)
60. Bellantone, M., Williams, H.D., Hench, L.L.: Broad-spectrum bactericidal activity of Ag_2O-doped bioactive glass. Antimicrob. Agents Chemother. **46**, 1940–1945 (2002)
61. Thamaraiselvi, T.V., Rajeswari, S.: Biological evaluation of bioceramic materials—a review. Trends Biomater. Artif. Organs **18**, 9–17 (2004)
62. Horton, J.A., Parsell, D.E.: Biomedical potential of a zirconium-based bulk metallic glass. Mater. Res. Soc. Symp. Proc. **754**, CC1.5.1 (2003)
63. Wang, W.H., Dong, C., Shek, C.H.: Bulk metallic glasses. Mater. Sci. Eng. R. Rep. **44**(2–3), 45–89 (2004)
64. Vallet-Regí, M., Izquierdo-Barba, I., Colilla, M.: Review: structure and functionalization of mesoporous bioceramics for bone tissue regeneration and local drug delivery. Philos. Trans. R. Soc. Lond. A **370**, 1400–1421 (2002)
65. Yan, X., Yu, C., Zhou, X., Tang, J., Zhao, D.: Highly ordered mesoporous bioactive glasses with superior in vitro bone-forming bioactivities. Angew. Chem. Int. Ed. Engl. **43**, 5980–5984 (2004)
66. Vallet-Regi, M.: Ordered mesoporous materials in the context of drug delivery systems and bone tissue engineering. Chem. Eur. J. **12**, 5934–5943 (2006)
67. Hench, L.L.: The story of Bioglass Hench LL. The story of BioglassVR. J. Mater. Sci. Mater. Med. **17**, 967–978 (2006)

68. Jones, J.R.: Review of bioactive glass: from Hench to hybrids. Acta Biomater. **9**, 4457–4486 (2013)
69. Goel, A., Kapoor, S., Rajagopal, R.R., Pascual, M.J., Kim, H.W., Ferreira, J.M.F.: Alkali-free bioactive glasses for bone tissue engineering: a preliminary investigation. Acta Biomater. **8**, 361–372 (2012)
70. Liu, X., Huang, W., Fu, H., Yao, A., Wang, D., Pan, H., Lu, W.W.: Bioactive borosilicate glass scaffolds: improvement on the strength of glass-based scaffolds for tissue engineering. J. Mater. Sci. Mater. Med. **20**, 365–372 (2009)
71. Liu, X., Pan, H., Fu, H., Fu, Q., Rahaman, M.N., Huang, W.: Conversion of borate-based glass scaffold to hydroxyapatite in a dilute phosphate solution. Biomed. Mater. **5**, 15005 (2010)
72. Fu, Q., Rahaman, M.N., Bal, B.S., Bonewald, L.F., Kuroki, K., Brown, R.F.: Silicate borosilicate, and borate bioactive glass scaffolds with controllable degradation rate for bone tissue engineering applications. II. In vitro and in vivo biological evaluation. J. Biomed. Mater. Res. A **95A**, 172–179 (2010)
73. Vitale-Brovarone, C., Baino, F., Bretcanu, O., Verne, E.: Foam-like scaffolds for bone tissue engineering based on a novel couple of silicate-phosphate specular glasses: synthesis and properties. J. Mater. Sci. Mater. Med. **20**, 2197–2205 (2009)
74. Abou Neel, E.A., Chrzanowski, W., Pickup, D.M., O'Dell, L.A., Mordan, N.J., Newport, R. J., Smith, M.E., Knowles, J.C.: Structure and properties of strontium-doped phosphate-based glasses. J. R. Soc. Interface **6**, 435–446 (2009)
75. Cai, S., Xu, G.H., Yu, X.Z., Zhang, W.J., Xiao, Z.Y., Yao, K.D.: Fabrication and biological characteristics of b-tricalcium phosphate porous ceramic scaffolds reinforced with calcium phosphate glass. J. Mater. Sci. Mater. Med. **20**, 351–358 (2009)
76. Luderer, A.A., Borrelli, N.F., Panzarina, J.N., Mansfield, G.R., Hess, D.M., Brown, J.L., Barnett, E.H., Hawn, E.W.: Glass-ceramic-mediated, magnetic-field-induced localized hyperthermia: response of a murine mammary carcinoma. Radiat. Res. **94**(1), 190–198 (1983)
77. Singh, K., Bala, I., Kumar, V.: Structural, optical and bioactive properties of calcium borosilicate glasses. Ceram. Int. **35**, 3401–3406 (2009)
78. Singh, K., Bahadur, D.: Characterization of $SiO_2 \pm Na_2O \pm Fe_2O_3 \pm CaO \pm P_2O_5 \pm B_2O_3$ glass ceramics. J. Mater. Sci. Mater. Med. **10**, 481–484 (1999)
79. Fu, Q., Saiz, E., Tomsia, A.P.: Direct ink writing of highly porous and strong glass scaffolds for load-bearing bone defects repair and regeneration. Acta Biomater. **7**, 3547–3554 (2011)
80. Navarro, M., Ginebra, M.P., Clement, J., Martínez, S., Avila, G., Planell, J.A.: Physico-chemical degradation of soluble phosphate glasses stabilized with TiO_2 for medical applications. J. Am. Ceram. Soc. **86**, 1345–1352 (2003)
81. Hiromoto, S., Tsai, A.P., Sumita, M.: Effects of surface finishing and dissolved oxygen on the polarization behavior of Zr65Al7.5Ni10Cu17.5 amorphous alloy in phosphate buffered solution. Corros. Sci. **42**(12), 2167–2185 (2000)
82. Hiromoto, S., Tsai, A.P., Sumita, M.: Effects of surface finishing and dissolved oxygen on the polarization behavior of Zr65Al7.5Ni10Cu17.5amorphous alloy in phosphate buffered solution. Corros. Sci. **42**(12), 2167–2185 (2000)
83. Horton, J.A., Parsell, D.E.: Biomedical potential of a zirconium-based bulk metallic glass. Mater. Res. Soc. Symp. Proc. **754**, CC1.5.1 (2003)
84. Wang, W.H., Dong, C., Shek, C.H.: Bulk metallic glasses. Mater. Sci. Eng. R. Rep. **44**(2–3), 45–89 (2004)
85. Wang, W.H., Dong, C., Shek, C.H.: Bulk metallic glasses. Mater. Sci. Eng. R. Rep. **44**(2–3), 45–89 (2004)
86. Lopez-Noriega, A., et al.: Ordered mesoporous bioactive glasses for bone tissue regeneration. Chem. Mater. **18**, 3137–3144 (2006)

87. Yan, X., Yu, C., Zhou, X., Tang, J., Zhao, D.: Highly ordered mesoporous bioactive glasses with superior in vitro bone-forming bioactivities. Angew. Chem. Int. Ed. Engl. **43**, 5980–5984 (2004)
88. Lei, B., Chen, X.F., Wang, Y.J., Zhao, N.: Synthesis and in vitro bioactivity of novel mesoporous hollow bioactive glass microspheres. Mater. Lett. **63**, 1719–1721 (2009)
89. Li, X., Wang, X., He, D., Shi, J.: Synthesis and characterization of mesoporous CaO–MO–SiO_2–P_2O_5 (M = Mg, Zn, Cu) bioactive glasses/composites. J. Mater. Chem. **18**, 4103–4109 (2008)
90. Hong, Y., et al.: Preparation, bioactivity, and drug release of hierarchical nanoporous bioactive glass ultrathin fibers. Adv. Mater. **22**, 754–758 (2010)
91. Hong, Y.L., et al.: Fabrication and drug delivery of ultrathin mesoporous bioactive glass hollow fibers. Adv. Funct. Mater. **20**, 1503–1510 (2010)
92. Wu, X., et al.: Chemical characteristics and hemostatic performances of ordered mesoporous calcium-doped silica xerogels. Biomed. Mater. **5**, 035006 (2010). (9 pp)
93. Zhu, M., et al.: Mesoporous bioactive glass-coated poly(L-lactic acid) scaffolds: a sustained antibiotic drug release system for bone repairing. J. Mater. Chem. **21**, 1064–1072 (2001)
94. Yun, H.S., Kim, S.E., Hyun, Y.T.: Preparation of bioactive glass ceramic beads with hierarchical pore structure using polymer self-assembly technique. Mater. Chem. Phys. **115**, 670–676 (2009)
95. Kang, X., et al.: Preparation of luminescent and mesoporous Eu^{3+}/Tb^{3+} doped calcium silicate microspheres as drug carriers via a template route. Dalton Trans. **40**, 1873–1879 (2011)
96. Zhao, S., Li, Y.B., Li, D.X.: Synthesis and in vitro bioactivity of CaO–SiO_2–P_2O_5 mesoporous microspheres. Microporous Mesoporous Mater. **135**, 67–73 (2010)
97. Rahaman, et al.: Bioactive glass in tissue engineering. Acta Biomater. **7**, 2355–2373 (2011)
98. Oki, A., Parveen, B., Hossain, S., Adeniji, S., Donahue, H.: Preparation and in vitro bioactivity of zinc containing sol-gel-derived bioglass materials. J. Biomed. Mater. Res. A **69**(2), 216–221 (2004)
99. O'Donnell, M.D., Watts, S.J., Hill, R.G., Law, R.V.: The effect of phosphate content on the bioactivity of soda-lime-phosphosilicate glasses. J. Mater. Sci. Mater. Med. **20**, 1611–1618 (2009)
100. Courtheoux, L., Lao, J., Nedelec, J.M., Jallot, E.: Controlled bioactivity in zinc-doped sol-gel-derived binary bioactive glasses. J. Phys. Chem. C **112**, 13663–13667 (2008)
101. Yang, X., et al.: Incorporation of B_2O_3 in CaO-SiO_2-P_2O_5 bioactive glass system for improving strength of low-temperature co-fired porous glass ceramics. J. Non Cryst. Solids **358**, 1171–1179 (2012)
102. Li, H.C., Wang, D.G., Hu, J.H., Chen, C.Z.: Crystallization, mechanical properties and in vitro bioactivity of sol-gel derived Na_2O–CaO–SiO_2–P_2O_5 glass–ceramics by partial substitution of CaF_2 for CaO. J. Sol-Gel. Sci. Technol. **67**(1), 56–65 (2013)
103. Doostmohammadi, A., et al.: Bioactive glass nanoparticles with negative zeta potential. Ceram. Int. **37**, 2311–2316 (2011)
104. De Oliveira, A.A.R., et al.: Synthesis, characterization and cytocompatibility of spherical bioactive glass nanoparticles for potential hard tissue engineering applications. Biomed. Mater. **8**, 025011 (2011). (14 pp)
105. Du, R.L., Chang, J., Ni, S.Y., Zhai, W.Y.: Characterization and in vitro bioactivity of zinc-containing bioactive glass and glass-ceramics. J. Biomater. Appl. **20**, 341–360 (2006)
106. Jones, J.R., Ehrenfried, L.M., Hench, L.L.: Optimising bioactive glass scaffolds for bone tissue engineering. Biomaterials **27**, 964–973 (2006)
107. Agathopoulos, S., et al.: Formation of hydroxyapatite onto glasses of the CaO–MgO–SiO_2 system with B_2O_3, Na_2O, CaF_2 and P_2O_5 additives. Biomaterials **27**, 1832–1840 (2006)
108. Pazo, A., Saiz, E., Tomsia, A.P.: Silicate glass coatings on Ti-based implants. Acta Mater. **46**, 2551–2558 (1998)
109. Saiz, E., Goldman, M., Gomez-Vega, J.M., Tomsia, A.P., Marshall, G.W., Marshall, S.J.: In vitro behavior of silicate glass coatings on Ti6Al4V. Biomaterials **23**, 3749–3756 (2002)

110. Boyd, D., Towler, M.R.: The processing, mechanical properties and bioactivity of zinc based glass ionomer cements. J. Mater. Sci. Mater. Med. **16**, 843–850 (2005)
111. Oudadesse, H., et al.: Apatite forming ability and cytocompatibility of pure and Zn-doped bioactive glasses. Biomed. Mater. **6**, 035006 (2011)
112. Uo, M., et al.: Properties and cytotoxicity of water soluble Na_2O–CaO–P_2O_5 glasses. Biomaterials **19**, 2277–2284 (1998)
113. Aina, V., et al.: Cytotoxicity of zinc containing bioactive glasses in contact with human osteoblasts. Chem. Biol. Interact. **167**, 207–218 (2007)
114. Aina, V., Malavasi, G., Pla, A.F., Munaron, L., Morterra, C.: Zinc-containing bioactive glasses: surface reactivity and behaviour towards endothelial cells. Acta Biomater. **5**, 1211–1222 (2009)
115. Goel, A., et al.: Structural role of zinc in biodegradation of alkali-free bioactive glasses. J. Mater. Chem. B **1**, 3073–3082 (2013)
116. Kapoor, S., et al.: Role of glass structure in defining the chemical dissolution behavior, bioactivity and antioxidant properties of zinc and strontium co-doped alkali-free phospho-silicate glasses. Acta Biomater. **10**, 3264–3278 (2014)
117. Murphy, S., Wren, A.W., Towler, M.R., Boyd, D.: The effect of ionic dissolution products of Ca-Sr-Na-Zn-Si bioactive glass on in vitro cytocompatibilty. J. Mater. Sci. Mater. Med. **21**, 2827–2834 (2010)
118. Murphy, S., Boyd, D., Moane, S., Bennett, M.: The effect of composition on ion release from Ca–Sr–Na–Zn–Si glass bone grafts. J. Mater. Sci. Mater. Med. **20**, 2028–2035 (2009)
119. Fredholm, Y.C., Karpukhina, N., Law, R.V., Hill, R.G.: Strontium containing bioactive glasses: glass structure and physical properties. J. Non Cryst. Solids **356**, 2546–2551 (2010)

Structure and Percolation of Bioglasses

Antonio Carlos da Silva

Abstract The bioactive glasses are functional materials with large and growing technological applications in the production of implantable devices in living organisms as well as bone tissue lesions filling or in some applications in soft tissue. Anyway, play a key role in repair and functional recovery surgical techniques for different host organism parts (human organisms in general, but extends to other organisms, especially mammals). As the first commercial bioglass, the 45S5 still represent the primary focus of study and applications for this type of material and hence it and other similar compositions it will be the reference used in present discussion because in general, the bioglass structure understanding and it's dissolution and ionic transport mechanisms comprehension is applicable to other bioactive materials.

1 Introduction About Bioglass

So the main representative of the bioactive phosphosilicate glass group is the 45S5 which is a materials belonging to the system SiO_2:CaO:Na_2O:P_2O_5 of which typical composition is given by 45.0SiO_2:24.5Na_2O:24.5CaO:6.0P_2O_5, wt%. Containing only 6.0 weight percent of P_2O_5 it is clear it's affinity with soda-lime glasses system (SiO_2:CaO:Na_2O) and therefore may also be classified as a "soda-lime phosphosilicate" glass. Given this kinship the 45S5 guard strict structural similarity and dissolution kinetics with soda-lime glasses especially when these glasses have its composition modified by R_xO_y secondary formers. In turn the soda-lime is the glass composition that have higher production volume (almost the whole of the production of all kinds of glass) because among other features it has sufficient chemical stability for the large majority of everyday applications and supports compositional modifications that make it relatively simple to manage its chemical inertness or

A.C. da Silva (✉)
São Paulo, Brazil
e-mail: dasilva.ac@uol.com.br

J. Marchi (ed.), *Biocompatible Glasses*, Advanced Structured Materials 53,
DOI 10.1007/978-3-319-44249-5_3

allow the easy introduction of other oxides than your basic triad (CaO, Na_2O and SiO_2) factors that also open up a wide range of technological applications.

The major use of this type of glass has led over the history that it was even for accidental reasons introduced into the human body and remaining there in many cases presenting minimal inflammatory response. One cannot say that such cases are related to the choice of the use of glass as materials for prostheses and incipient implants, however one of the oldest cases of soda-lime glass applications are aesthetic ocular prostheses, better known as "glass eye ". Such prostheses have been initially prepared by Egyptians and Romans from fifth century BC, in order to cover the anophthalmic cavities [1]. Despite some earlier dental applications, only in the twentieth century second half many "high tech" bioceramics became available for biomedical purposes [2–5]. However, although compatible with human tissues, such materials exhibit bioinert behavior after implantation, in other words, the low interaction with the host organism physiological processes and therefore their potential in illness or injury lesions repair is limited or null. Serious injuries in soldiers during the Vietnam War emphasized the fact that despite all the advances in existing medicine at that time the available reconstructive implants, based mostly in Rod's and metal plates were unable to offer therapeutic alternative to amputation members in many cases where there was a significant bone loss, or even when it was avoided, the overall functionality of the limb resulted compromised. It was clearly a need for a material which allows the growth of living tissue as a substitute of missing tissue, preferably the implanted material over time could absorbed by the host organism without significant toxicological damage thereto. Such demand at the end of the 60s brought significant changes in implantable material concept and application with the bioactive glass advent [6].

Despite the mineral component of the bone tissue has no defined composition and show variations between stages of maturation and aging, it tends to a crystalline structure, and Ca/P ratio resembling those of hydroxyapatite (HA), so in a simplistic way, can be said that for the growth of bone tissue, the stem cells require that the chemical elements are provided for forming the mineral phase of bone tissue, i.e., calcium and phosphorus ions from which calcium phosphate based phases will be formed and are relevant to each new bone growing stage. However, these ions should be supplied in amounts compatible with cell growth needs with the risk of not being quantity sufficient or conversely become toxic to the cells. Clearly this process is much more complex, involving osteoblasts stimulation by free silica, such as will be treated in more detail below.

Considered this, the glass lime-soda is a natural candidate as alkaline earth cation supplier (Ca^{2+}). Under certain composition conditions in this group of glasses it is possible the Ca^{2+} release by ion exchange (glass ion exchange with body fluid medium, e.g.) in a controlled dissolution process. Furthermore the glass dissolution rate and specific cation percolation to medium may also be "programmed" through its composition. The phosphorus ions supply may also be achieved since this is provided in the glass composition so that it remains loosely associated or unstably in the structure. These processes are the result well known transport phenomena and ion exchange facility to occur when such glasses are brought in contact with aqueous media [7, 8] especially the exchange between alkali and alkaline earth cations by middle H^+ cations. To be facilitated these calcium transport phenomena two conditions are proposed: (1) The presence of R^{2+} cations unstably associated in the glass network and therefore susceptible to exchange with the H^+ cations; and, (2) The percolation channels formation from the surface toward the inside of the glass. Both conditions are glass structure distribution dependent and of course, is a composition consequence. The 45S5 bioglass is the composition which achieve all behaviors required to obtain a bioactive implant which when absorbed by the body medium will stimulate bone tissue formation. The mechanisms involved in this process has been extensive research object. Other derivatives glasses and glass ceramics also feature varied bioactivity in material nature according. The bioactivity index is defined by the time required to be established the 50 % binding to implant material surface with host organism tissue ($BI = 100/t_{0,5bb)}$. The 45S5 bioglass is considered as high bioactivity (BI = 12.5) when compared to hydroxyapatite (BI = 3.1) [9], i.e., under the same experimental conditions Bioglass® 45S5 would take approximately 8 days for 50 % of its surface was bound to tissue cells, while HA would take about 32 days.

The special properties of bioactive compositions should reflect their ability to release a critical amount of sodium ions, calcium and silica in the body environment, creating favorable conditions for the cellular processes and stimulating osteogenesis [10, 11]. In this way the activity, and by consequence, the BI will be different according to the bioglass composition whose rate of silica release is different for each of them [12, 13]. The initial contact of the bioactive glass with a physiological environment directly determines the rate and manner in which Na^+, Ca^{2+} and silicate ions are dissolved and penetrate into the surrounding environment, promote the deposition of apatite on the surface of the implant and in addition affect the cells activity in a way that is favorable to bone growth. It is accepted that the dissolution products of these materials may also exercise a genetic control of osteoblasts cycle in the cell. In this way the seven groups of genes that regulate osteogenesis and production of growth factors in osteoprogenitor cells are stimulated by bioactive glass product dissolution ionic exposure [2, 6]. Apparently, silicon has great significance for tissue mineralization both by promoting cell differentiation as the collagen type I formation stimulus [2, 14].

As discussed above, an appreciable bioactivity is achieved only under strict glass composition. The relationship between bioactivity and composition of glass system SiO_2–CaO–Na_2O–P_2O_5 obtained by melting/solidification process is shown in Fig. 1, for a P_2O_5 constant concentration of 6 wt% [4, 15]. Note that the delimited fields, do not represent specific stages, but rather the material behavior with respect to bioactivity.

In accordance to the diagram shown in Fig. 1 where we have a cut to P_2O_5 6 wt% in the CaO–SiO_2–Na_2O–P_2O_5 quaternary system the compositions indicated by ***I*** (45S5) and ***II*** represent glasses which exhibit the highest bioactivity index for this system, making connections with both the bone tissue and connective tissue. With these glasses dissolution specified amounts of Si, P, Na and Ca ions are released from the glass, creating local concentration gradients in the physiological

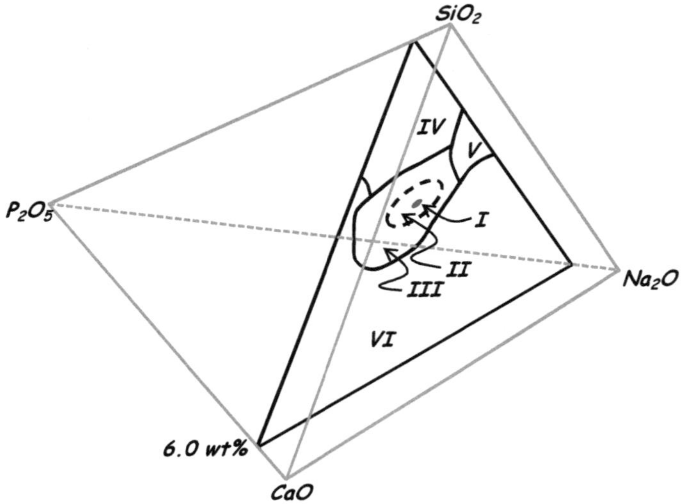

Fig. 1 Bioactivity kinetic diagram schematic representation for the SiO_2–CaO–Na_2O–P_2O_5 system (cut into 6.0 wt% P_2O_5) where: *I* bioglass 45S5; *II* bioactive compositions which form bonds with bone and connective tissues, *III* bioactive compositions which form only bonds with bone tissue; *IV* low reactivity bio-inactive compositions (poorly soluble) which does not form bonds with living tissues; *V* compositions with high reactivity (highly soluble) which are reabsorbed without forming tissues bonds; and *VI* compositions that do not form glass and do not form tissues bonds

environment which may approach the critical value required to stimulate cell activity [10, 16, 17]. The partial glass dissolution with the ions associated release drives both the deposition of apatite as the gene activation processes so it is interesting the bioglasses studies mainly broach aspects related to its dissolution. The compositions of the region ***III*** exhibit similar behavior, but the released ion gradients only stimulate binding to bone tissue. Compositions containing SiO_2 from 52 to 60 wt% have slower binding rates with bone tissue. The region ***IV*** represents compositions that are less soluble due to the high SiO_2 gradient and therefore show low reactivity. The compositions represented by region ***V*** are rich in alkalis, (R^+; Na^+) and impoverished in R^{2+} (Ca^{2+}) which makes them highly soluble (reactive) and they are rapidly reabsorbed. In addition, such compositions do not provide sufficient amounts of Ca^{2+} for the formation of calcium phosphate compounds. Finally the region ***VI*** compositions do not favor glass formation and also in which is not observed bioactivity for formed materials (crystalline phases). Above 60 wt% in SiO_2 there is no tissue link assuming the called bioinert material behavior. Having bioinert behavior these compositions when implanted in the body show minimal interfacial response which does not form connections with the host tissue. Furthermore these materials also generally are not rejected after implantation and it was observed the formation of a fibrous tissue membrane around the material in order to insulate it thus preventing possible additional interactions [2, 4, 15, 18, 19]. Some bioactivity in these materials may be induced by surface area increasing, different morphologies or by sol–gel synthesis process [5, 6, 9, 14, 15, 17].

We must consider primarily the glass interaction with the tissues around (with tissues bonds formation occurrence or absence) is surface reactions rate associated.

Although presenting general structure similar to bulk glass, surface reactions and reaction products precipitation regulate how and with what intensity the reactions and bioactivity will occur.

Taking into account the dissolution in aqueous solutions the soda-lime silicate glass and their SiO_2–CaO–Na_2O–R_xO_y derivatives can be classified in five distinct behaviors. The dissolution will always occur from glass surface and each behavior will depend on both the initial glass composition as the etching solution composition and pH [8]. According to this classification, a "Type ***A***" dissolution behavior is one where the attack and hydration occurs only in a thin layer from the surface (with a thickness of around 50 Å). In these glasses no significant change in surface composition or by alkali ions exchange or silica network dissolution is observed, since the pH of the solution is near neutrality. The fine hydrated layer formed has practically the same composition and the original mass of the glass composition. This behavior is mainly observed in the case of vitreous silica or glasses containing predominantly silica in its composition [8].

The dissolution behavior rating of "Type ***B***" is attributed primarily to glass compositions which after contact for a sufficient time with the etching solution is formed a film (surface layer) passivating which progressively hinders ion exchange and continuity the solution for glass attack. The passivating film formation is a result of alkali ions removing from glass surface [8]. In this class of glasses because they have relatively low alkali ions concentrations the rapid surface layer enrichment in silica is quickly reached. A glass having such a composition results in a fairly durable surface particularly in attack solutions where the pH is below to 9.0. This is the case with most commercial use soda-lime compositions [8].

The dissolution behavior classified as "Type ***C***" has the peculiarity that when the glass is subjected to contact an aqueous solution whose pH is near neutrality a double surface layer is formed as chemical interaction result. The double surface layer formation (it may be passivating or not) occurs when a secondary former such as Al_2O_3 or P_2O_5 is present in glass composition. The secondary former presence in small amounts in relation to main former (SiO_2) is a necessary but not sufficient condition for single or double surface layer formation (as will be treated throughout this text). In glasses that exhibit this type of behavior the outer layer is aluminum-silicate or calcium-phosphate composition in accordance to glass initial composition for example. Between the outer layer and the original glass will exist an enriched silica layer (as a result of alkaline and alkaline earth ion exchange in addition of secondary forming presence and subsequent silanol groups condensation) in most cases this layer consist in silica-gel [8]. Glasses of this type may have high chemical durability in both acidic and alkaline solutions. This is the composition group to which it belongs the SiO_2:CaO:Na_2O:P_2O_5 system bioactive glasses. In the bioactive glasses specific case the amorphous calcium phosphate outer layer is formed from previously released ions into the solution re-precipitation.

The dissolution behavior classified as "type ***D***" is observed for those glasses whose relative composition is poor in silica. In general way this group of glasses also forms the silica rich film on its surface like as "type ***B***" dissolution behavior glasses however due to its poor silica original composition the formed layer is unable to passivate the etching. Thus the exchange of alkali ions and the silica network hydrolyzing remains continuous and these glasses exhibit poor durability against solutions attack contact. In this dissolution behavior the attacked layer when it became thick enough will have little strength and little adherence with remaining virgin glass surface and will become detached, exposing the virgin glass directly to chemical attack [8]. Finally the "Type ***E***" dissolution behavior is observed when there is congruent dissolving from the glass surface with proportional loss by alkali ion exchange and silica hydrolyzing breaking the glass network. Due to uniform attack the surface composition of an "Type ***E***" glass is equivalent to its original composition. Thus, there is little difference in SiO_2 surface between a "Type ***E***" and "Type ***A***" dissolution behavior profile [8]. However, a "Type ***E***" behavior loses considerable ions amounts to solution. In this dissolution behavior the surface layer also can become detached exposing the virgin glass directly to chemical attack. Thus, the etching solution chemical analysis after the corrosion process distinguishes the two behavior types. This corrosion behavior may be heterogeneous over the etched glass surface when the pH is less than 9.0. The heterogeneity of such attack will result from local pH solution fluctuations with solution alkalinity increase. In its turn the solution alkalinity increasing will occur due to local glass composition variations throughout its surface. On the other hand when any silicate glass is exposed to attack solutions with pH > 9.0–10.0 the dissolution will tend to "Type ***E***" behavior. Although the bioactive glasses behavior was indicated as the close to "Type ***C***" other behaviors can be associated and this helps to understand at least partially the Fig. 1 diagram. In Fig. 2 we seek to associate only for illustrative purpose the 6 wt% P_2O_5 section in $CaO–SiO_2–Na_2O–P_2O_5$ quaternary system with the possible regions of each dissolution process predominant occurrence in approximate pH 7.5.

In this context, following will be discussed aspects about these glasses structure as well as their dissolution and ions transport mechanisms, using soda-lime glass as comparison to aid the subject understanding.

2 Soda-Lime Silicate and Bioactive Soda-Lime Phosphosilicate Glasses Structure

Usually a glass belonging to the soda lime silicate system (SiO_2:CaO:Na_2O) is presented as a material that can be obtained from the fusion of a mixture of silicon oxide with alkali and alkaline earth metal oxides (Na_2O and CaO) ranging in composition in according to the author that deals with the theme. In addition to the fusion process the glass can also be obtained by sol–gel process (which will not be

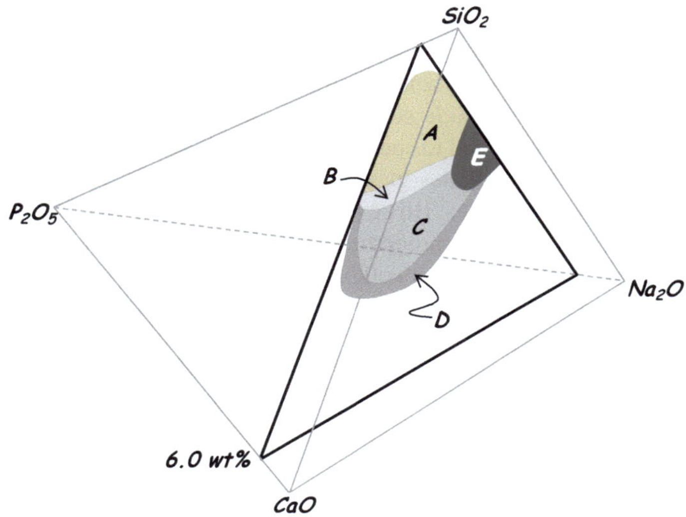

Fig. 2 $SiO_2-CaO-Na_2O-P_2O_5$ quaternary system 6 wt% P_2O_5 section, where are represented each possible dissolution process at pH about 7.5. Where *A* and *B* represent passivating layer forming behaviors; *C* represents bioactive glasses; and, *D* and *E* highly soluble glass

covered in this text) and obtained also adding a multitude of other oxides (P_2O_5, Al_2O_3, MgO, TiO_2, K_2O, Fe_2O_3, etc.), each with a specific function in the structural arrangement in material and giving rise to quaternary systems such as SiO_2:CaO: Na_2O:P_2O_5 in which forms part the 45S5 bioglass and derivative compositions.

The glass can be considered an amorphous material but it is not actually a completely holder this characteristic material. As an amorphous material the glass does not has long-range organization but in spite of that in the short-range order has any organization which postulated by Zachariasen [20] in the 1930s. Macrometric or more often nanometric crystalline phases can be observed in vitreous materials like process failures unless intentionally produced by heat treatment.

The glass formation by the melting process and quenching is widely studied and described in the literature [21] so we will not treat in detail here but it is important to point out that the glassy network disorganization degree will be not just from composition dependent but also the quenching and cooling rate that the liquid glass precursor can be subjected which may be checked by volume specific variations of a same composition materials. Although not present crystalline planes such as other materials to define the glass just as amorphous material is insufficient. The vitrification phenomenon is involved oxides interaction and their molecular characteristics dependent.

The glass structural arrangement began to be studied more closely from X-ray diffraction techniques improving. Since then several theories have been proposed to explain its structure. However all of them are based on the early theory presented by Zachariasen and formulated in 1932 [20]. This theory and its postulates although it was fundamental to understanding the glass structure basically describes those oxides which are able to form the skeleton of the glass network and therefore are called "*formers*" as discussed below. However it is less usual glasses that are composed only by formers oxide such as pure silica glass. In general for various reasons such glasses are limited to specific, noble or scientific research applications. The bioglass is a multiple oxides glass which obviously part of these oxides not fully meet the Zachariasen rules. However in despite this take place in structure and play a key role in bioglass final properties. In this way we can intuit that agreement in its role played in the glassy network each kind of employee oxide will exert a specific function in the structural network and in accordance with the performed function can be classified into groups. From author to author this classification may have some variation but in general they are restricted to formers, intermediate formers and modifiers, however, seeking to facilitate this understanding will be adopted an expanded classification shown below:

(1) Primary formers or formers;
(2) Secondary formers or intermediaries;
(3) Intermediate modifiers; and,
(4) Terminal modifiers.

The function that each oxide plays in the glass structure formation is better understood through of interatomic binding energies and their coordination number study. It must be noted that some oxides may perform more than one function in the vitreous network depending upon their coordination number and the vitreous system considered [22]. For example in lime-soda glass the alumina (Al_2O_3) may be either network former when in tetrahedral coordination as an intermediary oxide when in the trigonal coordination being able to occur in both within the same glass system as, for example, when the charge compensation is needed to achieve the structure stability.

The primary glass formers oxides or simply "formers oxides" are vitreous networks forming capable without presence of any heterogeneous oxide. Fully comply with Zachariasen rules and in general they are responsible for glassy network skeleton [22]. The cations of this oxides group are typically small size (compared with oxygen) present valence equal to or greater than three and Pauling electronegativity between 1.5 and 2.1 [22]. These oxides form covalent bonds (Cation-Oxygen) having interatomic bonding forces higher than 335 kJ/mol (80 kcal/mol). The SiO_2, P_2O_5, B_2O_3 oxides and some Al_2O_3 forms are examples of formers oxides which show all these characteristics. The cohesion of material formed bay this oxide kind is ensured by covalent bonds (Si–O, B–O, P–O, etc.) [23–25]. Covalent bonds are considered strong and markedly directional bonds thus favoring the tetrahedral structure formation as in the case of the Si–O bond [26] (Fig. 3).

The bonds covalent nature and their binding energies (high for the glass-network systems) will require higher activation energies to occur any transformation, hence, it is explained to be these oxides groups accountable for characteristics in glasses

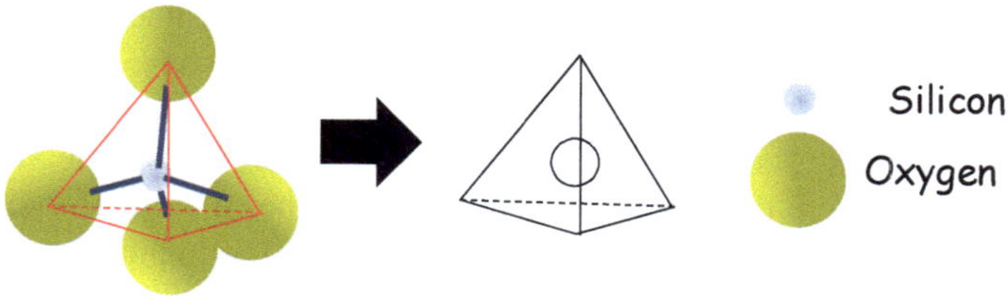

Fig. 3 SiO_4 tetrahedron representative scheme showing their atoms arrangement

such as high-melting temperatures (in the pure SiO_2 system this can overcome 2000 °C) or high chemical resistance.

Taking for example the pure silica glass in it all tetrahedra are connected by the vertices through sharing an oxygen atom with two silicon atoms. In most tetrahedrons all the four oxygen atoms can be shared with up to four other tetrahedra forming a three-dimensional network where the short-range arrangement or atom by atom is very similar to that of crystalline silica but without structural periodicity [23].

The oxygen atoms shared between the tetrahedra of equal nature are called "Bridging Oxigens" (BO). The oxygen sharing between two silica tetrahedra is schematically shown in Fig. 4.

The secondary formers oxides or simply intermediaries oxides are by definition the ones capable of forming glass but only if it is associated with a primary former. In other words, they can participate directly in the glass network forming covalent bonds and composing arrangements with primary formers oxides. It is in fact a group of vitreous network structural units in "transition" between the "primary formers" and "intermediate modifiers". With few exceptions another striking feature of this group is that generally they have more than one coordination in glassy systems in according the other oxides associated. Such possibility of associating the glass network with different coordination reinforces the transient character of this group and this way it is possible to find, for example, alumina as much as primary former (tetrahedral) as a secondary former (trigonal). Often it is observed over a single coordinating an oxide on a vitreous system, one being predominant and the other tending to be residual. In a coarse approach from a scientific point of view

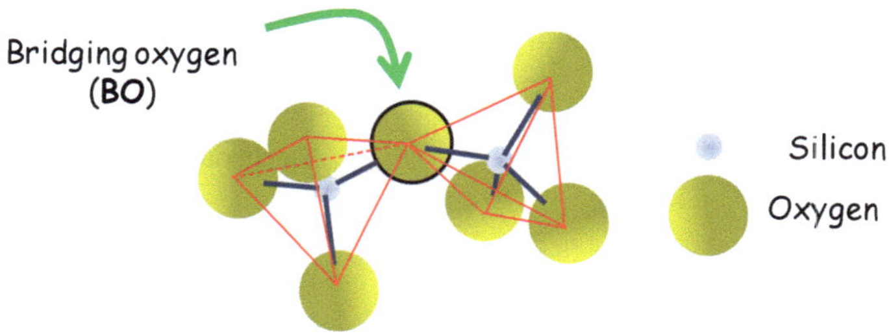

Fig. 4 Scheme exemplifying the oxygen atom sharing between two silica tetrahedral

because it is based only on empirical observations it is possible to adopt the following practical rule; a composition among the oxides who have a higher binding energy associated with a higher molar fraction will be preferred to adopt coordination that gives it the “best sites” in glass network. Thus, for example, in silica and alumina mixture where the silica molar fraction is higher than that of the alumina will be prevail the silica tetrahedral coordination (which has higher binding energy) and alumina tend to trigonal coordination. The occurrence of tetrahedral alumina only will be favored by increasing the relative fraction of this oxide. This can occur either by increasing the alumina content in the overall glass composition or by the compositional heterogeneities occurrence in any local site that causes a punctual enrichment of alumina content. Similar behavior occurs for the P_2O_5 determining its position and interaction form with the silica main network or their segregation in “clusters” in which are commonly associated with Ca^+.

One consequence of the secondary formers presence is that in glass network formation the oxygens sharing will occur among covalent bonds with cations of two different chemical elements, e.g., oxygen atom shared between tetrahedral silica and tetrahedral or trigonal alumina, as shown in Fig. 5.

The modifier oxides are generally regarded as a single group called “network modifiers” because of their similarity, but there are two clearly cations functions for these oxides group as its valence, i.e., in despite both act as charge compensating in glass structure the R^{2+} cations (intermediate modifiers that are in general alkaline earth metals oxides) performing the connection between forming oxide clusters while keeping the glass structure. In contrast the R^{1+} cations (terminal modifiers that are in general alkaline metal oxides) possesses the primarily role as charge compensator in former oxides glass network unconnected and/or terminal points.

Of course this is a brief description of these oxides functions in glass structure which will be better understood with the following discussion.

The modifiers group represent the oxides with cation-oxygen bond energy less than 200 kJ/mol (CaO, PbO, MgO, Na_2O, K_2O, etc.) which participate in glass structure by bonding it’s cation with oxygen atoms located at silica tetrahedron edges. The oxygen atoms associated with these cations are referred “non-bridging oxigens” (**NBO**). The **NBO**’s represent formers network discontinuity points where

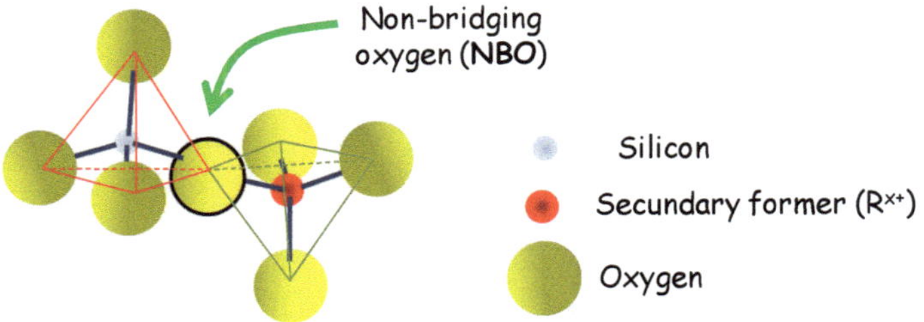

Fig. 5 Demonstrative sharing scheme of one oxygen atom between two different nature formers oxides where are formed only covalent bonds

there is the necessity of the oxygen negative charge compensation to achieve glass structure charge stability. The charge stability is achieved with former oxides association with different nature cations (usually R^+ and R^{2+}) where R^+ cations form ionic bonds [27–29] and it is considered in similar way that the R^{2+} cations also form ionic bonds, however, for this last case the references in literature about what kind of bond is formed are general way inconclusive.

This means that each added modifier oxide to the silica network may inhibit one Si–O–Si binding which allows oxygen to incorporate additional radical (Si–O–R binding) thus resulting in a modified glassy network [21, 28]. Thus the glassy structure can incorporate increasing amounts of modifier oxides until it reaches a ratio at which it is no longer possible to keep structural cohesion [30]. This will occur because clearly a massive modifiers cations incorporation will discontinue the glassy network covalent bonds sequence (composed by pure silica or combined with other formers) and for each bond formed with a modifier cation will always represent a new **NBO** with a lower energy binding than a **BO** between formers oxides. The ways by which the modifiers are incorporated into the glass network as its intermediate or terminal nature are shown schematically in Fig. 6.

As a result the glass final characteristics changes depending on the modifier oxides presence and content increase. Because of the weak links (NBO), in general way "modified glass" will present lower chemical resistance and lower hardness. These effects are more intense with network terminals modifiers (R^+) addition than that observed for the intermediate modifiers (R^{2+}) thus in glass formulation when is desired a glass specific dissolution rate are used proportions adjustments between the two natures modifier oxides (bioactive glasses and glass with biocide activity for example).

However we should avoid a simplistic view where the addition of monovalent modifier oxides to silica glass will only act on the charge compensation in glass network terminals sites. These oxides are used to lower the melting temperature because this R^{x+} possess the ability to contribute to the disruption of the bonds

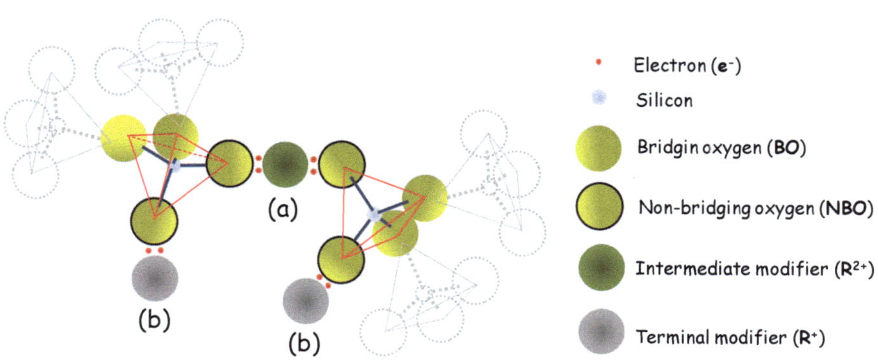

Fig. 6 Demonstrative scheme of one former oxide oxygen atom being shared with a modifier cation; **a** a terminals modifiers where R^+ represents Na^+, K^+, etc.; and, **b** a intermediary cation where R^{2+} represents Ca^{2+}, Mg^{2+}, etc.

between existing formers in oxides used as raw material already in melted glass liquid precursor. By this way will be promoted the association between “former” and “modifier” oxides. As a result there will be a “recombination” of raw materials constituent oxides to form the structure of a specific glass. In other words, the R^+ are associated with network termination points not only because charge balance opportunity but in fact are these cations that cause the occurrence of these discontinuities in glass network during raw materials melting. Owning this concept clearly in mind it is important to understand the bioglass dissolution mechanisms that control their bioactivity degree. Figure 7 schematically illustrates the structure of a glass composed only by a primary former (SiO_2) and a terminal modifier (Na_2O). This kind glass can be obtained at temperatures of a few hundred Celsius degrees, however have a reduced chemical resistance so that in general will dissolve with the existing moisture in the atmospheric air in short time.

The influence of the alkali oxide (R^+) as fluxing (reducing the melting temperature) increases with the cation atomic radius which is constituted, i.e., with increasing modifier radius/charge ratio and consequently network polarization enhances the ease of glass liquid precursor formation. The phase separations occur when little polarized cations are present [22].

On the other hand, if the modifier oxide is bivalent (intermediate modifiers, e.g. Ca^{2+}) there is the possibility of the cation associate two distinct segments of the SiO_2 network and consequently the effects observed by the presence of divalent modifier oxides (R^{2+}) will be less intense when compared to the effects caused by the monovalent oxide (R^+). In general modifiers cations to complete their coordination will form so many bonds with oxygen atoms as necessary. In addition alkaline earth oxides and some other cations may also cause a formers network breakdown but the discontinuity of the network is partly offset by the double

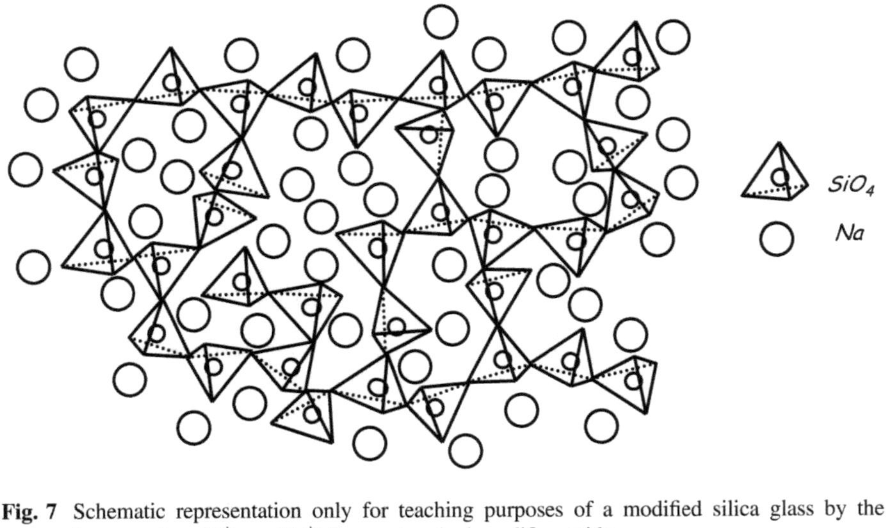

Fig. 7 Schematic representation only for teaching purposes of a modified silica glass by the cations incorporation (R^+, ex: Na^+) from a terminal modifier oxide

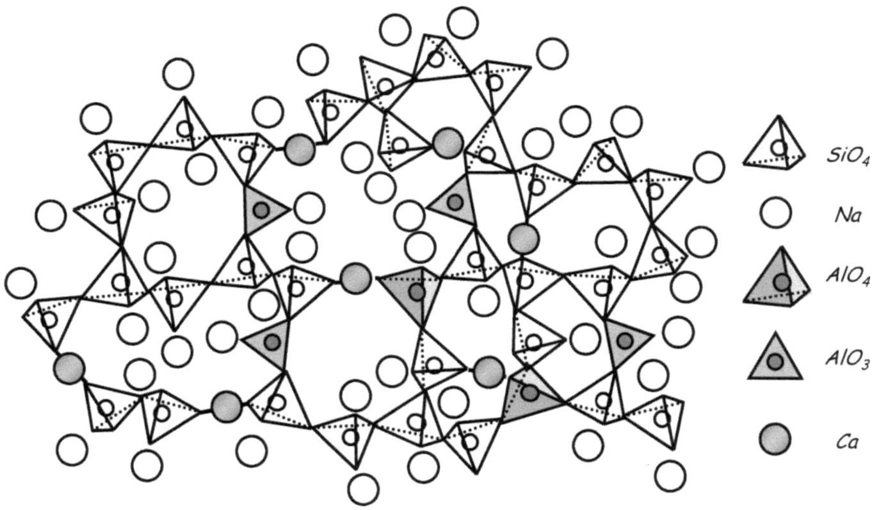

Fig. 8 Schematic representation only for didactic purposes of a glass silicate containing Na_2O, CaO and Al_2O_3

positive charge of these cations that come to act as bridges between two atoms oxygen [21]. The glasses with divalent cations modifier have higher melting temperatures and chemical resistance, generally higher when compared to the bond with the monovalent cations. Figure 8 shows a schematic representation of a glass composed by primary formers (tetrahedral silica and alumina), secondary formers (trigonal alumina), intermediate modifiers (CaO) and terminal modifiers (Na_2O).

In any glass network arrangement the SiO_2 tetrahedra oxygens can not be shared with other SiO_2 tetrahedra, i.e., some oxygen atoms are shared with otherwise formers cation or even with modifiers cations. These unshared oxygens, as we treat earlier are called "non-bridging oxigen" (**NBO**) [27]. Evidently as more complex is the glass composition and/or greater is the other oxides mole fraction more **NBO**'s will occur. Even though pure oxides glasses due to glass structure distortion if compared with a crystalline order, some oxygens are not shared. Taking as an example the silica primary forming the silica tetrahedra NBO's occurrence may be represented as follows: Q^4, Q^3, Q^2, Q^1, Q^0 (0, 1, 2, 3 and 4, **NBO**'s respectively), i.e., one silica tetrahedron Q^4 will be associated directly to four other silica tetrahedra by sharing oxygens with them; one silica tetrahedron Q^3 will be associated directly to three other silica tetrahedra; and so on until a silica tetrahedron Q^0 is not directly associated with any other silica tetrahedron. This notation consequently indicates the manner in which the glass network is organized as well as its structural coherence and can be represented as shown in Fig. 9.

As shown above as higher is the **BO**'s number in a glass structure as higher is its melting temperature and chemical resistance. Thus, a structure mainly formed with Q^4 species melt at a higher temperature and will have higher chemical resistance than other glass where the structure mainly formed with Q^2 species, for example.

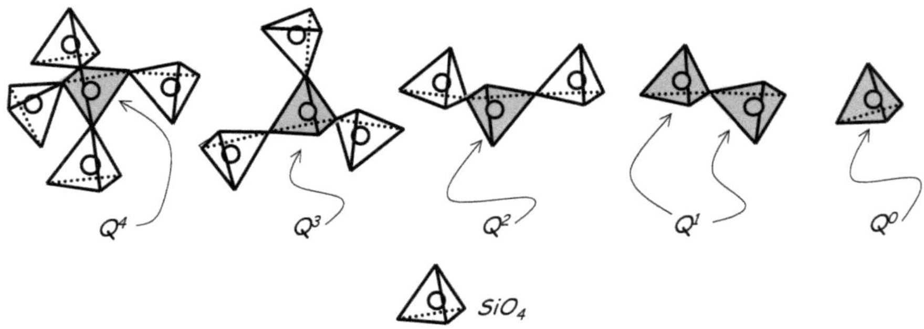

Fig. 9 Schematic representation only for didactic purposes of the possible "Q^x" silica species in a glass

In practical terms, viable silicate glass will be mainly formed by Q^4 Q^3 and Q^2 species and those whose are mostly formed by Q^1 and Q^0 species are unstable and have almost any application. The soda-lime silicate glass (including the soda-lime phosphosilicate glass group which include bioactive glass) are usually formed by combination of Q^2 and Q^3 species with a lower incidence of other species. Rarely a glass network is comprised of only a single species. Usually in a glass network a Q^x species predominant will be accompanied mainly by Q^{x-1} and/or Q^{x+1} variations since $x - 1$ is greater than or equal to zero and $x + 1$ is less than or equal to four. Q^x other species should be present in lesser amount. A glass whose structure that defers of this distribution will probably present fluctuations in their structural distribution arrangement and/or is formed by at least two glass phases. The same notation can be applied by analogy to other formers such as phosphorus oxide, for example, as their coordination. Even though secondary formers can form homogeneous regions to one another as a cluster in a silica network, where this study is also valid.

In general Q^4 species associations form three-dimensional clusters (Fig. 10) the Q^3 species associations form "sheet shape" or tetrahedral surfaces which must not be confused with crystalline planes (Fig. 11) because these surfaces are highly distorted in accordance with the tetrahedron free corner random distribution. Such configuration in surfaces is also characterized by the occurrence of silica tetrahedra rings (di-silanol and silanol-tri rings among others). In its turn Q^2 species form linear chains or "wires" of silica tetrahedrons (Fig. 12). Depending on other structural present groups in neighborhoods these filaments may be sufficiently distorted to result in di-silanol rings formation. The intersection of Q^2 chains also results in a occasional Q^3 or Q^4 silica (intersections between filaments) and several intersections not infrequently contribute to silica rings formation. The Q^1 species form simple dimers dispersed throughout the glass network (Fig. 13) and finally the Q^0 species constitute isolated monomeric tetrahedral from vitreous silica network (Fig. 14), although they can be united indirectly to it through a intermediary modifier or secondary former. In the glass network all these structures are also directly or indirectly attached. As an example of direct associations we can mention that from Q^3 surfaces may be emanating Q^2 straight chains and the shared

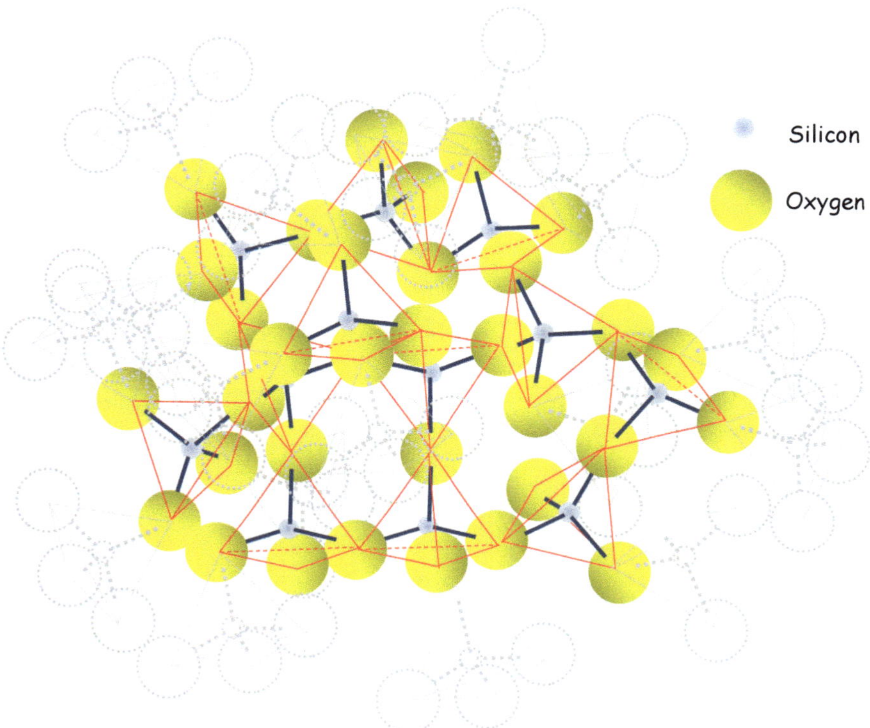

Fig. 10 Schematic representation just for didactic purposes of a glass where the structure is composed of silica species "Q^4"

tetrahedron that intersects both structures will be a Q^4 specie. An indirect association occurs when any of two silica tetrahedra groups are joined by "bridges" occurrence that are result of one or more intermediate former or secondary modifier oxides sharing. We must remember also that these species distribution and resulting structures organization gradient are due to the chemical composition and the super-cooling rate during glass casting (quenching).

Therefore, the units Q^x describe not only the glass network but also the **NBO**'s distribution and indirectly the alkali metal (R^+) sub-networks. Given the ionic bonds association between alkali metals and **NBO**'s the R^+ can easily migrate around the sub-networks [29].

A simplified form of the Q^n species study is to count the **BO**'s average number that are connected with a network forming atom [31] indicating in this way the glass network connectivity (**NC**). Lower **NC** values indicate a fragmented structure. The overall empirical correlation between the **NC** and bioglass bioactivity [31, 30] has a limiting value of about **NC** = 3.25 and essentially reflects the higher solubility in less interconnected glass structural distributions.

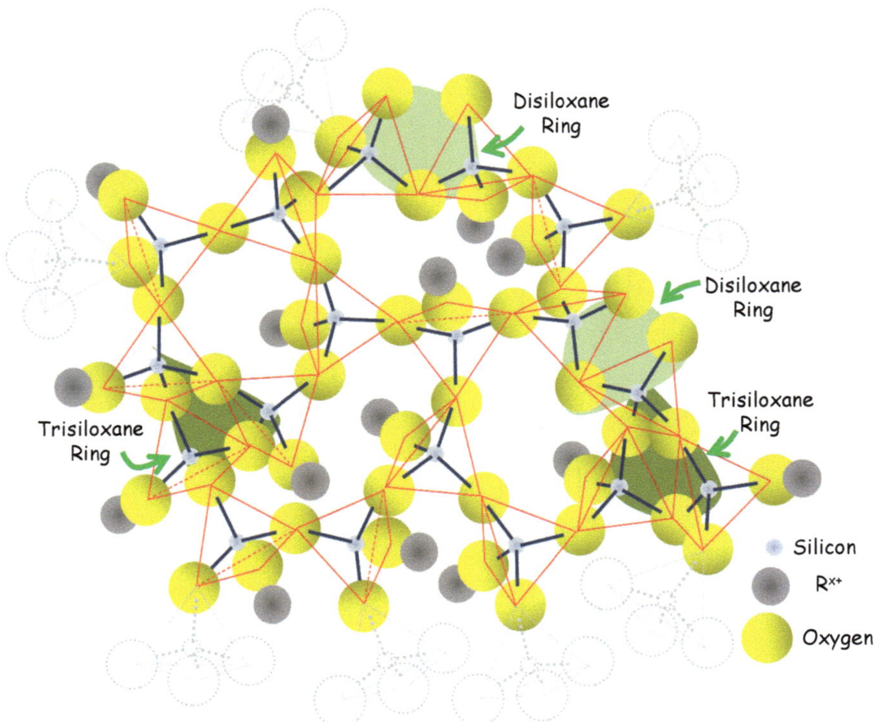

Fig. 11 Schematic representation just for didactic purposes of a glass where the structure is composed of silica species "Q^3". In the figure it can be observed the silica rings arrangement and are marked the di-siloxane and tri-siloxane rings

Have knowledge about the Q^n species distribution is important to understand the phosphate soda-lime glass bioactivity. For instance the soluble silica release in solution improves the gene activation properties. This release is facilitated when the majority of silicates chains (Q^2) do not intersect. In this case for breaking Si–O–Si bridges the dissolution of the silica will require less energy and will reflect the fragmentation of the chains for Q^1 species which reduce the required Si–O bonds number that are to be broken to separate these fragments from the matrix. Subsequently they are transported to the surface, and finally released in solution. On the other hand in a structure with an upper **NC** Q^2 silicate chains are intersecting each other to form rings of different sizes from the chains linked by Q^3 and/or Q^4 tetrahedrons in intersections. Thus the condensation is indicated in closed chain rings of different sizes which decelerates the dissolution and reduces the bioactivity [17, 32].

Returning to intermediate formers oxides discussion the P_2O_5 is soluble in the soda-lime silicate glass precursor liquid and can be added in varying amounts, depending on the glass composition before nucleation occurs. This oxide rarely crystallizes as separate oxides in the beginning of the crystallization, usually

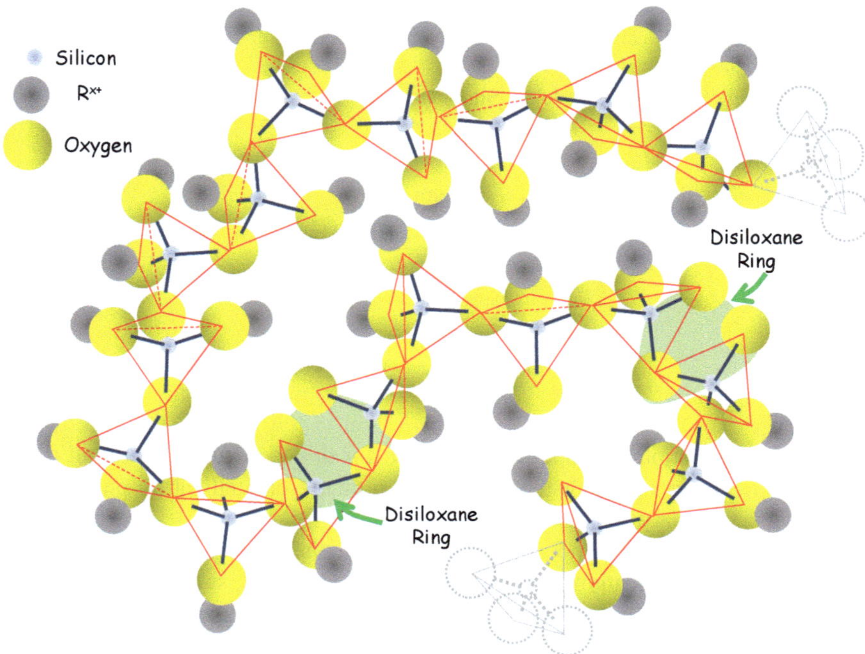

Fig. 12 Schematic representation just for didactic purposes of a glass where the structure is composed of silica species "Q^2". In the figure are marked the di-siloxane rings

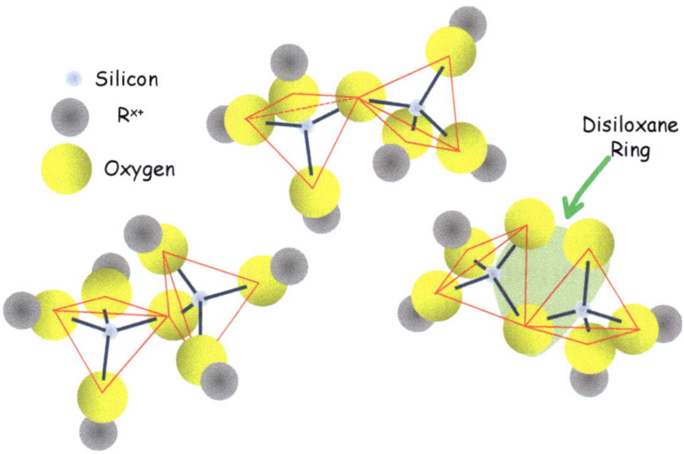

Fig. 13 Schematic representation just for didactic purposes of a glass where the structure is composed of silica species "Q^2". In the figure are marked the di-siloxane rings

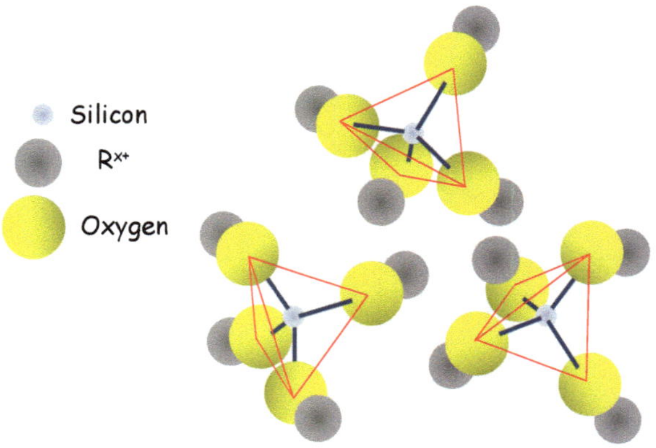

Fig. 14 Schematic representation just for didactic purposes of a glass where the structure is composed of silica species "Q^1"

precipitate as a complex compound. However, for this to occur are required one or more heat treatments at high temperature to promote crystallization phase(s) and growth of the primary microstructure [33].

Because of the high temperatures involved in the glass melting [34, 35] the intermediates formers cations presents in a precursor liquid, such as P_2O_5, may be form oxides with different coordination numbers that participate in the glass network making links with two or more structural units (silica tetrahedrons) and thus contributing to increase the structural cohesion which in the end affects the characteristic properties of glasses. At concentrations lower than <5 mol% secondary formers ions interact with the glass network in a way similar to alkali metals and alkaline earth metals [36], i.e. at low concentrations the R_xO_y acts as a network modifier.

The structural function of the secondary former in glasses depends on its valence and local coordination. So the glass network structural integrity and chemical stability are directly associated with the interaction between secondary ions formers and structure, that is, his ability as a glass former [37]. The presence of other elements, are modifying the network and/or intermediate formers, influence this balance and secondary former coordination. This behavior has relation with the ionic field, $\mathbf{Z/r^2}$ [36], which favors the intermediate former to join with the silica network when the **BO/NBO** relationship increases as the glass transition temperature (**Tg**) also increases [38] while the thermal expansion coefficient (**TEC**) decreases with the SiO_2 substitution by R_xO_y, i.e., the glass network increases its rigidity.

The R–O–Si bond energy is greater than the Na: O–Si due to the R–O is a covalent bond which is characteristic of an intermediate former. If a polyhedron R_xO_y replace a SiO_4 tetrahedron in the glass, a negative charge will be form due to the difference between the valence of Si^{4+} and R^{y+}. This negative charge is compensated by the proximity of Na^+ [36].

3 Interaction Mechanisms Between Living Tissue and Glasses Soda-Lime Phosphosilicate

The bioglass dissolution mechanism and it's interaction with living tissue study is particularly important in predicting bioglasses performance. In soda-lime phosphosilicate system this mechanism has six processes that can be identified. The first three process keep strict similarity with ordinary glasses (soda-lime silicate) dissolution process in an aqueous medium. The bioglass interaction with the living tissue properly so called will occur because the last two stages, with the formation of calcium phosphate compounds on the surface of these materials.

The glass dissolution rate is the measure of its chemical resistance which is defined through the trouble of removal of their constituents in according to their interaction with the environment where it is located, being an irreversible process [39, 40].

The complexity composition and the presence of inhomogeneities in a glass accentuate the character and difficult metastable thermodynamic equilibrium with water or with any means which is exposed [41–43]. By heterogeneities can be understood other components oxides, manufacturing defects (cracks, bubbles and contamination), changes in the vitreous nature of the material (crystallization seeds and crystals) or even local composition fluctuations and/or Q^x silica distribution, the latter being very important for bioglasses performance such as 45S5 because R^+ (Na^+) local concentrations are essential for the percolation channels formation and ion exchange in these materials, as will be discussed below. The glasses have a thermodynamic energy as high as the crystalline materials of the same composition. However, for being in metastable equilibrium materials tend to react with aqueous solutions to form more stable hydrated phases [44]. The variation of hydration free energy ($\Delta G_{Hidr.}$) in a tetrahedral silica glass structure can be estimated as the free energies of hydration sum and are proportional to the molar mass of its constituents [44–46]. The glass durability is primarily a result by the ratio with former elements and network modifiers.

The silicate bioglass dissolution occurs in general by a limited number of processes that are influenced by the attack medium pH [2, 41, 43, 46, 47]. The dissolution mechanism may be divided in steps, as the dominant dissolution process at a given time. Considering a bioglass system SiO_2–CaO–Na_2O–P_2O_5 briefly it may be description six stages:

(1) Cations and anions diffusion through the glass matrix;
(2) Glass network hydrolysis;
(3) Silica enriched layer formation on the glass surface;
(4) Glass network attack by OH^- ions;
(5) Ca^{2+} and PO_4^{3-} rich film formation in material surface; and,
(6) HA precipitation on the material surface.

From the kinetic standpoint of glass dissolution these steps can be respectively described as [47]: 1 and 2, selective dissolution; 3, 5 and 6, secondary phases formation at the interfaces between the glass surface and the solution; and, 4, glass matrix dissolution. Each numbered step is described below.

3.1 Cations and Anions Diffusion Through the Glass Matrix

It should initially consider that any body fluid contact with a bioglass implant is essentially an aqueous solution in which naturally occurs H^+ cation and OH^- anions by simple water dissociation to form solution. The diffusion of these ions through the bioglass surface will result in immediate ion exchange with its components and percolation channels formation that will further facilitate diffusion processes through the bulk bioglass. At this bioglass dissolution stage the first absorption process by the host organism has mainly the diffusion of H^+ and/or H_3O^+ cations through the glass matrix where to find favorable energy conditions such as R^+ attractions or ionic bonds with non-bridge oxygen (**NBO**) sites which are energy weaker than covalent oxygen bridge bonds (**BO**). The **NBO**'s generally form silica tetrahedron associations with intermediates and terminals modifiers, namely the Na^+ and Ca^{2+} cations. With the rapid exchange of these cations by H^+ they will be transported to the etching solution. This process also leads to the formation of silanol groups (Si^{3+}–OH) and by this way will occur the hydrated layer formation. At the attack beginning due to its weak ionic bond would be mainly affected the network terminal modifiers R^+ (Na^+ in Bioglass case) which will be initially removed (Eqs. 1 and 2).

$$\left(Si^{3+}-O-R\right)_{Glass}+H_3O^+ \leftrightarrow \left(Si^{3+}-OH\right)_{Glass}+R^+ +H_2O(R^+ = Na^+) \quad (1)$$

or

$$\left(Si^{3+}-O - R\right)_{Glass}+H^+ \leftrightarrow \left(Si^{3+}-OH\right)_{Glass}+R^+ \quad (2)$$

As can be seen in the above equations, due to charge compensation mechanisms, the H^+ protons will not only remove alkali cations, but also occupy the sites formerly belonging thereto. This removal and exchange mechanism is favored by a neutral pH or slightly alkaline, characteristic of bodily fluids. The removal of the alkali ions is facilitated by these showed good mobility and high diffusion coefficients. However, this diffusivity decreases due to depletion in the alkali concentration in glass surface which forms a barrier to the continued reaction (Fig. 15) [43, 45, 46, 47, 48, 49, 50, 51, 52, 53].

The glass surface region will then result depleted in alkali (Na^+) and the removal rate thereof is becoming smaller due to the diffusion barrier itself that this region will offer. The alkali replacement finally result in Si^{3+}–OH groups in vitreous subnets terminal positions. The R^+ original function is stabilizing the charges to maintain the glass subnet stable. Of course, for various reasons the H^+ will not fulfill this function identically to the original Na^+. In this manner it has been accentuated load instabilities in the above-described sub-networks and the two

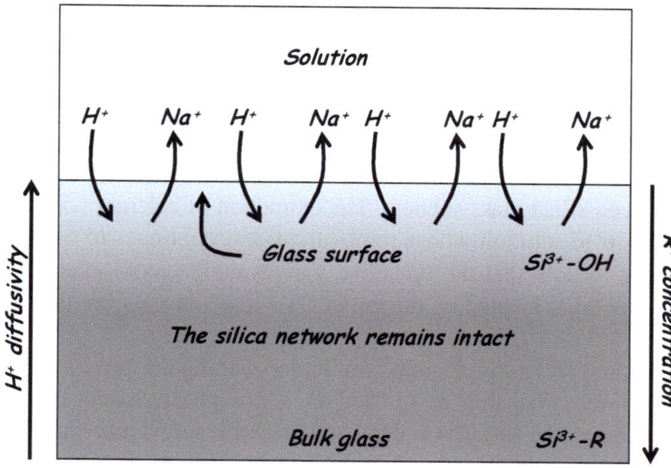

Fig. 15 Schematic representation of H^+ cations diffusion and Na^+ cations removal through the glass matrix from the surface

BO's connections formed by R^{2+} (Ca^{2+}, alkaline earth cations) will become non-equivalent energetically, this being sufficient condition so that they can be easily broken by anion attack H^+ and thus occurs the Ca^+ cations removal as shown in Eqs. 3 and 4 and in Fig. 16.

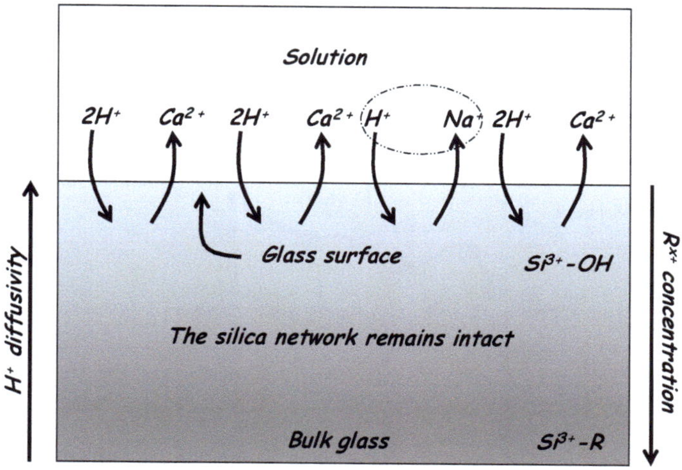

Fig. 16 Schematic representation of H^+ cations diffusion and Ca^{2+} and Na^+ cations removal through the glass matrix from the surface

$$\left(Si^{3+}-O-R-O-Si^{3+}\right)_{glass} + 2H_3O^+ \leftrightarrow 2\left(Si^{3+}-OH\right)_{glass} + R^{2+} + 2H_2O \quad \left(R^{2+} = Ca^{2+}\right) \quad (3)$$

or

$$\left(Si^{3+}-O-R-O-\ Si^{3+}\right)_{glass} + 2H^+ \leftrightarrow 2\left(Si^{3+}-OH\right)_{glass} + R^{2+} \quad (4)$$

As a result of calcium extraction are formed discontinuities that weaken the cohesion between silica glass subnets. The extraction of calcium will also facilitate the Na^+ transport to solution whose removal process continues to occur in parallel. It is interesting to note that the bioactive glasses antibacterial effect is due to the alkaline earth medium created by the initial Ca^{2+} ions release from the glass surface [54–59].

However, this is still a simplistic way of understanding this process. The bioactive glasses are mainly consisting of Q^3 and Q^2 silica groups which form structural sub-chains at disordered surfaces and twisted filaments forms respectively. Although of course there are interconnection points between these structures, the resulting arrangement will be fragmented and between them will exist sites where will be facilitated R^+ terminal modifiers allocation whose main function is the glass network charge compensation. The same regions also form the space required to accommodate most of the secondary Formers (e.g. phosphates) and intermediate modifiers (R^{2+}), which can also have interconnecting functions between glass subnet chains. Also these same regions will be those that will host the most of Q^1 and Q^0 silica species segregated from silica subnets. Indeed, the Na^+ is not distributed in a

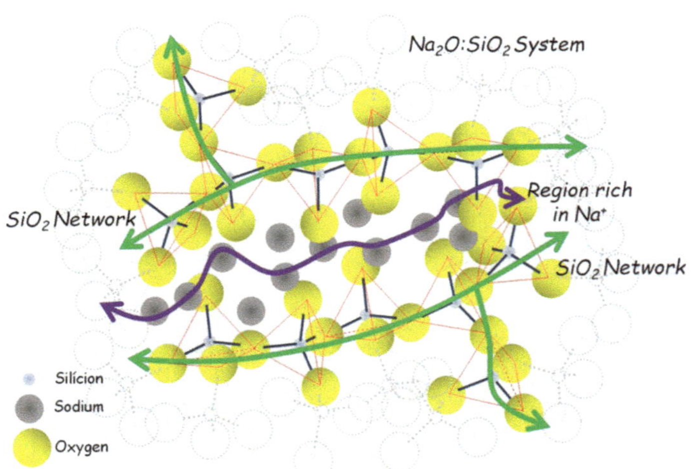

Fig. 17 Schematic representation of Na^+ cations enriched regions between the silica subnets in a glass

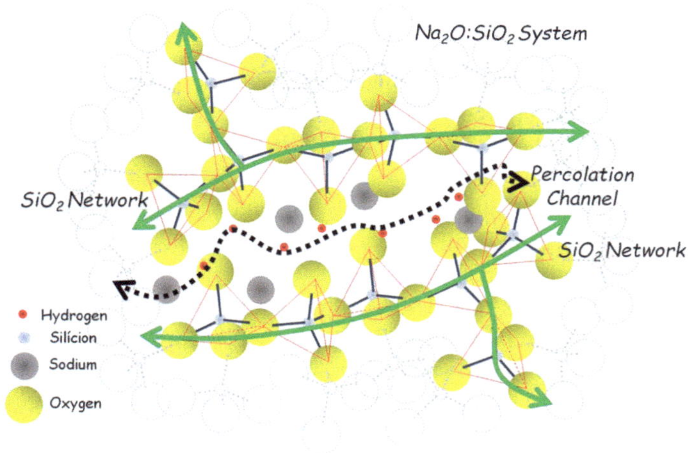

Fig. 18 Schematic representation of percolation channels formation by Na^{+} ion exchange in enriched regions between the silica subnets in a glass

homogeneous manner through the bulk glass, resulting in alkali cations enriched regions distributed among the glass network main arrangement (Fig. 17).

The high Na^{+} and Ca^{2+} modifier cations hydrophilicity in conjunction with the glass structure fragmented nature promote adequate mechanisms for surface water penetration into the bulk glass, i.e., the exchange of alkali cations by H^{+} cations in the abundant sodium regions. The alkali ions exchanging by H^{+} process leads to percolation channels formation through which the diffusion of cations from the solution is facilitated. Thus the H^{+}, H_3O^{+} and OH^{-} cations may penetrate and easily

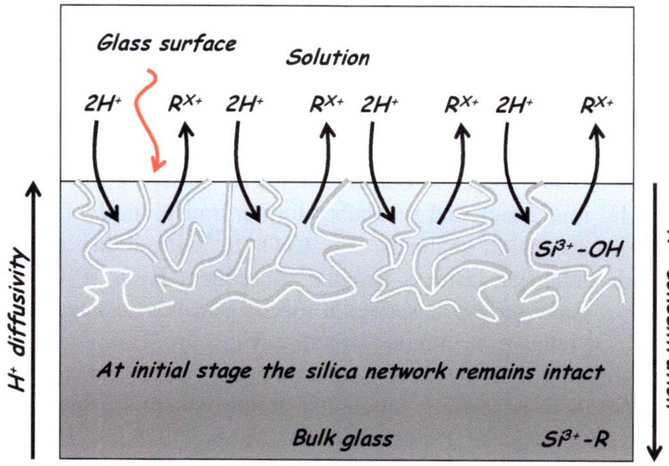

Fig. 19 Another schematic representation of percolation channels formation by Na^{+} ion exchange in enriched regions between the silica subnets in a glass

access the glass inner regions without significantly Si–O–Si bonds distorting or breaking near the surface (Figs. 18, 19).

The alkali ion concentration gradients in glasses are dependent also to its thermodynamic historical and thus the "quenching" cooling rate and subsequent heat treatment will affect the distribution of R^+. In the case of a glass subjected to "annealing" the best glass network accommodation will tend to segregation of the alkali, benefiting the percolation channels formation, on the other hand, when it accommodates the structure will be less spaced and which may hinder the transport ionic. The percolation channels formation play a key role in the bioglass dissolution and subsequent processes that define it's bioactivity. The Na^+ and Ca^{2+} cations strong hydrophilicity equilibrates the exposed siloxane fragments low water affinity [17, 60, 61]. The dissociated water penetration facilitates and helps to fast initial bioglass dissolution. The substantial Ca^{2+} removal in these early stages gives the biocide characteristic of this biomaterial. Therefore, the Na^+/H^+ ion exchange mechanism which is the first stage of the glass surface degradation engages in a dominant way the Na^+–H_2O interactions establishing through the surface and sodium enriched regions, which promotes the percolation channels formation and the dissociated water transport inside the glass structure. Considering the occurrence of interfacial ion exchange, it is preferred to lower binding energies, in this way the R^+ will initially be changed and when it becomes scarce, the R^+ will be more required for charge compensation and will become more strongly attracted to the network glass, in this way R^{2+} cations become released more easily. Only in longer time scales and after partial Na^+ removal the interactions between water and network's phosphosilicate will be established.

A secondary former (R_2O_n; P_2O_5, for example) when present in glass will compete with the silica to form the network. The preference for placement form in the vitreous network will be determined by the binding energies and the relative concentrations. For small concentrations the silica primary former replacement by R_2O_n is hindered and these oxides generally tend to take different coordination of the tetrahedral. In this case, the secondary former oxide (R_2O_n) plays a role similar to R^{2+} modifier ions and compete with them by the NBO's. In a glass network in these conditions, the R_2O_n will contribute to the network charge imbalance being compensated by alkaline and/or alkaline cations. Therefore with the exchange H^+/Na^+ will result unstably Si–O–R bonds in the glass network, making thus more susceptible to H^+ ions attack and secondary former transportation (PO_4^{3-}) to glass surface through percolation channels. The CaO (R^{2+}) instability and consequent Ca–NBO bonds breakage easiness and the subsequent R_2O_n (P_2O_5, in bioglass case) removal to glass surface describes a mechanism whose intensity is proportional to the R_xO_y relative in vitreous structure (Figs. 20, 21).

It is also interesting to note that in a soda-lime glass the phase separation results in regions where there is calcium cations clustering which is generally associated with dissolution rate increase. However, in bioglasses where also PO_4^{3-} is present this one has a strong affinity for Ca^{2+}. As a result may form calcium phosphate enriched nanodomains [62] which induce to dissolution rate reduction. In this case the loss of bioactivity is characterized by the formation of calcium phosphate

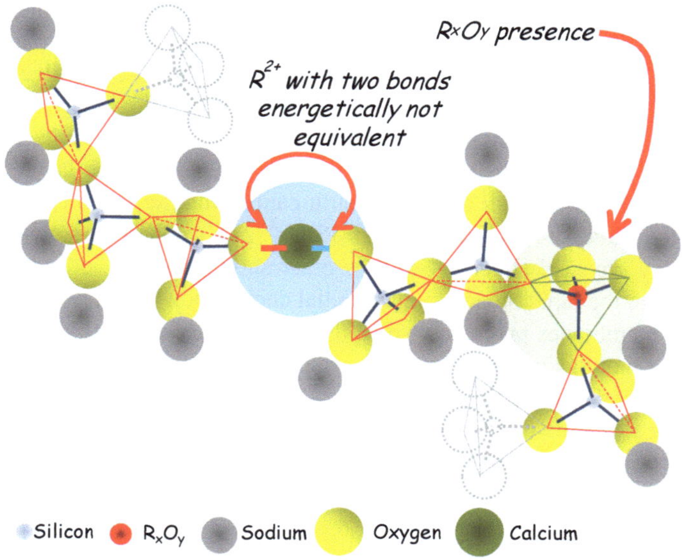

Fig. 20 Schematic representation of the R^{2+} with energetically unstable bonds due to the R_xO_y group proximity in the silica network

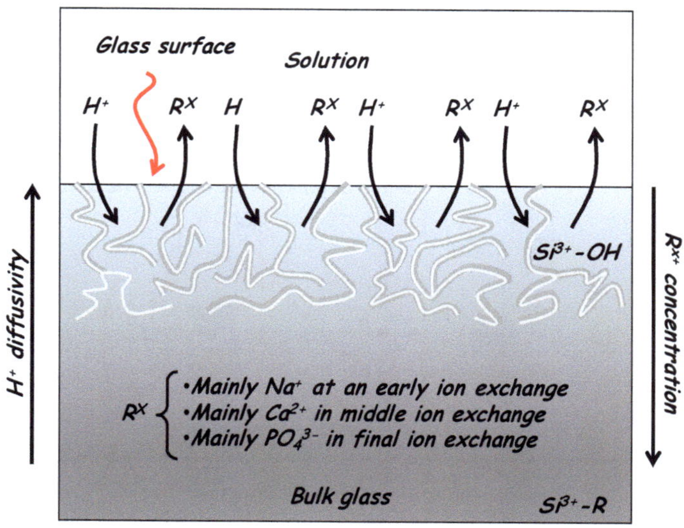

Fig. 21 Schematic representation of the R^x ions transport to glass surface

nanoclusters which are segregated from those other regions enriched in silica. The calcium phosphate segregation is a consequence of the P_2O_5 concentration increase in basic composition. This greater dissolution resistance in a phase segregated glass [63, 64] can be interpreted due to the lower mobility of ions trapped in isolated regions [65] which reduces the regions filled by primary modifier which favor the percolation channels formation which constitute the ions migration paths through the glass structure [17, 62, 64, 66, 67, 68]. Thus the increase in calcium concentration from the 45S5 composition gradually reduces the bioactivity.

The R^+ and R^{2+} cations removal from the surface layers results in a higher isolated orthosilicate tetrahedra (SiO_4^{4-}) fraction in these surface layer than in the bulk glass. Due to the alkali and alkali earth cations intense ion exchange with the medium, the direct free silicate species (SiO_4^{4-}, Q^0) release to solution will be enhanced (by physical effect) as well as other short chain (Q^1 or even some Q^2) contributing to the rapid bioactive glass initial degradation that may affect the living tissues cell membranes processes which the free silicate are quickly transported. Is worth noting that this removed free silica fraction does not reflect the dissolution of the silica network core, i.e., they are released isolated tetrahedrons (Q^0) or small tetrahedrons segments due to their silica network attachment was dependent upon the modifiers which were involved in ion exchange (Fig. 22).

To the dissolved silica has been attributed to osteoblasts stimulation property and to promote quick bone growth [69, 70]. The bone tissue growth from the bioglass particles surface, filling the space between them, will lead to residual bioglass encapsulation where several small clusters of this material are dispersed in a new bone matrix. Although dependent on other bioglass dissolution, which will be discussed below, this behavior called osteoproduction is taken as a result of improved osteoblasts activity due to dissolved silica stimulation at this stage, being unique to bioglasses among other bioactive materials. In fact the bioactive glasses

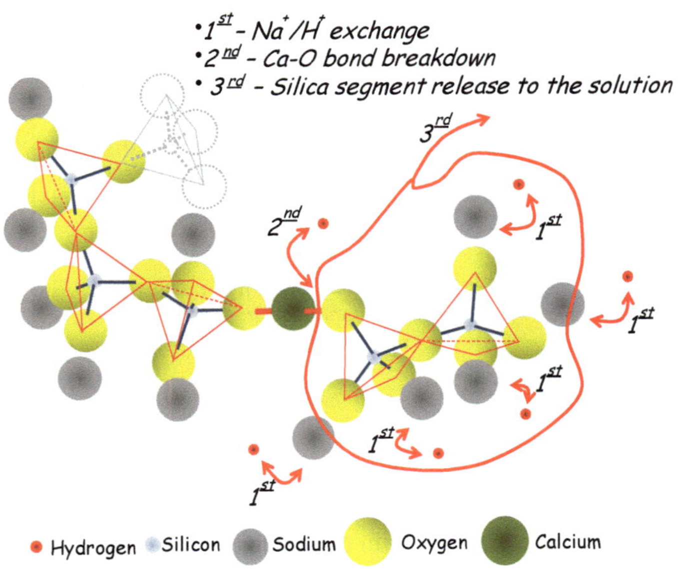

Fig. 22 Schematic representation of the silica segments to solution release mechanism by R^{x+}/H^+ ion exchange effect

combine osteoconductive properties, i.e. the ability to produce a biocompatible interface which stimulate links with the living tissues, with the increasing of osteogenic cell activity in the surrounding environment, which allows to the newly formed bone growth will drive to far from the surface of the bone-implant interface [71]. The ability to release silica in rates and/or amounts capable to osteoblasts stimulating is associated with a small range of bioglass compositions close to 45S5. These compositions also exhibit the ability to form bonds with soft tissues such as muscles and ligaments, which is exploited in some clinical applications [6]. The combination of these properties in the 45S5 composition or other very similar brings a greater possibility of surgical implant success [17, 72].

3.2 Glass Network Hydrolysis

The second bioglass dissolution process is the glass network hydrolysis. In reality this is not exactly a second step since it occurs in parallel to the ion diffusion and exchange. However the hydrolysis process is enhanced with the occurrence of alkali ion exchange. This process occurs by silica network siloxane bonds (Si^{3+}–O–Si^{3+}) rupture with continuous formation of silanol groups. As a result the glass dissolution mechanisms are accelerated and occurs the soluble silica hydroxides release from the material to the solution in the $Si(OH)_4$ form.

During hydrolysis the silica oxides network formers are hydrated by the oxygens bridge bonds rupture. The adsorbed water dissociates spontaneously forming a silanol group by direct OH^- association with silicon. Whereas with the breaking of the bond will be two reactive points resulting in one of them will form the silanol group by adding OH^- while the other network segment will be formed a NBO which be available to accept the proton from the water forming a second silanol group. With the breakdown of BO bonds the network continuity is affected and a Si^{n+}–OH rich layer over the glass surface is formed [21, 52] (Fig. 23).

In a simplified way the hydrolysis reaction can be expressed in accordance with the following Eqs. 5, 6 and 7 [43, 51]:

$$\left(Si^{3+}-O-Si^{3+}\right)_{Glass}+H-OH \leftrightarrow \left(^{3+}Si - OH\right)_{soluble}+\left(Si^{3+}-O-\right)_{Glass}+H^{+} \tag{5}$$

$$\left(Si^{3+}-O-\right)_{Glass}+H^{+} \leftrightarrow \left(Si^{3+} - OH\right)_{Soluble} \tag{6}$$

or

$$\left(Si^{3+}-O-Si^{3+}\right)_{Glass}+H_2O \leftrightarrow 2\left(Si^{3+}-OH\right)_{Soluble} \tag{7}$$

These reactions illustrate the glass surface dissolution sequence by intermediate formers oxides hydrolysis in solution. The glass dissolution rate is determined by

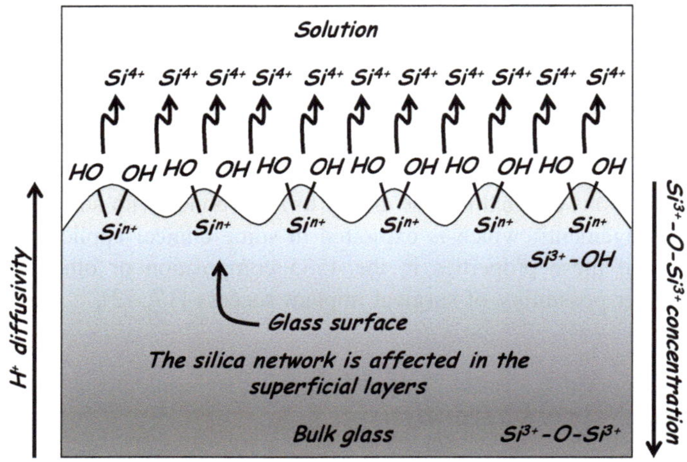

Fig. 23 Silica network hydrolysis on the glass surface schematic representation

the less resistant former removal [41]. That is, in bioglass the phosphorus oxide is strongly associated with the silica network and usually it remaining after the protonic attack, by another hand in this step it can be easily removed.

In the silica network hydrolysis reactions must be considered that the bioglass is formed in its silica network mainly by Q^2 and Q^3 species. The Q^3 silica is responsible for the structural sub-networks formation. These Q^3 sub-networks has as characteristic a highly distorted plans shape that are composed by different sizes silicon rings. The bioactive silicate glasses surface is the key region for interactions with the surroundings body fluids and living tissues and it is characterized by small stretched silica rings such as the trisiloxane and disiloxane type (Figs. 11, 12, 13). These two silica rings types are highly reactive. The di-siloxane rings hydrolysis, for example, results in its openness to the linear form [73–76]. In another aspect, due to the tri-siloxane rings high internal stress its hydrolysis due to dissociated water adsorption constitutes a very small barrier energy even when only a single water molecule is involved [77].

With the network hydrolysis process on the largest rings Si^{3+}–O–Si^{3+} bonds not all Si–O bonds created by the network fracture will be passivated by surface relaxation and some are left exposed or incorporated into small stretched rings. With the condensation of silanol groups (Si–OH) [78] and new trisiloxane and siloxane rings can be formed leading to an surface reactivity increase. However, having highly distorted shape Q^3 plans may also take the geometric dependence for the hydrolysis occurrence that in many instances difficult and it thus constituting a kinetic barrier to small rings hydrolytic opening. Anyway network silica rings take an important role in both the bioactive glass reactivity as in its living tissues adhesion [79].

The bioglass surface reactivity is locally dependent of chemical concentration fluctuations and local structural arrangement variation along the glass surface that may have significantly different behavior in different points of the surface.

3.3 Silica Enriched Layer Formation on the Glass Surface

With the occurrence of the earlier steps will be formed a hydrolyzed silica gel layer on the glass surface and involving the percolation channels. This layer is amorphous, porous and silica rich. The gel layer will not be directly overlaid on the virgin glass, between them there will be a thin layer of exhausted Na^+ and Ca^+ cation [2, 17, 57] (leached layer) as shown in Fig. 24.

The gel layer formation results from the polycondensation of in previous step formed silanol groups as the reaction 8:

$$Si^{3+}{-}OH + OH{-}Si^{3+} \leftrightarrow Si^{3+}{-}O{-}Si^{3+} + H_2O \tag{8}$$

With the gel layer formation as hydrolysis result there is increased the water diffusion difficulty and ion modifiers extraction progressively slowing the bioglass degradation. This surface gel layer when it becomes sufficiently thick, it can be detached exposing a new virgin glass surface exposed to the medium which will be attacked by both process: by the modifiers cations extraction and by network hydrolysis. The progress of this process leads to glass dissolution [7, 41, 44, 52]. In bioactive glasses this layer must be stable (type C, as described above, Fig. 2).

Cations acting as secondary formers, such as phosphorus, may be chemically stabilized during the process favors the secondary products nucleation which will inhibit future attack [39, 40, 44, 80].

Thus an effective stable state can be reached and the thickness of this layer becomes constant. However in soda-lime glasses, such as bioglass, crack formation

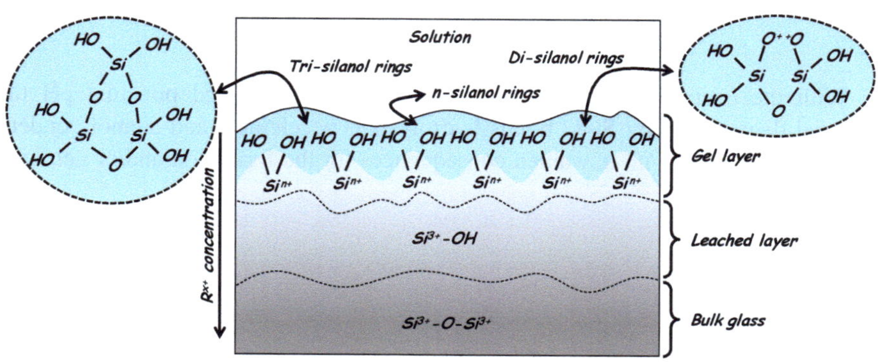

Fig. 24 Hydrolyzed silica gel layer formed by silanol groups poly-condensation schematic representation

and percolation channels through the leached layer can occurs and will facilitate the dissolution process progress (approximately linearly with time) probably by the water move forward underneath the layer leached and reacting with virgin glass.

3.4 Glass Network Attack by OH^- Ions

This is not strictly considered a stage of absorption and bioactivity process of 45S5 bioglass however appears as a complication in the use of this material and other glass and/or bioabsorbable material.

Possibly due to both the composition fluctuations in body fluids or by the free ions concentration (Na^+ and Ca^{2+}) resulting from the progressive dissociation of water particularly in the earlier described cases, where in general the dissolution rate is fast without the interference of other degradation factors. Soluble species biological effects, its toxicity and the process by which the ions are dispersed are not clearly understood. However in these conditions the ion exchange may not follow a proper dispersion of these cations through body fluids and so result in solutions with highly alkaline hydroxides which has significantly influence to the biological microenvironment at the implant interface with living tissue site [81–84]. When these alkaline hydroxides are not readily dispersed in the body fluid solution will be able to take place a rapid increase in the pH beyond 7.5 the (approximate pH of body fluids). These pH fluctuations do not occur homogeneously over the bioactive glass implantation surface. As a result of medium alkalinity raising the glass silica network hydrolysis reaction with OH^- groups will be accelerated causing intense bridging oxygen rupture process with consequent glass network destruction (reactions 9 and 10) [35, 47].

$$(\equiv Si{-}O{-}Si\equiv)_{Glass} + OH^- \rightarrow (\equiv Si{-}O{-})_{Soluble} + (\equiv Si{-}OH)_{Soluble} \quad (9)$$

$$(\equiv Si{-}O{-}) + H_2O \rightarrow (\equiv Si{-}OH) + OH^- \quad (10)$$

With the occurrence of processes which lead to increased punctual pH the material degradation by Si–O bonds hydrolysis is accelerated and silanol condensation is difficulted with unwanted consequences for the formation and/or gel layer stability.

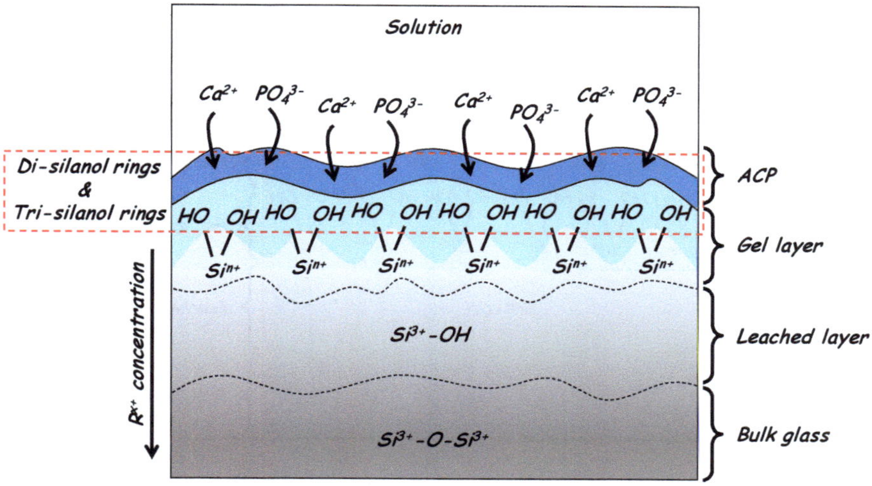

Fig. 25 Ca^{2+} and PO_4^{3-} deposition on the gel layer schematic representation

3.5 Ca^{2+} and PO_4^{3-} rich film formation in material surface

Once formed the silica gel layer on the glass surface this in its turn provides a high roughness and porosity surface favorable for heterogeneous film nucleation from Ca^{2+} and PO_4^{3-} ions present in the solution. In reality the gel layer surface has defects that promote the energy barrier lowering and the nucleation is facilitated and Ca^{2+} and PO_4^{3-}, (ACP) amorphous film growth which will progressively cover the entire silica gel layer. In this case the di-siloxane and tri-siloxane rings are hydrolyzed by body fluid without the subsequent occurrence of silica polycondensation (since the pH in physiological medium is approximately neutral) [17] and therefore these rings come to attract and guide the calcium phosphate deposition on the silica gel surface. Note that in spite of ions precipitation this gel is amorphous and especially is not a stoichiometric calcium phosphate compound being only a crystalline hydroxyapatite precursor (Fig. 25).

3.6 HA Precipitation on the Material Surface

The biological bone-bonding mechanisms are not fully disclosed, but apparently these mechanisms involve the adsorption of growth factors, followed by attachment, proliferation and differentiation of osteoprogenitor cells [16, 82]. The osteoblasts (bone forming cells) induce the formation of an extracellular matrix of collagen in which the ACP film mineralize in nanocrystalline hydroxyapatite form. So finally the Ca^{2+} and PO_4^{3-} ions rich amorphous film will crystallize with the initial formation of a HA layer due to the interaction of these ions with OH^- and

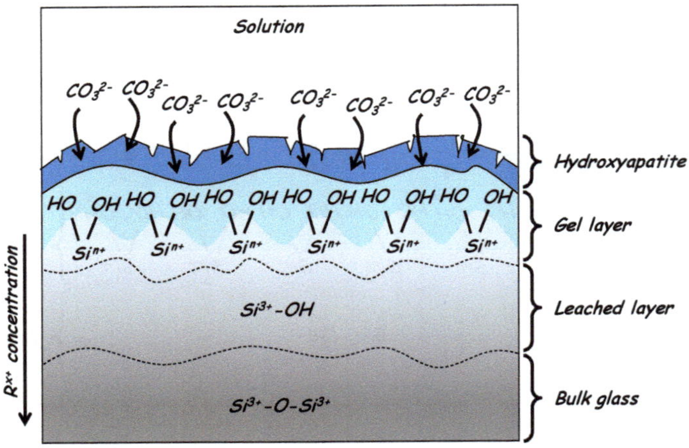

Fig. 26 Hydroxyapatite film on the gel layer formation schematic representation

CO_3^{2-} present in the gel and solution respectively (Fig. 26). The growing apatite layer acts as glass passivating face further degradation preventing its immediate complete resorption: in this way, a stable interface is maintained long enough to promote the subsequent interaction with collagen and biomolecules that ultimately results in an strong bond interface between the implanted glass and the living tissues [85, 86]. Obviously the glass conversion will continue over the time however with progressively reduced rates [87].

The bioactive glass conversion mechanism is a pseudomorphic reaction (the external dimensions of the product are nearly identical to the starting material). If the reaction time is sufficiently long to occur complete crystallization of the product will obtain HA, $Ca_{10}(PO_4)_6(OH)_2$ [81–84]. However, the Ca/P ratio of converted materials often varies from the interface with living tissues to residual matrix glass which may cause compositional fluctuations across the HA film [88].

The bioglass conversion hydroxyapatite resulting layer in general consists in a mesoporous structure and nanoparticles with a high surface area [89]. Only in a few cases the bioglass will be fully absorbed and replaced by precipitated hydroxyapatite. In a more common way is obtained a residual bioglass matrix covered by hydroxyapatite layer. The result therefore is a layered and not homogeneous structure and may be highly complex and may present porosity and calcium phosphate clusters not yet fully converted [81, 82, 90, 91, 92, 93, 94]. Generally the outermost layer (or surface) is less porous. The porosity will increase toward the residual glass matrix.

References

1. Sperb, L.C.M., Neves, A.C.C., et al.: Considerações Sobre Prótese Ocular Sua Importância na Odontologia Atual. RGO **49**, 202 (2001)
2. Siqueira, R.L., Zanotto, E.D.: Biosilicato®: Histórico de uma vitrocerâmica brasileira de elevada bioatividade. Quim. Nova **34**, 1231 (2011)
3. Boccaccini, A.R., Gough, J.E.: Tissue Engineering Using Ceramics and Polymers. CRC Press, New York (2007)
4. Hench, L.L.: Bioceramics. J. Am. Ceram. Soc. **81**, 1705–1728 (1998)
5. Salinas, A.J., Vallet-Regí, M., et al.: Evolution of ceramics with medical applications. Z. Anorg. Allg. Chem. **633**, 1762–1773 (2007)
6. Hench, L.L.: The story of bioglass. J. Mater. Sci. Mater. Med. **17**, 967–978 (2006)
7. Paul, A.: Chemistry of Glasses. Chapman and Hall, Londres (1982)
8. Hench, L.L., Clark, D.E.: Physical chemistry of glass surfaces. J. Non Cryst. Solids **28**, 83–105 (1978)
9. Hench, L.L.: Biomaterials: a forecast for the future. Biomaterials **19**, 1419–1423 (1998)
10. Xynos, I.D., Edgar, A.J., et al.: Gene-expression profiling of human osteoblasts following treatment with the ionic products of Bioglass 45S5 dissolution. J. Biomed. Mater. Res. **55**, 151–157 (2001)
11. Tsigkou, O., Jones, J., Polak, R., et al.: Differentiation of fetal osteoblasts and formation of mineralized bone nodules by 45S5 Bioglass conditioned medium in the absence of osteogenic supplements. Biomaterial **30**, 3542–3550 (2009)
12. Hench, L.L., Wheeler, D.L., et al.: Greenspan, molecular control of bioactivity in sol–gel glasses. J. Sol Gel. Sci. Technol. **13**, 245–250 (1998)
13. Bosetti, M., Cannas, M.: Bioactive glasses induces bone marrow stromal cells differentiation. Biomaterials **26**, 3873–3879 (2005)
14. Jones, J.R., Gentleman, E., et al.: Bioactive glass scaffolds for bone regeneration. Elements **3**, 393–399 (2007)
15. Kokubo, T.: Bioceramics and Their Clinical Applications. CRC Press, Boca Raton (2008)
16. Hench, L.L., Polak, J.M.: Third generation biomaterials. Science **295**, 1014–1017 (2002)
17. Tilocca, A.: Models of structure, dynamics and reactivity of bioglasses: a review. J. Mater. Chem. **20**, 6848–6858 (2010)
18. Chevalier, J., Gremillard, L.: Ceramics for medical applications: a picture for the next 20 years. J. Eur. Ceram. Soc. **29**, 1245–1255 (2009)
19. Kawachi, E.Y., Bertran, C.A.: Biocerâmicas: Tendências e perspectivas de uma área interdisciplinar, Quim. Nova **23**, 518–522 (2000)
20. Zachariasen, W.H.: The atomic arrangement in glass. J. Am. Chem. Soc. **54**, 3841–3851 (1932)
21. Navarro, J.M.F.: El Vidrio, 3ª ed. Madrid, Consejo Superior de Invest. Científicas - Fundacion Centro Nacional del Vidrio (2003)
22. Kirk and Othmer (1994) In: Boyd, D.C., Danielson, P.S., et al. (eds.) Glass Encyclopedia of Chemical Technology, vol. 12, pp. 555–627
23. Van Vlack, L.H.: Princípios de Ciências dos Materiais. Edgard Blücher Ltda, São Paulo (1998)
24. Delaye, J.M., Ghaleb, D.: Molecular dynamics Simulation of $SiO_2 + B_2O_3 + Na_2O + ZrO_2$ glass. J. Non-Cryst. Solids **195**, 239–248 (1996)
25. Jiawei, S., Kwansik, C., et al.: Vitrification of liquid waste from nuclear power plants. J. Nucl. Mater. **297**, 7–13 (2001)
26. Kingery, W.D., Bowen, H.K., et al.: Introduction to Ceramics, 2nd edn. John Wiley & Sons, New York (1976)
27. Mysen, B.O.: Transport and configurational properties of silicate melts: relationship to melt structure at magmatic temperatures. Phys. Earth Planet. Inter. **107**, 23–32 (1998)

28. Sen, S., Youngman, R.E.: NMR study of Q-speciation and connectivity in K_2O-SiO_2 glasses with high silica content. J. Non-Cryst. Solids **331**, 100–1007 (2003)
29. Gedeon, O., Liska, M., et al.: Connectivity of Q-species in binary sodium-silicate glasses. J. Non Cryst. Solids **354**, 1133–1136 (2008)
30. Hill, R.G.: An alternative view of the degradation of Bioglass. J. Mater. Sci. Lett. **15**, 1122–1125 (1996)
31. Strnad, Z.: Role of glass phase in bioactive glass-ceramics. Biomaterials **13**, 317–321 (1992)
32. Arcos, D., Greesnpan, D.C.: Influence of the stabilization temperature on textural and structural features and ion release in SiO_2–CaO–P_2O_5 sol–gel glasses. Chem. Mater. **14**, 1515–1522 (2002)
33. Beall, G.H., Pinckney, L.R.: Nanophase glass-ceramics. J. Am. Ceram. Soc. **82**, 5–16 (1999)
34. Calas, G., Cormier, L.: Structure–property relationships in multicomponent oxide glasses. Chimie **5**, 831–843 (2002)
35. Silva, A.C.: Vidros e vitrocerâmicos com alta concentração de metais a partir de resíduos industriais (Doctoral tesis, Universidade de São Paulo), Brazil (2008)
36. Holland, D.Mekki, et al.: The structure of sodium iron silicate glass—a multi-technique approach. J. Non-Cryst. Solids **253**, 192–202 (1999)
37. Pinakidou, F., Katsikini, M., et al.: Structural role and coordination environment of Fe in Fe_2O_3–PbO–SiO_2–Na_2O composite glasses. J. Non-Cryst. Solids **354**, 105–111 (2008)
38. Mekki, A., Holland, D., et al.: An XPS study of iron sodium glass surfaces. J. Non-Cryst. Solids **208**, 267–276 (1996)
39. Bevilacqua, A.M., Bernasconi, N.B., et al.: A. Immobilization of simulated high-level liquid wastes in sintered borosilicate, aluminosilicate and aluminoborosilicate glasses. J. Nucl. Mater. **229**, 187–193 (1996)
40. Abraitis, P.K., Mcgrail, B.P., et al.: Single-pass flow-though experiments on a simulated waste glass in alkaline media at 40 °C. I—Experiments conducted at variable flow rate to glass surface and ratio. J. Nucl. Mater. **280**, 196–205 (2000)
41. Eaz-Eldin, F.M.: Leaching and mechanical properties of cabal glasses developed as matrices for immobilization high-level wastes. Nucl. Instrum. Methods Phys. Res. **183**, 285–300 (2001)
42. Erol, M., Kucukbayrak, S., et al.: Crystallization behavior of glasses produced from fly ash. J. Eur. Ceram. Soc. **21**, 2835–2841 (2001)
43. Sheng, J., Lou, S., et al.: The leaching behavior of borate waste glass SL-1. Waste Manag **19**, 401–407 (1999)
44. Peret, D., Crosivier, J.L., et al.: Thermodynamic stability of waste glasses compared to leaching behavior. Appl. Geochem. **18**, 1165–1184 (2003)
45. Newton, R.G., Paul, A.: A new approach to predicting the durability of glasses from their chemical compositions. Glass Techol. **21**, 307–309 (1980)
46. Newton, R.G.: The durability of glass. Glass Techol. **26**, 21–38 (1985)
47. Spence, R.D., Gilliam, T.M., et al.: Laboratory stabilization/solidification of surrogate and actual mixed-waste sludge in glass and grout. Waste Manag. **19**, 453–465 (1999)
48. Feng, X., Pegg, I.L.: A glass dissolution model for the effects of S/V on leachate pH. J. Non-Cryst. Solids **175**, 281–293 (1994)
49. Hamilton, J.P., Pantano, C.G.: Effects of glass structure on the corrosion behavior of sodium-aluminosilicate glasses. J. Non-Cryst. Solids **222**, 167–174 (1997)
50. Koenderink, R.H., Brzesowsky, R.H., et al.: Effect of the initial stages of leaching on the surface of alkaline earth sodium silicate glasses. J. Non-Cryst. Solids **262**, 80–98 (2000)
51. Sigoli, F.A., Kawano, Y., et al.: Phase separation in pyrex glass by hydrothermal treatment: Evidence from micro-raman spectroscopy. J. Non-Cryst. Solids **284**, 49–59 (2001)
52. Cooper, C.I., Cox, G.A.: The aqueous corrosion of potash-lime-silica glass in the range 10–250 °C. Appl. Geochem. **11**, 511–521 (1996)
53. Yan, J., Neretnieks, I.: Is the glass phase rate always a limiting factor in the leaching processes of combustion residues? Sci. Total Environ. **172**, 95–118 (1995)

54. Zamet, S., Darbar, U.R., et al.: Particulate bioglass as a grafting material in the treatment of periodontal intrabony defects. J. Clin. Periodontol. **24**, 410–418 (1997)
55. Allan, I., Newsam, H., et al.: Antibacterial activity of particulate bioglass against supra- and subgingival bacteria. Biomaterials **22**, 1683–1687 (2001)
56. Moya, J.S., Esteban-Tejeda, L., et al.: Glass powders with a high content of calcium oxide: a step towards a "green" universal biocide. Adv. Eng. Mater. **13**(6), B256–B260 (2011)
57. Moya, J.S., Cabal, B., et al.: Mechanism of calcium lixiviation in soda-lime glasses with a strong biocide activity. Mater. Lett. **70**, 113–115 (2012)
58. Silva, A.C.: Incorporação de resíduo galvânico em vidro silicato obtido a partir de finos de sílica (Master degree dissertation, Universidade de São Paulo), Brazil (2004)
59. Esteban-Tejeda, L., Silva, A.C., et al.: Kinetics of dissolution of a biocide soda-lime glass powder containing silver nanoparticles. J. Nanopart. Res. **15**(2), 1–6 (2013)
60. Bolis, V., Fubini, B., et al.: Hydrophilic and hydrophobic sites on dehydrated crystalline and amorphous silicas. J. Chem. Soc., Faraday Trans. **87**, 497–505 (1991)
61. Hassanali, A.A., Singer, S.J.: Model for the water-amorphous silica interface: the undissociated surface. J. Phys. Chem. B **111**, 11181–111193 (2007)
62. Tilocca, A., Cormack, A.N.: Structural effects of phosphorus inclusion in bioactive silicate glasses. J. Phys. Chem. B **111**, 14256–14264 (2007)
63. Wu, H.F., Lin, C.C., et al.: Structure and dissolution of CaO-ZrO_2–TiO_2–Al_2O_3–B_2O3–SiO_2 glass (II). J. Non-Cryst. Solids **209**, 76–86 (1997)
64. Tilocca, A., Cormack, A.N., et al.: Structure and dynamics of bioactive phosphosilicate glasses and melts from ab initio molecular dynamics simulation. Chem. Mater. **19**, 95 (2007)
65. Jund, P., Kob, W.: Channel diffusion of sodium in a silicate glass. Phys. Rev. B: Condens. Matter **64**, 134303–134313 (2001)
66. Mead, R.N., Mountjoy, G.: A molecular dynamics study of the atomic structure of (CaO)x $(SiO_2)_{1\text{-}x}$ glasses. J. Phys. Chem. B **110**, 14273–14278 (2006)
67. Huang, C., Cormack, A.N.: Structural differences and phase separation in alkali silicate glasses. J. Chem. Phys. **95**, 3634–3642 (1991)
68. Tilocca, A., Cormack, A.N.: The effect of nano scale inhomogeneity and silicate network connectivity on the activity of glasses with biological applications. Nuevo Cimento B **123**, 1415–1423 (2008)
69. Oonishi, H., Hench, L.L., et al.: Comparative bone growth behavior in granules of bioceramic materials of various sizes. J. Biomed. Mater. Res. **44**, 31–43 (1999)
70. Oonishi, H., Hench, L.L., et al.: Quantitative comparison of bone growth behavior in granules of bioglass, AW glass-ceramic, and hydroxyapatite. Biomed. Mater. Res. **51**, 37–48 (2000)
71. Wilson, J., Yli-Urpo, A., et al.: In: Hench, L.L., Wilson, J. (eds.) An Introduction to Bioceramics. World Scientific, Singapore, pp. 63–73 (1993)
72. Cao, W., Hench, L.L.: Bioactive materials. Ceram. Int. **22**, 493–507 (1996)
73. Mischler, C., Horbach, J., et al.: Water adsorption on amorphous silica surfaces: a Car-Parrinello simulation study. Phys. Condens. Matter. **17**, 4005–4013 (2005)
74. Masini, P., Bernasconi, M.J.: Ab initio simulations of hydroxylation and dehydroxylation reactions at surfaces: amorphous silica and brucite. Phys. Condens. Matter. **14**, 4133–4144 (2002)
75. Bunker, B.C., Haaland, D.M., et al.: Kinetics of dissociative chemisorption on strained edge-shared surface defects on dehydroxylated silica. Surf. Sci. **222**, 95–118 (1988)
76. Walsh, T.R., Wilson, M., et al.: Hydrolysis of the amorphous silica surface. II. Calculation of activation barriers and mechanisms. J. Chem. Phys. **113**, 9191–9201 (2000)
77. West, J.K., Wallace, S.: Interactions of water with trisiloxane rings. I. Experimental analysis. J. Non-Cryst. Solids **152**, 101–108 (1993)
78. Wallace, S., West, J.K., et al.: Interactions of water with trisiloxane rings II. J. Non-Cryst. Solids **152**, 109–117 (1995)
79. Hench, L.L., West, J.K.: Molecular orbital models of silica. Annu. Rev. Mater. Sci. **25**, 37–68 (1995)

80. Nogues, J.L., Vernuz, E.Y., et al.: Nuclear glass corrosion mechanism applied to the French LWR reference glass. Mater. Res. Soc. **44**, 89–98 (1985)
81. Huang, W., Day, D.E., et al.: Kinetics and mechanisms of the conversion of silicate (45S5), borate, and borosilicate glasses to hydroxyapatite in dilute phosphate solution. J. Mater. Sci. Mater. Med. **17**, 583–596 (2006)
82. Rahaman, M.N., Day, D.E., et al.: Bioactive glass in tissue engineering. Acta Biomater. **7**, 2355–2373 (2011)
83. Yao, A., Wang, D.P., et al.: In vitro bioactive characteristics of borate based glasses with controllable degradation behavior. J. Am. Ceram. Soc. **90**, 303–306 (2007)
84. Fu, Q., Rahaman, M.N., et al.: Bioactive scaffolds with controllable degradation rates for bone tissue engineering applications. I. Preparation and in vitro degradation. J. Biomed. Mater. Res. **95A**, 164–171 (2010)
85. Hench, L.L., Splinter, R.J., et al.: Bonding mechanisms at the interface of ceramic prosthetic materials. J. Biomed. Mater. Res. **5**, 117–141 (1971)
86. Kokubo, T., Kim, H.M., et al.: Novel bioactive materials with different mechanical properties. Biomaterials **24**, 2161–2175 (2003)
87. Duccheyne, P., Qiu, Q.: Bioactive ceramics: the effect of surface reactivity on bone formation and bone cell function. Biomaterials **20**, 2287–2303 (1999)
88. LeGeros, R.Z., LeGeros, J.P.: Phosphate minerals in human tissues. In: Nriogu, J.O., Moore, P.B. (eds.) Phosphate Minerals, p. 351. Springer-Verlag, Berlin (1984)
89. Rahaman, M.N., Day, D.E., Brown, R.F., Fu, Q., Jung, S.B.: Nanostructured bioactive glass scaffolds for bone repair. Ceram. Eng. Sci. Proc. **29**, 211 (2008)
90. Day, D.E., White, J.E., et al.: Transformation of borate glasses into biologically useful materials. Glass Technol. Part A **44**, 75–81 (2003)
91. Conzone, S.D., Day, D.E.: Preparation and properties of porous microspheres made form borate glass. J. Biomed. Mater. Res. **88A**, 531–542 (2009)
92. Wang, Q., Huang, W., et al.: Preparation of hollow hydroxyapatite microspheres. J. Mater. Sci. Mater. Med. **17**, 641–646 (2006)
93. Huang, W., Rahaman, M.N., et al.: Strength of hollow hydroxyapatite microspheres prepared by a glass conversion process. J. Mater. Sci. Mater. Med. **20**, 123–129 (2009)
94. Fu, H., Rahaman, M.N., et al.: Effect of process parameters on the microstructure of hollow hydroxyapatite microspheres prepared by a glass conversion method. J. Am. Ceram. Soc. **93**, 3116–3123 (2010)

The Evolution, Control, and Effects of the Compositions of Bioactive Glasses on Their Properties and Applications

Breno Rocha Barrioni, Agda Aline Rocha de Oliveira and Marivalda de Magalhães Pereira

Abstract Bioactive glasses have been extensively studied for several applications, and understanding their structures is very important for the design of alternative materials and comprehension of the behaviors of these materials. The dissolution products of bioactive glasses are critical for their performance and application and heavily depend on the bioactive glass network. The incorporation of physiologically active ions into their structures and the controlled ion release can lead to therapeutic benefits, such as cell differentiation, antibacterial action, and anti-inflammatory effects, improving the properties of the bioactive glasses. This chapter covers literature reports that have investigated the physicochemical and biological properties of bioactive glasses based on their structures. In particular, recent advances in the understanding of the effects of bioactive glasses with different compositions, which are fabricated via the incorporation of several different ions, on their biological properties and applications are summarized and discussed. This chapter provides an overview of new tissue engineering approaches based on therapeutic ion release, which aids in understanding how the chemical composition can be tailored according to each application.

1 Introduction

Biomaterials for use in the body were first suggested to be as inert as possible when exposed to a physiological environment because it was accepted that any material applied in the human body would result in the formation of non-adherent scar tissue on the material interface as a consequence of a foreign body reaction. Corrosion resistant metals and insoluble non-toxic polymers became the standard first

B.R. Barrioni · M.de MagalhãesPereira (✉)
Department of Metallurgical Engineering and Materials, School of Engineering, Federal University of Minas Gerais (UFMG), Av. Antônio Carlos, 6627 - Pampulha, Belo Horizonte 31270-901, MG, Brazil
e-mail: mpereira@demet.ufmg.br

A.A.R. de Oliveira
JHS Biomateriais, Rua Ouro Branco, 345, Sabará 34650-120, MG, Brazil

J. Marchi (ed.), *Biocompatible Glasses*, Advanced Structured Materials 53,
DOI 10.1007/978-3-319-44249-5_4

generation biomaterials [1]. Nonetheless, the failure of devices made from bio-inert materials was common, causing tissue breakdown and loosening over time. Incompatibilities between the mechanical properties of biomaterials and bone also led to resorption of bone and long term implant failure, necessitating revision surgeries [1, 2].

The second generation of biomaterials for the replacement of tissues emerged when a special composition of soda-lime-phosphate-silicate glass was made by Hench and implanted in the femurs of rats at the University of Florida in 1969 [2, 3] as an alternative to bio-inert materials. The glass composition contained 45 % SiO_2, 24.5 % Na_2O, 24.5 % CaO, and 6 % P_2O_5, in weight %. The Phase Diagram for Na_2O–CaO–SiO_2 Ceramic was used by Hench [3] to design this first composition, which was selected to provide a large amount of CaO with some P_2O_5 in a Na_2O–SiO_2 matrix and produce a composition very close to a ternary eutectic, making it easy to melt. Bioglass® appeared as an alternative for inert materials, forming an interfacial bonding between the implant (bioactive glass) and the host tissue so strong that it could not be removed without breaking the bone [3–5]. The high amounts of Na_2O and CaO, as well as the relatively high CaO/P_2O_5 ratio, make the glass surface highly reactive in physiological environments [5].

Compositions such as 45S5, which have high rates of bioactivity and good biocompatibility, induce the rapid regeneration of trabecular bone with an amount, architecture and bio-mechanical quality of bone that matches that originally present in the site [1]. Additionally, they could degrade over time, allowing for the controlled release of therapeutically active ions and enabling bone regeneration rather than replacement, thereby restoring the original bone state and function [6]. The bonding of bioactive glasses with bone occurs as a result of a rapid sequence of chemical reactions on the surface of the implanted material in living tissues [3]. The first five steps lead to a rapid release of soluble ion species and the formation of a hydroxy-carbonate apatite (HCA) layer, and the glass composition has a great influence on the ion dissolution rate and consequently on the HCA layer formation and bone bond. Briefly, the five proposed stages of HCA formation are [4, 7–10]: I—formation of silanol bonds (Si–OH) on the glass surface due to rapid cation exchange (Na^+ and/or Ca^{2+}) with H^+ from solution; II—breakage of Si–O–Si bonds due to loss of soluble silica in the form of $Si(OH)_4$ into the solution, leaving more silanols at the glass-solution interface; III—condensation of Si–OH groups near the glass surface and repolymerization of SiO_2-rich layer; IV- migration of PO_4^{3-} and Ca^{2+} groups to the surface through the SiO_2-rich layer and from the solution, forming a film rich in amorphous CaO–P_2O_5 on top of the SiO_2-rich layer; V-incorporation of OH^- and CO^{-3} anions from the solution and crystallization of the CaO–P_2O_5 film to HCA. The HCA layer interacts with collagen fibrils of damaged bone, which are responsible for bone bonding [11]. After the HCA layer formation, the next steps are thought to involve the agglomeration and chemical bonding of biological moieties in the HCA layer, such as protein adsorption, incorporation of collagen fibrils and the action of macrophages, followed by the attachment of bone progenitor cells, cell proliferation, differentiation and excretion of the bone extracellular matrix [3, 4, 8].

Mineralization of the matrix is the last stage, and mature osteocytes, encased in a collagen-HCA matrix, are the final product [3].

The name "Bioglass®" is a trademark from the University of Florida related to the original 45S5 composition developed by Hench [3] to distinguish the material from other bioactive glass and glass-ceramic products being developed world wide. This discovery initiated a new era in the field of bioactive ceramics, with many other new materials being formed from variations of bioactive glasses, glass-ceramics and ceramics, such as synthetic hydroxyapatite (HA) and other calcium phosphates, that also stimulated beneficial responses from the body and bonding to host tissue [1, 3, 4, 6, 12]. Others bioactive glass compositions developed over the years contain no sodium, as it is has the primary role of lowering the melting temperature in melt-derived bioactive glasses, whereas it is not required in processes that use lower processing temperatures, such as the sol–gel method, which is a method based basically on polycondensation reactions from organic precursors, such as metal alkoxides [13–17]. Additional elements can also be incorporated in the silicate network [5], or silicate can be replaced, forming phosphate and borate-based glasses with different physicochemical properties and biological responses in bone tissue regeneration [4]. Therefore, it is essential to study how bioactive glasses can actively stimulate and enhance new tissue formation, and the relation between different compositions of bioactive glasses and their physicochemical and biological properties. This knowledge can be used to design bioactive glasses tailored for specific required properties.

1.1 Glass Structure

Glasses are characterized by their amorphous structures and are typically brittle. The atoms in a glass are arranged in a random manner similar to that of a liquid; glasses are essentially super-stiff liquids and exhibit time-dependent glass transformations [18]. This behavior is known as their glass transition range (T_g), the temperature interval in which a system transforms from a supercooled liquid to a solid glass. Glasses have no long-range order, and when heated, they show a smooth decrease in their viscosity by a few orders of magnitude, which is the reason that glasses can be synthesized in various shapes [6] using both traditional melting methods and sol–gel techniques, which plays an important role in the bioactive glass structure and composition [5, 8, 19]. In a typical melt-quenching process, the precursor oxides are melted together at high temperatures, usually between 1200 and 1500 °C, depending on the composition, and the formed liquid is quenched in a graphite mold (for rods or monoliths) or in water (frits) [4, 20]. In the sol–gel method, bioactive glasses are prepared basically by polycondensation reactions from organic precursors, such as metal alkoxides (e.g., tetraethylorthosilicate) [13–16]. Melt-derived bioactive glasses are dense, whereas sol–gel glasses tend to have an inherent nanoporosity, which can result in improved cellular response due to nanotopography and larger surface area and favor HCA nucleation [21–24].

The network formers are the main components of the glass structure; they are able to form glasses without the need for additional components. Commonly used network formers for bioactive glass synthesis are silica (SiO_2), phosphorus pentoxide (P_2O_5) and boron trioxide (B_2O_3) [6]. Among these networks, silicate bioactive glasses are the most popular, normally using silica oxide as the precursor in melt-derived glass, whereas tetraethyl-orthosilicate (TEOS) is the most common precursor for sol–gel derived bioactive glass, but other metal alkoxides, such as tetramethyl-orthosilicate (TMOS), are also related [8]. The silica network is formed from multiple silica tetrahedral units connected by –Si–O–Si– bridging oxygen bonds. Each oxygen anion is coordinated by two Si cations, corresponding to corner sharing of the oxide tetrahedral, preventing the close-packing of anion layers and resulting in relatively open structures [18]. The silica tetrahedron and its associated bonds can be referred as Q^n units, indicating silicon that connects to n bridging oxygen [25]. ^{29}Si solid-state NMR suggests that the host silica network of Bioglass® primarily consists of 69 % chains and rings of Q^2 SiO_4, and 31 % Q^3 units, which provide some degree of crosslinking [26]. Dietary intake of silicon has been shown to increase bone mineral density, which is essential for the formation and calcification of bone tissue [27]. Moreover, $Si(OH)_4$ in physiological concentrations stimulates collagen type I synthesis in human osteoblast-like cells, and could also enhance osteoblastic differentiation [28].

In addition to SiO_2, many bioactive glasses contain a second network former: P_2O_5. In sol–gel synthesis, triethyl orthophosphate (TEP) and phosphoric acid (H_3PO_4) are usually employed as phosphorous precursors [20, 29, 30], and in melt-derived glasses the typical phosphorous precursor is phosphorous pentoxide [31–33], but others, such as ammonium phosphate monobasic ($NH_4H_2PO_4$) [34], sodium dihydrogenphosphate [35], and sodium metaphosphate ($NaPO_3$) [36, 37], are also used. Several works show that phosphorus is present in an orthophosphate form rather than taking part in the silicate network, and ^{31}P NMR indicates that the orthophosphate (PO_4^{3-}) groups are surrounded by the modifier cations for charge-balancing purposes [38] and that there are no Si–O–P bonds [26, 39]. However, Si–O–P bonds are not impossible. A recent study showed that, while the majority of phosphorous atoms are present as orthophosphate, small amounts of Si–O–P bonds (8 %) are also present [40]. Phosphate is rapidly lost from the glass on exposure to aqueous environments [21], mainly because it is isolated from the silica network and removes sodium and calcium cations from their network-modifying role [4, 41]. In addition, the release of the phosphate ions from these glasses will quickly form an amorphous calcium phosphate layer that crystallizes and gives rise to a hydroxyapatite layer [36]. Phosphorus is not essential for bioactive glass bioactivity, but when it is present, the apatite layer formation is faster, consequently affecting bioactivity [42]. The presence of orthophosphate in bioactive glass can cause phase separation depending upon the phosphate content and play a significant role in nucleation and crystallization. The phosphate-rich regions increase in size and number as the phosphate content increases, thus allowing for nucleation and crystallization of orthophosphate species. The phase separation depends on various factors, including composition, network connectivity, phosphate content, type of

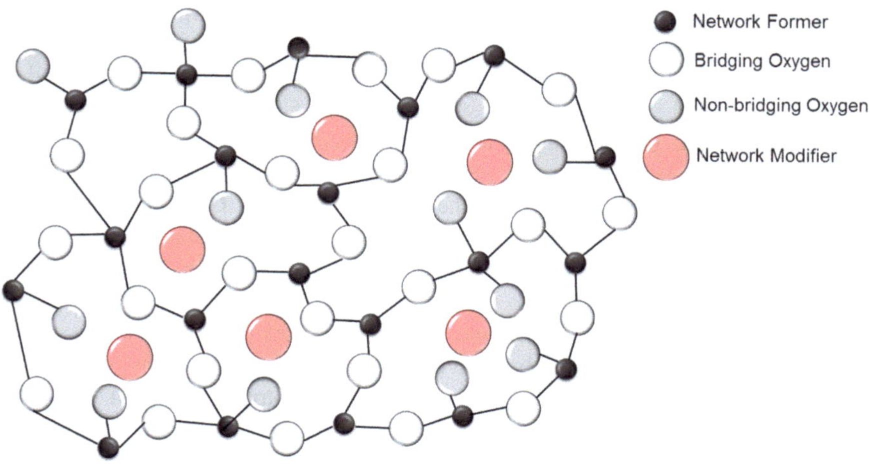

Fig. 1 Structure of a bioactive glass network

modifiers, and glass synthesis process and may be important on controlling or preventing crystallization [6, 40]. Figure 1 shows the structure of a bioactive glass composed of an interconnected near-random distribution of covalently-bonded network formers, for example silicate chains, whose negative charges are balanced by coordination with network modifiers.

Bioactive borate glasses are formed by incorporating B_2O_3 as a network former in SiO_2-free or P_2O_5-free glasses as well as others that contain certain amount of SiO_2 or P_2O_5. These materials normally use boron trioxide (B_2O_3) [43, 44] or boracic acid (H_3BO_3) as the precursor [45–48], which is often used as an additive to enhance the workability of bioactive glasses [6, 49]. Due to the complicated structural behavior of B_2O_3 in the glass, including BO_3 and BO_4 units, processing seems to vary depending on the composition, and further studies are still needed to fully understand the mechanism of how B_2O_3 improves the processing of bioactive glasses [6, 34]. However, the biological effects of boron have also been reported, including improvement of wound healing, actions in reproduction and embryogenesis and bone health [49], enhancing proliferation and the expression of collagen type I and runt-related transcription factor 2 (Runx2) of osteoblasts [50]. Boron has also been shown to enhance the total functional RNA-molecules that produce vascular endothelial growth factor (VEGF) and transforming growth factor beta (TGF-β)—in fibroblasts and the secretion of protein from chick embryo cartilage and human fibroblasts in culture [51]. VEGF is a sub-family of growth factors that stimulates vasculogenesis and angiogenesis, while TGF-β is vital for new bone formation and wound healing.

Bioactive, biodegradable and fully densified borate glass ceramics ($CaO–SiO_2–B_2O_3$ system) containing up to 8.4 % B_2O_3 showed higher mechanical strengths than other commercial bioactive glasses, with an HCA layer formed earlier on the surface when the amounts of calcium metaborate and amorphous borosilicate matrix increased [44]. Bioactive glasses in the $CaO–SiO_2–P_2O_5–B_2O_3$ system used to coat cancellous screws inserted into dogs presented directly bond to cancellous bone, improving the bone-implant osteointegration [52]. The biodegradation rate was based on the boron content in the quaternary system, which also helped increase the mechanical properties and lower the melting temperature of bioactive glass [45]. The presence of boron in the glass networks of $CaO–P_2O_5–B_2O_3$ systems also favored bioactivity when compared to the performance of the bioinert pure calcium phosphate glass [34], and it was also observed when Na_2O is replaced by B_2O_3 in the quaternary system [53].

Sodium and calcium are typical examples of network modifiers in glass structures. They disrupt the network by converting bridging oxygen atoms (mostly with covalent chemical bonds) into nonbridging oxygen atoms ($Si–O–M^+$ linkages, predominantly ionic in character, where M^+ is a modifier cation), altering the glass structure. Network formers cations are typically threefold or fourfold coordinated, while network modifiers usually show high coordination numbers according to neutron diffraction and molecular dynamics (MD) simulation experiments [6].

Knowing the structure of bioactive glasses is very important when designing alternative compositions and for understanding their behavior. Network connectivity (NC) is an important tool that can predict properties such as bioactivity, surface reactivity, solubility, and glass transition temperature [54]. This value is defined as the average number of bridging oxygens bonded to a network-forming atom, with lower NC values denoting a more fragmented structure. The release of soluble silica in solution plays a significant role in bone mineralization along with gene-activation properties [18] and occurs more easily when most Si are incorporated in silicate chains that do not intersect. Silica dissolution requires less energy to break Si–O–Si bridges in the presence of network modifiers when compared with a structure with a higher NC (or a more compact structure), where silicate chains are crosslinked to each other, forming rings of different sizes [55]. Bioactive glasses with high silica contents present large proportions of bridging oxygen bonds, resulting in a highly connected network and, consequently, low dissolution and low bioactivity [4]. Vitreous silica has a network connectivity of four, while bioactive glasses usually have network connectivities between 2 and 3, but glasses with NC greater than 2.6 may have reduced bioactivity due to their resistance to dissolution [36]. The NC decreases due to the addition of more network-modifying cations, such as calcium and sodium [6, 56, 57]. Phosphorous is located in the interstices of the silica network and extracts some modifier cations around phosphate complexes to counter-balance the charges due to phosphorus addition, involving a repolymerization of the silicate network, thus increasing NC [36].

The bioactivity of melt-derived glasses is limited to compositions of up to 60 mol % SiO_2, whereas sol–gel glasses allow for the expansion of bioactive compositional range up to 90 mol% silica [29] due to their inherent nanoporosity in combination with a reduction in network connectivity. During the drying of sol–gel glasses, water and alcohol evaporate, leaving behind an interconnected network. The pores formed are interstices between the coalesced nanoparticles, and sol–gel derived glasses present pores diameters typically on the order of 1–30 nm, depending on the precursor used and the glass composition [4, 58]. This ordered mesoporous bioactive glass (MBG) is of interest in several biomedical applications, such as drug delivery, as drug can be delivered within mesoporous network [59–61].

The drying process removes water from sol–gel bioactive glasses, but some hydroxyl (OH) groups are left on the pore walls [4, 21, 25]. Thermal stabilization removes most of the hydroxyl content, forming O–Si–O bonds, but some remain, and the final sol–gel glass composition also contains OH groups [62], reducing the network connectivity as the bridging oxygen bonds decrease. The sintering temperature should be kept below the crystallization temperature, preventing the formation of a glass-ceramic. Sintering sol–gel glasses above their T_g causes a reduction in the porosity and densification of the silica network [4, 25].

1.2 Therapeutic Ion Release

The outstanding behavior of bioactive glasses in bone repair can primarily be attributed to the high reactivity of its surface in body fluids via the release of critical concentrations of soluble Si, Ca, P, and other ions, that can lead to favorable intracellular and extracellular responses promoting rapid bone formation [63]. The HCA layer forms following solution-mediated dissolution of the glass in which the accumulation of dissolution products causes changes in the chemical composition and pH of the solution, providing surface sites and a pH conducive to HCA nucleation [3, 64]. Nevertheless, recent evidence has indicated that the ionic dissolution affects not only the mineralization but also appears to stimulate the growth and differentiation of osteoblasts at the genetic level, an effect that has been found to be dose dependent [65–68].

Glass structures allow for large flexibility in composition, as they are not dependent on a specific stoichiometry, which permits the incorporation of various concentrations of ions with physiological activities and therapeutic properties [6, 59, 69] that are released during the dissolution process. Ions acting as network modifiers (ionically linked to nonbridging oxygen atoms) can be released easily and rapidly by ion exchange with the surrounding body fluid and thus be available in the body because they are released in the exact site where they are needed, optimizing the therapeutic effect and minimizing the side effects providing a significant advantage over the systemically administered medication [6]. Additionally, bioactive glasses can allow for continued ion release, with a sustained therapeutic effect through glass degradation, and the release rate can be optimized through variations in the glass network connectivity and the type of modifier or intermediate ion [6].

The ionic dissolution product from bioactive glasses are very important to understand the behavior of these materials in vitro and in vivo in the context of tissue engineering applications [70]. There is a need to develop materials that are not only biocompatible and osteoconductive but also possess controllable degradation rates, antibacterial effects, promote angiogenesis and osteogenesis, and have other therapeutic effects to aid in the regeneration of diseased or damaged tissue [65]. Thus, research efforts have been made to incorporate ions, including Sr, Co, Mg, Ag, Zn, Cu and others, in calcium phosphates, hydroxyapatite, bioactive silicate glasses and phosphate glasses, resulting in the altered dissolution behavior of these materials and their modified (usually improved) biological performance [18, 70].

2 Composition Effects on Properties and Applications of Bioactive Glasses

In designing bioactive glasses, the understanding of how the physicochemical structures of these materials can affect their properties is of great importance, allowing the material to be tailored for specific applications. Each component has a role on the bioactive glass functionality. For example, calcium can favor osteoblast differentiation and apatite precipitation [71], while strontium can also stimulate bone-forming cells and also prevent osteoclasts from resorbing bone [72]. Similar properties are also observed in magnesium-doped bioactive glass [73, 74]. Vascularization can also be enhanced when using bioactive glass by using ions such as cobalt [75] or copper [76]. Other ions also show good antibacterial properties, such as silver [77] and gallium [78]. The use of these ions can improve the bioactive glass performance in vitro and in vivo, and the effect of different ions on bioactive

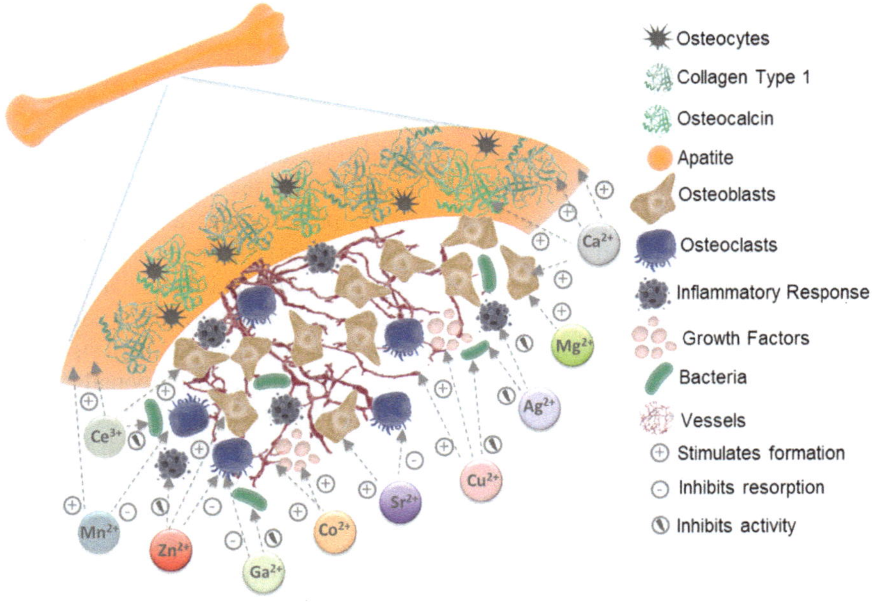

Fig. 2 Biological response to metallic ion-substituted silicate based bioactive glasses

Table 1 Summary of the biological responses of some ions

Ion	Function	Reference
Ca	Favor osteoblast differentiation and apatite precipitation	[6, 70]
	Increase extracellular matrix mineralization	[71]
	Regulator of bone cells through the activation of extracellular calcium-sensing receptors	[79]
	Up-regulate collagen type I and osteocalcin mRNA expression	[80]
F	Accelerate the formation of apatite in bone and mineralized tissue, increase tissue stability and stimulate cell proliferation	[81, 82]
	Reduce the demineralization of enamel and dentin, preventing dental decay	[54]
	Favor the formation of fluorapatite, preventing dental caries	[57, 83]
Sr	Regulates bone resorption and osteoclastogenesis	[49, 84, 85]
	Possible agent for treating osteoporosis	[86, 87]
Zn	Stimulates osteoblastic bone formation and inhibit osteoclastic bone resorption	[88]
	Protect against inflammatory responses	[89, 90]
	Important to metalloenzymes that are vital for new bone formation	[49, 88]
Mg	Essential in bone metabolism, stimulating new bone formation	[49, 91]
	Improve cell adhesion and stability, by interacting with integrin of osteoblast cells	[73]
	Stabilizes enzymes and is involved in lipid, protein, nuclei acid and coenzymes synthesis	[92]
Mn	Cofactor of enzymes involved in extracellular matrix remodeling, necessary for constituents of skeletal and cartilages structures	[93]
	Influence the inhibition of bone resorption induced by free radicals	[94]
	Mn deficiency could lead to a reduction in calcium incorporation in bone tissue	[93, 95]
Co	Promote angiogenesis via activation of hypoxia inducible factor	[35, 96–98]
	Can accelerate development and regeneration of bone tissue and stem cell differentiation	[35, 75]
Cu	Antibacterial activity	[99–101]
	Increase the differentiation of mesenchymal stem cells towards the osteogenic lineage	[102]
	Enhance vascularization, triggering endothelial cells towards angiogenesis	[76, 103]
Ag	Potent antibacterial activity	[6, 49, 104, 105]
	Reduce the inflammatory and granulation tissue phases of healing	[77]
Ga	Modulate osteoclastic response without affecting osteoblasts	[106]
	Treatment of osteoporosis and hypercalcemia associated with tumor metastasis to bone	[107]
	Antibacterial activity	[33, 107, 108]
Ce	Antioxidant properties, acting as a neuroprotective agent	[109, 110]
	Broad spectrum of antibacterial activity	48, 111, 112]
	Enhance osteoblastic differentiation and production of collagen	[113]

(continued)

Table 1 (continued)

Ion	Function	Reference
Si	Essential for the formation and calcification of bone tissue	[27]
	Stimulate collagen type I formation and enhance osteoblastic differentiation	[28]
P	Regulates bone formation proteins expression in osteoblasts	[114]
B	Enhance total of functional RNA in fibroblasts	[51]
	Improve proliferation and expression of collagen type I and runt-related transcription factor 2 (Runx2) of osteoblasts	[50]

glass properties. Figure 2 and Table 1 give a summary of the biological responses of different ions, and the next topics will present further discussions about the effects of different ions on the properties of bioactive glasses.

2.1 *Effect of Sodium*

Most research on bioactive glass until the late 1980s were based on 45S5 Bioglass®, which contain Na_2O in its composition, incorporated with the primary role of improving processability, as it can lower the melting-point of melt-quenched bioactive glasses [62]. The rapid rate of HCA formation was attributed to the presence of Na_2O and other alkali and alkali earth ions in the glass compositions [115], but other works have already demonstrated that bioactive glasses produced by the sol–gel method with no Na_2O content showed more bioactivity than melt-derived bioactive glasses with the same composition [57]. Therefore, the Na_2O content is not a critical component of the bioactive glass compositions [115], and its incorporation in sol–gel derived bioactive glass is not common. Bioactivity is actually more dependent on size and volume of the pores in the gel than on the Na_2O content [57]. Although sodium-based bioactive glasses show good bioactivity and biocompatibility, high Na_2O contents can present a cytotoxic response [7].

Bioactive glasses were synthesized to study the influence of sodium oxide contents on the glass properties while keeping the network connectivity constant by systematically replacing calcium oxide with sodium oxide. Linear decreases in the glass transition temperature and peak crystallization were observed with increasing sodium content [7]. The addition of Na_2O is referred as a network disrupter because the glass network expands with increasing Na_2O content. Reductions in the glass transition temperature were observed with increasing sodium content, as it is an expression of the network disruption of a glass [57]. By increasing the Na_2O content in bioactive glasses as a substitute for CaO, the silicate network is widened (i.e., the packing density decreased), due to the replacement of one Ca^{2+} ion by two Na^+ ions, which reduces the glass density and can also reduce the glass hardness, as the network becomes less compact [31].

2.2 Effect of Calcium

Calcium ions constitute one of the main components of many bioactive glasses; calcium is an almost universal intracellular messenger that has effects on a wide range of target proteins and regulates an enormous range of cellular processes [116]. In bone metabolism, calcium acts as a signaling molecule that affects cell functions and gene expressions via the activation of extracellular signal-related kinases signaling pathways [80]. Because calcium is one of the main components of the inorganic phase of human bone, these ions play an essential role in bone formation and resorption, favoring osteoblast differentiation and apatite precipitation, and can also increase the expression of insulin-like growth factors, such as IGF-I or IGF-II, which regulate human osteoblast proliferation [6, 70]. In vitro data indicate that calcium is a physiological regulator of bone cells through the activation of extracellular calcium-sensing receptors (CaSRs), which regulate the recruitment, differentiation and survival of osteoblasts and osteoclasts [79].

The mechanism of interaction with bone cells and the stimulating effect of these ions, along with the specific extracellular matrix concentration information are important when producing advanced materials with tailored ion release kinetics and controlled biological response in the physiological environment [70]. Studies indicated that 2–6 mM of Ca^{2+} is suitable for survival and proliferation of osteoblast, whereas 6–10 mM of Ca^{2+} is suitable for osteoblast proliferation, differentiation and mineralization, while higher concentrations are cytotoxic [71]. Cell proliferation, alkaline phosphatase (ALP) activity and Prostaglandin E2 (PGE_2, a potent mediator of bone remodeling) level significantly improved in mesoporous silica xerogel with 5 % calcium when compared with silica xerogel with no calcium. Additionally, the collagen type I and osteocalcin mRNA expression were up-regulated [80].

A common source of calcium in sol–gel bioactive glasses is calcium nitrate ($Ca(NO_3)_2$); however, it requires heating to remove the toxic nitrate by-products [117]. Additionally, using calcium nitrate, the calcium only enter the silicate network above 400 °C [4, 25, 118]. Calcium ions are incorporated into the network of silica secondary particles as network modifiers on bioactive glass structures and also help in the fusion of secondary particles to become tertiary particles, adopting a role as a "fuser" in sol–gel derived bioactive glass [25]. The oxygen in the Si–O–Ca bonds is non-bridging oxygen, and calcium is loosely bound within the glass network; ion loss from these materials is facile: it is achieved via simple ion exchange with body fluid [119]. Inhomogeneity in the structure appears when using a conventional calcium source because $Ca(NO_3)_2$ is soluble in the pore liquor (the byproduct of the condensation reaction) that is expelled from the gel due to shrinkage. During drying, the pore liquor evaporates, leaving $Ca(NO_3)_2$ deposits that may diffuse a limited distance during thermal stabilization [118, 120]. To avoid the problem of nitrate toxicity, calcium chloride ($CaCl_2$) is also used as a calcium source, but studies have shown that calcium is not incorporated at any temperature into the bulk of the material [118].

The processing temperature makes the application of bioactive glasses in hybrid materials difficult, and most of them contain no incorporated calcium [4]. Calcium methoxyethoxide (CME) has been used in bioactive glass processing as an alternative calcium source because it was found to enter the glassy network at lower temperatures [4, 117, 118, 120, 121]; however, processing materials using CME is too difficult due to its sensitivity to water [4]. New calcium sources that do not release toxic by-products and are incorporated at lower temperatures are still needed for hybrid applications.

2.3 *Effect of Fluorine*

Fluorine is an essential microelement in the human body, and proper levels of fluorine can accelerate the formation of apatite in bone and mineralized tissue, increase tissue stability and stimulating cell proliferation, thus increasing the biocompatibility of glass ceramics [81, 82]. Nonetheless, higher concentrations (>500 ng ml^{-1}) can suppress osteoblast activity [70]. Fluoride is of particular interest in bioactive glasses for dental applications to prevent dental caries due to the formation of fluorapatite (FA) in physiological solutions, which is more acid-resistant than HCA [57, 83]. It can also reduce the demineralization of enamel and dentin, enhancing remineralization and inhibiting bacterial enzymes, consequently preventing dental decay [54]. Some works also relate fluoride ions with an increase in bone density and prevention of fractures, which is of interest in patients suffering from osteoporosis, but there is still some controversy over its effectiveness [70, 83, 122].

Fluoride ion complexes with modifier cations (Ca^{2+}, Na^{+}, etc.) in bioactive glasses lead to more ionic character in the chemical bonds due to the electronegativity of fluoride [6]. The fluoride environment in bioactive glasses shows similarities to the structure of fluorite (CaF_2), and the crystallization and glass transition temperatures can decrease with increasing fluoride content [6, 57, 83]. The substitution of CaF_2 for CaO cause the polymerization of the silicate network and increase NC significantly, and fluoride can be lost as SiF_4, especially in highly crosslinked silicate glasses [83]. However, the formation of SiF_4 is prevented as the affinity of silicon for oxygen anions is higher than the affinity for fluoride ion in highly disrupted glass, including bioactive glasses with higher concentration of non-bridging oxygen and no Si–F bonds [83].

Typical precursors of fluoride-containing bioactive glasses are CaF_2 and NH_4HF_2 as precursors [81, 83]. The addition of CaF_2 to bioactive glasses have shown a reduced reactivity, as F ions have been thought to act as a corrosion inhibitor and also promotes the formation of a thin surface gel layer with a high silica concentration [82]. Higher fluoride concentrations in doped bioactive glasses can favor the formation of fluorite and calcite instead of apatite formation [122]. Fluorite presents low solubility, but bioactive glass can readily release calcium and fluoride ions, favoring the formation of an FA surface layer [6]. This layer act as a protective material, which can be helpful in materials proposed to dentistry field. The release of calcium ions in solution plays a very important role in apatite formation, and a larger release of this ion is observed with the presence of fluoride.

Fluoride-doped bioactive glass favors a faster and higher degree of crystallization of FA (compared with the formation of pure HA) and/or can promote a partial substitution of fluoride for hydroxide ions in HA [82]. The formation of FA instead of HA is consequently favored for higher concentrations of this ion [82, 83].

Hemolysis tests, in vitro toxicity tests and systemic toxicity tests demonstrated that bioactive glasses derived from $CaO–Na_2O–SiO_2–P_2O_5$ systems doped with NH_4HF_2 or CaF_2 possess good biocompatibility and conform to the requirements of biological safety as well as good osseointegration of implants with animal bone tissue after implantation for 2 months, indicating that the material is promising for use as implants [81].

2.4 Effects of Strontium

Strontium is a non-essential element that is naturally present mainly in bone. Strontium ranelate (a strontium(II) salt of ranelic acid) has been used for the treatment of osteoporosis [86, 87]. Strontium is also present in the liver, muscles and physiological fluids [49, 123, 124]. It is more often found in new and cancellous bones than in old and cortical bones [123]. The biological functionality of strontium is related to its chemical similarity with calcium and other group 2A elements, which have strong affinities with bone cells. Strontium ions are thought to displace Ca^{2+} ions in osteoblast-mediated processes due to its similarity in charge and size with Ca^{2+} [49]. Strontium is incorporated in the bone matrix by surface exchange with the incorporation of Sr^{2+} into the lattice of the bone mineral or by ionic substitution with Ca^{2+} [61]. Strontium-substituted bioactive glasses have been shown to stimulate osteoblasts and prevent osteoclasts from resorbing bone [6]. Strontium activates the calcium sensing receptors (CaSRs) in osteoblasts, increasing the production of osteoprotegerin (OPG) while decreasing the expression of the receptor activator of nuclear factor kappa beta ligand (RANKL). The OPG/RANKL ratio regulates the bone resorption and osteoclastogenesis [49, 84, 85].

Strontium-doped materials are of great interest in the biomedical field because of their biological effects and are usually incorporated in bioactive glass networks using $SrCO_3$ (melt-derived glass) [123, 124] or $Sr(NO_3)_2$ (sol–gel derived) [61, 125] as the precursors. A series of bioactive glasses with the composition 49.46 SiO_2–1.07 P_2O_5–23.08 CaO–26.38 Na_2O (mol%) were produced via melt with strontium substituted for calcium with different ratios up to 1, and it was confirmed that the substitution results in little change in the chemical structure of the glass, but an expansion of the glass network was observed that is associated with the larger size of the Sr^{2+} cation, which causes a decrease in the glass transition temperature and dilatometric softening point [123, 126]. Nonetheless, strontium addition in bioactive glasses appears to decrease the apatite-forming ability, but the formation of a silica-rich gel-like layer and deposition of amorphous calcium phosphate was observed after 1 h of immersion in SBF, and chemical degradation in Tris-HCl was slower after the addition of strontium [124, 127].

The in vitro effects of bioactive glasses containing strontium were studied on osteoblasts and osteoclast cultures and demonstrated that these materials promote osteoblast proliferation and activity and decrease osteoclast activity and resorption [72, 125]. Bioactive glass formulations enhanced the metabolic activity in sarcoma osteogenic cell cultures (SAOS-2) compared with the control, and the MTT activity in cells treated with strontium substituted bioactive glass was significantly enhanced compared with non-strontium containing glasses [72]. Additionally, strontium increases ALP activity and inhibits Tartrate Resistant Acid Phosphatase (TRAP) activity on CaP films, which is a marker of osteoclast differentiation and resorbing activity [72]. Strontium substituted in binary sol–gel glasses had a beneficial effect on fetal mouse calvarial bone cells, as indicated by the greater ALP activity and osteocalcin secretion and the up-regulation of transcription factors strongly involved in skeletal formation and bone repair, as well as collagen type I, bone sialoprotein and osteocalcin mRNA levels [125].

The incorporation of strontium in mesoporous bioactive glass scaffolds was investigated for the healing of bone defects in the femurs of rats induced by ovariectomy and presents a reduced number of tartrate-resistant acid phosphatase-positive cells when compared to other materials, improving bone repair [86]. A Sr-substituted MBG scaffold demonstrated a similar ability to form new bone and inhibit osteoclast bioactivity for the regeneration of osteopenic bone defects compared with estrogen therapy [86], making strontium an important element in bone tissue engineering as a therapeutic agent.

2.5 *Effect of Zinc*

Zinc is an important essential trace element, and several metalloenzymes use zinc for structure, catalytic, or regulatory actions, such as ALP activity, which is vital for the maturation of new bone formations [49, 88]. ALP is responsible for creating an alkaline environment that allows precipitation and subsequent mineralization of inorganic phosphates onto the extracellular matrix (ECM) that osteoblasts produce [49]. Zinc plays an important role in bone metabolism, stimulating osteoblastic bone formation and inhibiting osteoclastic bone resorption, increasing bone mass, and supplementation of nutritional zinc has been shown to have preventive and therapeutic effects on bone loss caused by bone disorders [88]. Evidence for zinc activation of osteoblast bone formation was found in mouse osteoblastic cells, by stimulating protein tyrosine phosphatase activity [89]. Zinc deficiency was shown to attenuate osteogenic activity by decreasing bone gene transcription through reduced and delayed Runx2 expression, which is a bone-specific transcription factor, and also by decreasing ECM mineralization through inhibition of ALP activity in osteoblasts, retarding skeletal growth [89]. Additionally, zinc can present an anti-inflammatory effect by suppressing interleukin 6 (a pro-inflammatory cytokine) synthesis via the inhibition of phospholipase C and phospholipase D in osteoblasts [89, 90].

Zinc can be incorporated in melt-derived glasses using ZnO or $ZnCO_3$ as a precursor [32, 128, 129], whereas $Zn(NO_3)_2$ is the typical precursor for the sol–gel process [15, 130, 131]. A bioactive glass with a composition of 64 % SiO_2–26 % CaO–5 % P_2O_5–5 % ZnO (mol%) that was synthesized by the sol–gel method was compared to non-zinc-containing glass [15], and the bioactivity was not reduced after the incorporation of Zn, the cell attachment was improved, and Zn was beneficial for maintaining the pH of SBF within the physiological limit by forming zinc hydroxide in the SBF solution. Additionally, studies have also shown that limited amounts of Zn resulted in early cell proliferation and promoted differentiation in in vitro biocompatibility assessments [15, 131], but zinc addition can slow down the degradation profile of bioactive glasses [128, 132]. However, studies also show that the proliferation and osteogenesis of human adipose stem cells (hASCs) were inhibited by bioactive glass scaffolds containing zinc, as shown by Haimi et al. [132], but the author suggests that the hASCs proliferation and osteogenesis were not detected because the addition of zinc slowed down the degradation rate of the materials. More studies should be performed to confirm the osteogenic effect of Zn released as ionic dissolution product from Zn-doped bioactive glasses [70].

HA layer formation was observed during in vitro analysis of zinc-doped bioactive glasses, and the increase in zinc content decreased the surface area and pore size, related to the network modifier behavior of this cation [130]. A stable thermal behavior was also observed in samples with a high zinc content [130].

2.6 *Effect of Magnesium*

Magnesium is the tenth most abundant element in the human body, and almost 99 % of total body magnesium is located in bone, muscles and non-muscular soft tissue, whereas 50–60 % resides as surface substituents of the hydroxyapatite mineral component of bone [92]. Mg is essential to bone metabolism, and dietary Mg deficiency has been implicated as a risk factor for osteoporosis [133]. This ion is vital to all living cells, including osteoblasts and osteoclasts, having stimulating effects on new bone formation [49, 91]. Mg also stabilizes enzymes, including many ATP-generation reactions, required for glucose utilization and is involved in lipid, protein, nuclei acid and coenzyme synthesis [92]. Studies have shown that Mg deficiency caused impaired bone growth, decreased osteoblast number and increased osteoclast number in young animals, as well as the loss of trabecular bone with stimulation of cytokine activity in bone [133]. Magnesium may interact with the integrin of osteoblast cells, which are responsible for cell adhesion and stability, and therefore, the incorporation of Mg^{2+} in bioceramics improves integration of implants in orthopedic and dental surgeries [73]. Mg can also stabilize cell membranes due to its positive charge, and Mg homeostasis can impact cell and tissue functions [91]. In vitro studies also revealed that high levels of magnesium can induce the synthesis of nitric oxide in endothelial cells, enhance the response of angiogenesis factors and attenuate the response of lipopolysaccharide (LPS) [134].

Magnesium-doped bioactive glass can be synthesized using magnesium oxide (MgO) as a precursor in melt-derived glass [135, 136] or magnesium nitrate ($Mg(NO_3)_2$) in sol–gel procedures [30, 43]. Magnesium-doped bioactive glasses formed a Ca–P–Mg-rich layer during the growth of the apatite layer between the bone and the glass, with Mg entering in the forming hydroxyapatite nuclei, thus inhibiting their evolution into tiny apatite crystals because this element cannot be accommodated in the HA structure [136, 137]. The formation of amorphous calcium phosphate is consequently promoted because Mg^{2+} suppresses the crystallization of apatite at higher concentrations, promoting greater dissolution of the apatite precipitates in the bioactive glass [30, 135, 136]. However, Mg introduction disrupts the glass matrix network, creating nonbridging oxygen and indirectly increasing the bioactive glass dissolution [70, 135], which can also affect the silica gel layer thickness, formed prior to the apatite-like layer [135]. The presence of MgO in bioactive glasses can also inhibit osteoporosis and enhance bone restoration [91, 138].

Osteoblasts cultured on SiO_2–CaO–MgO pellets expressed higher ALP activity than those on the control after incubation for 7 days, and the biocompatibility was confirmed because the osteoblasts adhered, proliferated and spread well on the surface of the pellets [43]. Similar results were obtained by Saboori et al. [137], where sol–gel Mg-doped bioactive glasses presented significantly higher alkaline phosphatase expressions than polystyrene plates at 37 and 39.5 °C, temperatures at which cells should proliferate slower and start differentiation. This result indicates that magnesium in bioactive glass can stimulate early bone cell differentiation [137]. Mg-doped hydroxyapatite granulate showed greater osteoconductivity and higher material resorption when compared with non-doped hydroxyapatite tested in vitro in femoral defects of rabbits [139]. Clinical uses of magnesium phosphate bone cement are also discussed [49], and further studies should be performed to confirm its osteogenic effect.

2.7 *Effects of Manganese*

Manganese is a trace element that plays important roles in the metabolism of bone and muscle [49, 140, 141]. It is present in small amounts in several tissues and organs, such as bone, pancreas, liver, and intestinal mucosa [140]. This element is a cofactor for metalloenzymes (oxidases and dehydrogenases), DNA polymerases and kinases [142, 143], and enzymes, such as glycosyltransferases (or mucopolysaccharides), which are involved in the extracellular matrix (ECM) remodeling that is necessary for the production of proteoglycans, which are important constituent of skeletal and cartilage structures [93]. The most important ECM protein is collagen, which gives particular structural properties to connective tissues, and this protein is degraded in the bone tissue remodeling process, releasing essential constituents, such as prolidase, a metalloprotease that has a specific requirement for manganese [140]. Mn^{2+} strongly influences the activation of integrins, a family of receptors that mediate cellular interactions with the extracellular matrix and cell surface ligands, consequently influencing the cell adhesion [143, 144]. Manganese is also known to be an important element for the maintenance of the homeostasis of glucose and lipid metabolism [141].

Manganese can influence the inhibition of bone resorption induced by free radicals [94], and osteoporosis has been associated with prolonged Mn deficiency, and low serum Mn levels have been found in osteoporotic subjects [145]. Mn as supplement after ovariectomy in rats can be an effective inhibitor of bone loss, both on the axial and peripheral levels [94]. This diet can help increase bone mineral density through facilitation of bone formation regardless of ovariectomy, with significantly increase on serum osteocalcin levels, a more sensitive bone formation biomarker [141]. A low Mn diet also resulted in increased fractures in deer antlers, which reduced peak force, impact energy and possibly cortical bone density [146]. It was suggested that Mn deficiency may lead to a reduction in the incorporation of calcium in bone tissue, resulting in an antler bone material with reduced density and porosity [146]. The authors suggest that osteoporosis may be caused by a lack of Mn, with calcium loss as a consequence and not the origin [93, 95, 146], but further studies in this area should be performed to confirm this hypothesis.

Human osteoblastic cell cultures with directly addition of Mn^{2+} showed a reduced cell spreading and proliferation in a concentration-dependent manner; therefore, the release of manganese ions in a biomaterial should be thoroughly adjusted according to the tolerance levels [140, 143, 147]. A calcium phosphate solution doped with Mn was used to coat metallic substrates with Mn-containing hydroxyapatite and indicated that the presence of this ion could reduce the precipitation and dimension of spherical aggregates as well as the degree of crystallinity of the apatitic phase, but the osteoblast osteocalcin production was significantly enhanced [148]. Mn-tricalcium phosphate also had positive effects on MC3T3-E1 in vitro pre-osteoblastic proliferation and differentiation, with the incorporation of small amounts of Mn^{2+} effectively accelerating bone mineralization [93].

Mn-doping was also evaluated in bioactive glass with up to 0.5 % MnO, which was synthesized using $MnCO_3$ as the precursor and produced by melting and quenching; Mn did not influence the thermal glass stability, but a slightly decrease in the bioactivity kinetics of the glass were observed during the first steps of the process; however, at longer times, Mn resulted in higher bioactivity [140]. In the same study, Mn-doped sheets significantly increased osteoblast differentiation and mineralization compared to undoped samples, with beneficial effects on the expression of ALP and bone morphogenetic proteins (BMP) [140]. Therefore, manganese is a promising dopant for bioactive glasses.

2.8 *Effect of Cobalt*

Cobalt is a trace element naturally found in the human body, and an essential micronutrient in the form of vitamin B_{12} (hydroxocobalamin), but inorganic cobalt is not required in the human diet, and cobalt deficiency has never been described in humans [149]. After a single dose of cobalt (Co^{2+}) in humans, the cobalt concentration in blood and serum is initially high but decreases rapidly and gradually, due to tissue uptake, mainly in the liver and kidney, combined with urinary (and fecal) excretion, and reaches a low level by 24 h [149]. Cobalt is a known angiogenic agent due to a well-established stabilizing effect on Hypoxia Inducible Factor (HIF-1α). The HIF-1α pathway is activated by low oxygen pressure (hypoxia), which results in the activation of a cascade of pro-vasculogenic genes critical for angiogenesis, including VEGF, thus mimicking the normal regenerative response. The HIF-1 pathway plays an essential role in coupling angiogenesis with osteogenesis, accelerating the development and regeneration of bone tissue and is important for the development of angiogenesis, stem cell differentiation, and fracture repair [35, 97, 98]. Therefore, Co-releasing materials have been suggested as a potential strategy for the promotion of neovascularization [35, 97, 150, 151]. Cells adapt to hypoxia by expressing a number of genes that are related to angiogenesis mobility and glucose metabolism, all via the HIF-1α pathway [75].

Cobalt was shown to promote angiogenesis via activation of the HIF-1 pathway in a rat remnant kidney in vivo model by subcutaneous injections of cobalt [96]. Additionally, in an in vivo rat bladder model, an enhanced hypoxia response was observed. The stimulated expression of HIF-1α and VEGF lead to cell growth and angiogenesis [35, 152]. Although cobalt is naturally present in the human body, and the body is equipped to excrete moderate amounts of excess cobalt, too many cobalt ions are potentially toxic; therefore, a controlled ion release system is vital for any tissue engineering strategy involving the delivery of cobalt [97, 153].

A series of bioactive glasses (BG) prepared via the melt-quench route with up to 4 mol% of Co^{2+} were prepared to investigate the role of cobalt within bioactive glass networks [97]. In the orthophosphate phase of the BGs, Co^{2+} appears to charge balance the orthophosphate groups, while in the silicate phase, Co^{2+} seems to play a dual role, both entering the silicate network and disrupting it as a network modifier, depending upon the concentration. Glass dissolution, ion release and HCA formation are delayed by inclusion of Co^{2+} in the BG in a concentration-dependent manner [97]. Bioactive glass based on a 53 wt% SiO_2, 6 wt% Na_2O, 12 wt% K_2O, 5 wt% MgO, 20 wt% CaO and 4 wt% P_2O_5 composition were Co-doped by replacing the CaO content with up to 5 wt% CoO using cobalt nitrate as precursor, and its bioactivity was evaluated [35]. The samples were immersed in SBF for different periods of time, and Co ions appear to diffuse through the SiO_2 layer (which itself is depleted of Co) and are substituted in the calcium phosphate layer [35]. An ion release study showed that Co release can be adjusted within the therapeutic range by tailoring the glass composition [35]. Co-doped bioactive glass scaffolds with sustained release of Co^{2+} ions support the attachment and growth of bone marrow stromal cells (BMSCs), and no obvious cytotoxicity was found [75]. However, a higher Co concentration did have the effect of reducing the BMSC viability. Incorporating ionic Co into the bioactive glass scaffolds did not affect the ALP activity of BMSCs and induced a significant hypoxic cascade, including increased VEGF protein secretion and HIF-1a and VEGF gene expression in BMSCs [75]. Cobalt-doped materials have potential uses in bone tissue engineering, with excellent osteogenesis in combination with angiogenesis function.

2.9 *Effects of Copper*

Copper is known to play a significant role in endothelial cells with beneficial effects in the process of angiogenesis and blood vessel maturation [49, 102]. Cu ions are related to the activity of several transcription factors (via HIF-1 and proline hydroxylase) and bind to cell membrane releasing complex, favoring the release of growth factors and cytokines from producing cells [76]. It can enhance the formation of organized collagen fibrils and fibers, with fibroblasts and mesenchymal cells synergistically participating in the presence of copper towards collagen synthesis and deposition [76]. There is also evidence for the osteogenic potential of Copper; it has been shown to increase the differentiation of mesenchymal stem cells towards the osteogenic lineage [102]. Copper also shows antibacterial activity, suppressing a range of bacterial pathogens [99–101].

Copper can exist in its oxidized cupric (Cu^{2+}) or reduced cuprous (Cu^{+}) state, but the divalent form has received more attention due to its role in angiogenic processes [49]. Cu can be added as CuO [154] or as the basic Cu carbonate ($CuCO_3{\cdot}Cu(OH)_2$) [102] for the preparation of melt-bioactive glasses, and copper nitrate ($Cu(NO_3)_2$) [100, 101] is usually used for sol–gel derived glasses. Cu^{2+} acts as a network modifier and is incorporated in the glass network in octahedral coordination, surrounded by two non-bridging oxygen [102]. Higher connectivity in Cu-doped bioactive glass was observed, likely due to the more covalent character of the Cu–O bond compared to the Ca–O bond, allowing repolymerization of Si and non-bridging oxygen [102]. Increasing the concentration of CuO in bioactive glass to near the Bioglass® composition showed a decrease in its glass nucleation and crystallization temperature, which decreases the bioactivity but provides enhanced chemical durability, density, microhardness and flexural strength [154]. Cu was incorporated in the apatite layer in SBF studies and could be released in controlled ranges [102]. Hydroxyapatite scaffolds modified with cupper bioactive glass have shown good drug delivery capacities and antibacterial effects as the Cu ions are released [99]. Similar results were obtained in nano-Cu-doped bioactive glass, which effectively prevented bacterial colonization after 24 h [100].

2.10 *Effect of Silver*

Silver ions are well known for their antibacterial properties [6, 49]. The anti-bacterial properties of silver can be attributed to its very small size and therefore high surface to volume ratio, which allows the metal ions to interact very closely with the membranes of the bacteria [104]. The cell membrane interaction can cause leakage of intracellular substances and consequently causes cell death, and some silver nanoparticles may also penetrate into the cells [105]. Silver ions can also control the spread of infection around an implant by preventing bacteria from colonizing, but the concentration of silver should be controlled, as high levels can lead to cell toxicity [104]. Ag ions have been shown higher antibacterial activities than other metal ions, such as copper, because bacteria show a low propensity toward developing resistance to silver-based materials. Additionally, it is less toxic to animal cells [155]. Silver-doped materials are also of interest in wound repair applications because it can damage bacterial RNA and DNA when in contact with moisture on the skin surface or with wound fluids, inhibiting replication [77]. Silver can reduce the inflammatory and granulation phases of healing, and induce epidermal repair [77].

Silver presented better antimicrobial action than copper against *E. coli* and *S. aureus* in growth studies performed in the presence of nanoparticles to observe their effect on the growth profile [105]. The incorporation of Ag into glasses can be performed by ion exchange with a molten silver salt because their charge to size ratio is similar than that of sodium ions [6]. A silver ion exchange process in bioactive glass led to an increase in the compressive strength of scaffolds, and the addition of silver into the composition has not affected the formation of a hydroxyapatite layer on its surface, supported cell attachment and maintained cell viability [104].

Sol–gel derived SiO_2–CaO–P_2O_5–Ag_2O, prepared using silver nitrate ($AgNO_3$) as the Ag precursor, was also evaluated and compared with the silver-free bioactive glass system, and a slow release of silver in aqueous solution was observed when compared with other constituents of the glass, suggesting that it was strongly chelated by the silicate network and the release profile can be tailored to specific clinical applications [77]. Furthermore, silver ions presented bactericidal properties towards *E. coli*, and the silver-free bioactive glass did not affected the viability of the bacterial strain under investigation [77]. A similar result was obtained for nanoporous bioactive glass synthesized using obtained using cetyltrimethyl ammonium bromide as a template to produce a nanoporous structure, which presented an antibacterial rate reaching 75 % in 1 h and 99 % in 12 h against *E. coli* [156]. It also showed a clotting ability, decreasing prothrombin time (PT) and activating partial thromboplastin time (APTT), indicating that its higher surface area could promote blood clotting when compared to bioactive glass with the same composition but without nanopores. In vivo tests showed that nanoporous bioactive glass doped with silver could be a good dressing, with antibacterial and hemostatic properties, shortened wound bleeding time and controlled hemorrhaging [156].

Phosphate-based bioactive glass with up to 1 mol% of Ag_2O was studied to understand to its influence on serum albumin adsorption, which is the most abundant protein in plasma and the first to surround foreign bodies when they come in contact with blood; therefore, it is a good indicator of the inflammatory response [157]. Silver appears to increase the adsorption potential of albumin on the samples surface, but for higher Ag_2O concentrations an alteration in the protein secondary structure was observed, mainly due to the appearance of metallic Ag^0 with unfolding of the protein as a consequence [157]. It is important for bioactive glasses to obtain an optimal silver content to provide an increase in the amount of attached protein and lack of conformational changes in the protein structure.

Commercial sutures coated with silver-doped bioactive glass powders are another clinical application, and studies of silver-coated sutures showed the greatest limiting effect on bacterial attachment in experiments carried out using *Staphylococcus epidermidis* [155]. The incidence of biomaterial-centered infection often lead to revision surgery, which can be avoided by improving biomaterial properties [77], and silver-doped materials feature prominently in the avoidance and treatment of bacterial infections.

2.11 *Effects of Gallium*

Gallium ion is known to have a potent antibacterial effect [33, 78, 107, 108] and is a drug that is already approved for the treatment of osteoporosis and hypercalcemia associated with tumor metastasis to bone [107]. It modulates osteoclastic bone resorption without affecting osteoblasts [106]. A proposed mechanism of Ga^{3+} action against bacteria is that gallium can disrupt Fe^{3+}-dependent events, which increases the vulnerability of these microorganisms because iron is redox active but gallium is redox inactive and infecting bacteria are unable to differentiate between Ga^{3+} and Fe^{3+} [33, 107, 108].

Gallium-doped phosphate glasses have shown to have antibacterial properties, with the ability to prevent the growth of biofilms of *Pseudomonas aeruginosa*, a pathogen that can cause hospital-acquired infections [108]; in addition, it has antibacterial effects against *Staphylococcus aureus, Escherichia coli,* and a small effect on methicillin-resistant *Staphylococcus aureus* and *Clostridium difficile.* These glasses have excellent long-term release of Ga^{3+} ions into the medium [33]. The structural study of borate-based gallium-doped glasses (using Ga_2O_3 as pre-cursor) showed an increase in the stability of the structure after replacing Na_2O with Ga_2O_3 because GaO_6 octahedra were formed, blocking the migration of the Na^+ ions, affecting the concentration of Ga^{3+} ions available for release, the overall stability and the rate of degradation [106, 158]. The lower rate of dissolution could be due to the participation of gallium in the glass network along with borate, possibly acting as a network modifier and improving its chemical stability [106]. A composite scaffold made of Ga^{3+}-loaded Bioglass® and alginate showed antibacterial effects and improved mechanical properties without decreasing the high level of bioactivity provided by the bioactive glass [107].

2.12 *Effect of Cerium*

Cerium has a variety of biochemical and physiological effects, primarily based on its similarity to calcium [111]. Beneficial effects of cerium (Ce) and cerium oxide

(CeO_2) have been reported, such as antioxidant properties that promote cell survival under conditions of oxidative stress [109, 110] and influence the intracellular Ca^{2+} level [110]. Cerium act as a neuroprotective agent, behaving as an antioxidant to limit the amount of reactive oxygen required to kill cells [109]. Ce plays an important role in physiological functions related to bone metabolism [159], and in vitro tests showed positive effects of cerium on osteoblasts proliferation, differentiation and mineralization [109, 111]. Cerium also presents a broad spectrum of antibacterial activity, a quick in vitro bioactive response, and low toxicity [109, 111, 112, 160].

Cerium can exist in two oxidation states, Ce^{3+} and Ce^{4+}, originating two different oxide forms, Ce_2O_3 and CeO_2 in bulk material [161]. Studies suggest that the concentration of Ce^{3+} relative to Ce^{4+} increases as the particle size decreases, meaning that, at the nanoscale, Ce oxide has oxygen vacancies or defects caused by the charge deficiency due to the presence of Ce^{3+} [109]. These oxygen defects have significant catalytic activity, imbuing ceria oxide nanoparticles with improved redox properties compared with the bulk material [161]. They can also scavenge superoxide radicals efficiently, which is of interest in biomedical areas where pathologies are associated with excessive oxidative stress [161]. Nanocomposite scaffolds of bioactive glass containing nanoceria additives demonstrated to enhance the osteoblastic differentiation of human mesenchymal stem cells (HMSCs) and production of collagen (when compared to undoped bioactive glass scaffold), even in the absence of any osteogenic supplements [113], indicating that nanoceria may act as an oxygen buffer, regulating the differentiation of HMSCs.

Sol–gel bioactive glasses containing Ce_2O_3, using cerium nitrate ($Ce(NO_3)_3$) as a precursor, presented a delayed in vitro response, due to the affinity of cerium towards phosphate, giving rise to a mixed phase, but the hydroxyapatite layer formation ability was not lost [78]; this ability was also observed in other works [60, 159]. Other studies have presented mesoporous bioactive glasses modified with cerium oxide for use as drug delivery systems, and cerium-doped glasses improved drug loading and release within therapeutic limits [60]. CeO_2-doped melt bioactive glasses revealed that cerium is present mainly as Ce^{3+}, and the content increases as the % CeO_2 increases in the starting oxide mixtures [162]. The chemical durability improved at higher cerium concentrations due to the low solubility of the cerium oxides, hydroxides and phosphates, as well as the stabilization of the glass structure, which is related to the partial covalent character of the Ce–O bond compared with the ionic Na–O and Ca–O bonds [162].

Borate-based bioactive glass containing up to 5 wt% Ce_2O_3 revealed a slower degradation rate compared with bare borate glass, but cerium did not alter the hydroxyapatite formation in SBF, when cerium was incorporated at lower concentrations [106]. At higher cerium concentrations, cerium ions possibly acted as a network modifier in the glass structure, leading to an improvement of the chemical durability, similar to the silicate-based glass [78, 106, 162].

3 Summary and Outlook

Bioactive glasses have been extensively studied for several applications, especially in bone tissue engineering. The dissolution of the glass networks favors the development of silica-rich layers in physiological solutions, which form surface layers of biomimetic apatite that can strongly bond to bone, allowing for its regeneration rather than bone replacement. The dissolution products heavily depend on the bioactive glass network, and understanding its structure is critical for in vitro and in vivo applications.

Bioactive glasses allow for the incorporation of physiologically active ions into their structures, and the resulting controlled ion release can lead to therapeutic benefits, such as the activation of several genes that are associated with osteogenesis and angiogenesis, the promotion of antibacterial action and anti-inflammatory effects, and improvement of the bioactive glass properties. Indeed, as discussed in this chapter, the dissolution products of several ions, such as Cu^{+}, Co^{2+}, Zn^{2+}, and F^{-}, have been shown to have stimulating biological effects on specific host tissues that are of interest to regenerative medicine. However, more experimental tests should be performed to confirm the therapeutic efficacy of single biologically active ions released as dissolution products from these glasses. Additionally, a deep understanding that is based on more in vivo evidence of the systemic toxicity and carcinogenic effects of ions released from biomaterials, as well as the ways in which these ions directly affect both healthy and diseased cellular regulation and cell–cell signaling, is needed. Furthermore, the incorporation of different ions in bioactive glasses can alter the dissolution behavior of the glass, and this behavior should be considered when analyzing test results because it leads to a biological response that may be difficult to compare with unmodified control glass. It is important to achieve controlled ion dissolution and release kinetics in physiological environments and provide an ion concentration that stimulates the biological response desired for tissue regeneration without toxicity. Moreover, the fabrication process of a bioactive glass and the way in which the material is applied also influence its dissolution behavior and, consequently, its therapeutic effects. The fabrication of composite and hybrid polymer/bioactive glass scaffolds is a method for controlling the dissolution of the glasses while maintaining their bioactivities and improving their mechanical properties.

New tissue engineering approaches can be developed based on the therapeutic effects of ions released from bioactive glasses, but much effort is still needed; this research truly connects chemistry and medicine for the development of improved materials. A deeper understanding of the chemical pathways and molecular mechanisms of the interactions between the developed materials and the host tissue will allow for tailoring of the physicochemical and mechanical properties of biomaterials in a way that induces the desired biological response for each application.

Acknowledgments The authors gratefully acknowledge financial support from CNPq, CAPES, and FAPEMIG/Brazil.

References

1. Hench, L.L.: Chronology of bioactive glass development and clinical applications, pp. 67–73. (2013). doi:10.4236/njgc.2013.32011
2. Hench, L.L., Hench, J.W., Greenspan, D.C.: Bioglass(R): a short history and bibliography. Mater. Sci. **40**, 1–42 (2004)
3. Hench, L.L.: The story of Bioglass. J. Mater. Sci. Mater. Med. **17**, 967–978 (2006). doi:10.1007/s10856-006-0432-z
4. Jones, J.R.: Review of bioactive glass: From Hench to hybrids. Acta Biomater. **9**, 4457–4486 (2013). doi:10.1016/j.actbio.2012.08.023
5. Gerhardt, L.-C., Boccaccini, A.R.: Bioactive glass and glass-ceramic scaffolds for bone tissue engineering. Materials (Basel) **3**, 3867–3910 (2010). doi:10.3390/ma3073867
6. Brauer DS. bioactive glasses-structure and properties. Angew Chemie Int. Ed. (2015). doi:10.1002/anie.201405310
7. Wallace, K.E., Hill, R.G., Pembroke, J.T., Brown, C.J., Hatton, P.V.: Influence of sodium oxide content on bioactive glass properties. J. Mater. Sci. Mater. Med. **10**, 697–701 (1999). doi:10.1023/A:1008910718446
8. Gupta, R., Kumar, A.: Bioactive materials for biomedical applications using sol–gel technology. Biomed. Mater. **3**, 034005 (2008). doi:10.1088/1748-6041/3/3/034005
9. Pereira, M.M., Clark, A.E., Hench, L.L.: Calcium phosphate formation on sol–gel-derived bioactive glasses in vitro. J. Biomed. Mater. Res. **28**, 693–698 (1994)
10. Pereira, M.M., Hench, L.L.: Mechanisms of hydroxyapatite formation on porous gel-silica substrates. J. Sol–Gel. Sci. Technol. **7**, 59–68 (1996). doi:10.1007/BF00401884
11. Rabiee, S.M., Nazparvar, N., Azizian, M., Vashaee, D., Tayebi, L.: Effect of ion substitution on Properties of bioactive glasses: a review. Ceram. Int. **41**, 7241–7251 (2015). doi:10.1016/j.ceramint.2015.02.140
12. Kokubo, T.: Bioactive glass ceramics: properties and applications. Biomaterials **12**, 155–163 (1991). doi:10.1016/0142-9612(91)90194-F
13. Zhong, J., Greenspan, D.C.: Processing and properties of sol–gel bioactive glasses. J. Biomed. Mater. Res. **53**, 694–701 (2000). doi:10.1002/1097-4636(2000)53:6<694:AID-JBM12>3.0.CO;2-6
14. Lei, B., Chen, X., Han, X., Zhou, J.: Versatile fabrication of nanoscale sol–gel bioactive glass particles for efficient bone tissue regeneration. J. Mater. Chem. **22**, 16906 (2012). doi:10.1039/c2jm31384g
15. Balamurugan, A., Balossier, G., Kannan, S., Michel, J., Rebelo, A.H.S., Ferreira, J.M.F.: Development and in vitro characterization of sol–gel derived $CaO–P_2O_5–SiO_2–ZnO$ bioglass. Acta Biomater. **3**, 255–262 (2007). doi:10.1016/j.actbio.2006.09.005
16. Faure, J., Drevet, R., Lemelle, A., Ben Jaber, N., Tara, A., El Btaouri, H., et al.: A new sol–gel synthesis of 45S5 bioactive glass using an organic acid as catalyst Preparation of Powder Gel. Mater. Sci. Eng., C **47**, 407–412 (2015). doi:10.1016/j.msec.2014.11.045
17. De Oliveira, A.A.R., Gomide, V.S., Leite, M.D.F., Mansur, H.S., Pereira, M.D.M.: Effect of polyvinyl alcohol content and after synthesis neutralization on structure, mechanical properties and cytotoxicity of sol–gel derived hybrid foams. Mater. Res. **12**, 239–244 (2009). doi:10.1590/S1516-14392009000200021
18. Kaur, G., Pandey, O.P., Singh, K., Homa, D., Scott, B., Pickrell, G.: A review of bioactive glasses: their structure, properties, fabrication and apatite formation. J. Biomed. Mater. Res. A **102**, 254–274 (2014). doi:10.1002/jbm.a.34690
19. Hanson, E.T., Lewis, R.L., Auerbach, R., Thomson, J.A., Applica, B.: Third-generation biomedical materials, p. 295 (2002)
20. Siqueira, R.L., Zanotto, E.D.: The influence of phosphorus precursors on the synthesis and bioactivity of $SiO_2–CaO–P_2O_5$ sol–gel glasses and glass-ceramics. J. Mater. Sci. Mater. Med. **24**, 365–379 (2013). doi:10.1007/s10856-012-4797-x

21. Sepulveda, P., Jones, J.R., Hench, L.: Characterization of melt-derived 45S5 and sol–gel-derived 58S bioactive glasses. J. Biomed. Mater. Res. **58**, 734–740 (2001). doi:10.1002/jbm.10026
22. De Barros Coelho, M., Magalhães Pereira, M.: Sol–gel synthesis of bioactive glass scaffolds for tissue engineering: effect of surfactant type and concentration. J. Biomed. Mater. Res. B Appl. Biomater. **75**, 451–456 (2005). doi:10.1002/jbm.b.30354
23. Pereira, M.M., Clark, A.E., Hench, L.L.: Effect of texture on the rate of hydroxyapatite formation on gel-silica surface. J. Am. Ceram. Soc. **78**, 2463–2468 (1995)
24. Valerio, P., Guimarães, M.H.R., Pereira, M.M., Leite, M.F., Goes, A.M.: Primary osteoblast cell response to sol–gel derived bioactive glass foams. J. Mater. Sci. Mater. Med. **16**, 851–856 (2005). doi:10.1007/s10856-005-3582-5
25. Lin, S., Ionescu, C., Pike, K.J., Smith, M.E., Jones, J.R.: Nanostructure evolution and calcium distribution in sol–gel derived bioactive glass, pp. 1276–1282 (2009). doi:10.1039/b814292k
26. FitzGerald, V., Pickup, D.M., Greenspan, D., Sarkar, G., Fitzgerald, J.J., Wetherall, K.M., et al.: A neutron and X-ray diffraction study of bioglass® with reverse Monte Carlo modelling. Adv. Funct. Mater. **17**, 3746–3753 (2007). doi:10.1002/adfm.200700433
27. Jugdaohsingh, R., Tucker, K.L., Qiao, N., Cupples, L.A., Kiel, D.P., Powell, J.J.: Dietary silicon intake is positively associated with bone mineral density in men and premenopausal women of the Framingham Offspring cohort. J. Bone Miner. Res. **19**, 297–307 (2004). doi:10.1359/JBMR.0301225
28. Reffitt, D.M., Ogston, N., Jugdaohsingh, R., Cheung, H.F.J., Evans, B.A.J., Thompson, R.P.H., et al.: Orthosilicic acid stimulates collagen type 1 synthesis and osteoblastic differentiation in human osteoblast-like cells in vitro. Bone **32**, 127–135 (2003). doi:10.1016/S8756-3282(02)00950-X
29. Sopcak, T., Medvecky, L., Girman, V., Durisin, J.: Mechanism of precipitation and phase composition of $CaO–SiO_2–P_2O_5$ systems synthesized by sol–gel method. J. Non Cryst. Solids **415**, 16–23 (2015). doi:10.1016/j.jnoncrysol.2015.02.014
30. Vallet-Regí, M., Salinas, A.J., Román, J., Gil, M.: Effect of magnesium content on the in vitro bioactivity of $CaO–MgO–SiO_2–P_2O_5$ sol–gel glasses. J. Mater. Chem. **9**, 515–518 (1999). doi:10.1039/a808679f
31. Farooq, I., Tylkowski, M., Müller, S., Janicki, T., Brauer, D.S., Hill, R.G.: Influence of sodium content on the properties of bioactive glasses for use in air abrasion. Biomed. Mater. **8**, 065008 (2013). doi:10.1088/1748-6041/8/6/065008
32. Salih, V., Patel, A., Knowles, J.C.: Zinc-containing phosphate-based glasses for tissue engineering. Biomed. Mater. **2**, 11–20 (2007). doi:10.1088/1748-6041/2/1/003
33. Valappil, S.P., Ready, D., Abou Neel, E.A., Pickup, D.M., Chrzanowski, W., O'Dell, L.A., et al.: Antimicrobial gallium-doped phosphate-based glasses. Adv. Funct. Mater. **18**, 732–741 (2008). doi:10.1002/adfm.200700931
34. Saranti, A., Koutselas, I., Karakassides, M.A.: Bioactive glasses in the system $CaO–B2O_3–P2O_5$: preparation, structural study and in vitro evaluation. J. Non Cryst. Solids **352**, 390–398 (2006). doi:10.1016/j.jnoncrysol.2006.01.042
35. Hoppe, A., Jokic, B., Janackovic, D., Fey, T., Greil, P., Romeis, S., et al.: Cobalt-releasing 1393 bioactive glass-derived scaffolds for bone tissue engineering applications. ACS Appl. Mater. Interfaces **6**, 2865–2877 (2014). doi:10.1021/am405354y
36. Mercier, C., Follet-Houttemane, C., Pardini, A., Revel, B.: Influence of P_2O_5 content on the structure of $SiO_2–Na_2O–CaO–P_2O_5$ bioglasses by 29Si and 31P MAS-NMR. J. Non Cryst. Solids **357**, 3901–3909 (2011). doi:10.1016/j.jnoncrysol.2011.07.042
37. Lebecq, I., Désanglois, F., Leriche, A., Follet-Houttemane, C.: Compositional dependence on thein vitro bioactivity of invert or conventional bioglasses in the Si–Ca–Na–P system. J. Biomed. Mater. Res., Part A **83A**, 156–168 (2007). doi:10.1002/jbm.a.31228
38. Elgayar, I., Aliev, A.E., Boccaccini, A.R., Hill, R.G.: Structural analysis of bioactive glasses. J. Non Cryst. Solids **351**, 173–183 (2005). doi:10.1016/j.jnoncrysol.2004.07.067

39. Tilocca, A., Cormack, A.N.: Structural effects of phosphorus inclusion in bioactive silicate glasses. J. Phys. Chem. B **111**, 14256–14264 (2007). doi:10.1021/jp075677o
40. Fayon, F., Duée, C., Poumeyrol, T., Allix, M., Massiot, D.: Evidence of nanometric-sized phosphate clusters in bioactive glasses as revealed by solid-state 31P NMR. J. Phys. Chem. C **117**, 2283–2288 (2013). doi:10.1021/jp312263j
41. Pedone, A., Charpentier, T., Malavasi, G., Menziani, M.C.: New insights into the atomic structure of 45S5 bioglass by means of solid–state NMR spectroscopy and accurate first-principles simulations. Chem. Mater. **22**, 5644–5652 (2010). doi:10.1021/cm102089c
42. Padilla, S., Román, J., Carenas, A., Vallet-Regí, M.: The influence of the phosphorus content on the bioactivity of sol–gel glass ceramics. Biomaterials **26**, 475–483 (2005). doi:10.1016/j.biomaterials.2004.02.054
43. Chen, X., Liao, X., Huang, Z., You, P., Chen, C., Kang, Y., et al.: Synthesis and characterization of novel multiphase bioactive glass-ceramics in the CaO–MgO–SiO_2 system. J. Biomed. Mater. Res. B Appl. Biomater. **93**, 194–202 (2010). doi:10.1002/jbm.b.31574
44. Ryu, H.-S., Lee, J.-K., Seo, J.-H., Kim, H., Hong, K.S., Kim, D.J., et al.: Novel bioactive and biodegradable glass ceramics with high mechanical strength in the CaO–SiO_2–B_2O_3 system. J. Biomed. Mater. Res. A **68**, 79–89 (2004). doi:10.1002/jbm.a.20029
45. Yang, X., Zhang, L., Chen, X., Sun, X., Yang, G., Guo, X., et al.: Incorporation of B_2O_3 in CaO–SiO_2–P2O_5 bioactive glass system for improving strength of low-temperature co-fired porous glass ceramics. J. Non Cryst. Solids **358**, 1171–1179 (2012). doi:10.1016/j.jnoncrysol.2012.02.005
46. Fu, Q., Rahaman, M.N., Fu, H., Liu, X.: Silicate, borosilicate, and borate bioactive glass scaffolds with controllable degradation rate for bone tissue engineering applications. I. Preparation and in vitro degradation. J. Biomed. Mater. Res. A **95**, 164–171 (2010). doi:10.1002/jbm.a.32824
47. Liu, X., Huang, W., Fu, H., Yao, A., Wang, D., Pan, H., et al.: Bioactive borosilicate glass scaffolds: Improvement on the strength of glass-based scaffolds for tissue engineering. J. Mater. Sci. Mater. Med. **20**, 365–372 (2009). doi:10.1007/s10856-008-3582-3
48. Gu, Y., Wang, G., Zhang, X., Zhang, Y., Zhang, C., Liu, X., et al.: Biodegradable borosilicate bioactive glass scaffolds with a trabecular microstructure for bone repair. Mater. Sci. Eng., C **36**, 294–300 (2014). doi:10.1016/j.msec.2013.12.023
49. Bose, S., Fielding, G., Tarafder, S., Bandyopadhyay, A.: Understanding of dopant-induced osteogenesis and angiogenesis in calcium phosphate ceramics. Trends Biotechnol. **31**, 594–605 (2013). doi:10.1016/j.tibtech.2013.06.005
50. Wu, C., Miron, R., Sculean, A., Kaskel, S., Doert, T., Schulze, R., et al.: Proliferation, differentiation and gene expression of osteoblasts in boron-containing associated with dexamethasone deliver from mesoporous bioactive glass scaffolds. Biomaterials **32**, 7068–7078 (2011). doi:10.1016/j.biomaterials.2011.06.009
51. Dzondo-Gadet, M., Mayap-Nzietchueng, R., Hess, K., Nabet, P., Belleville, F., Dousset, B.: Action of boron at the molecular level: effects on transcription and translation in an acellular system. Biol. Trace Elem. Res. **85**, 23–33 (2002). doi:10.1385/BTER:85:1:23
52. Lee, J.H., Nam, H., Ryu, H.S., Seo, J.H., Chang, B.S., Lee, C.K.: Bioactive ceramic coating of cancellous screws improves the osseointegration in the cancellous bone. J. Orthop. Sci. **16**, 291–297 (2011). doi:10.1007/s00776-011-0047-1
53. Maheswaran, A., Hirankumar, G., Heller, N., Karthickprabhu, S., Kawamura, J.: Structure, dielectric and bioactivity of P_2O_5–CaO–Na_2O–B_2O_3 bioactive glass. Appl. Phys. A **117**, 1323–1327 (2014). doi:10.1007/s00339-014-8545-6
54. Ali, S., Farooq, I., Iqbal, K.: A review of the effect of various ions on the properties and the clinical applications of novel bioactive glasses in medicine and dentistry. Saudi Dent J **26**, 1–5 (2014). doi:10.1016/j.sdentj.2013.12.001
55. Tilocca, A.: Models of structure, dynamics and reactivity of bioglasses: a review, p. 20 (2010). doi:10.1039/c0jm01081b

56. Fu, Q., Saiz, E., Rahaman, M.N., Tomsia, A.P.: Bioactive glass scaffolds for bone tissue engineering: state of the art and future perspectives. Mater. Sci. Eng. C **31**, 1245–1256 (2011). doi:10.1016/j.msec.2011.04.022
57. Farooq, I., Imran, Z., Farooq, U., Leghari, A., Ali, H.: Bioactive glass: a material for the future. World J. Dent. **3**, 199–201 (2012). doi:10.5005/jp-journals-10015-1156
58. De Oliveira, A.A.R., De Souza, D.A., Dias, L.L.S., De Carvalho, S.M., Mansur, H.S., Magalhães Pereira, M.: Synthesis, characterization and cytocompatibility of spherical bioactive glass nanoparticles for potential hard tissue engineering applications. Biomed. Mater. **8**, 025011 (2013). doi:10.1088/1748-6041/8/2/025011
59. El-Fiqi, A., Kim, T.-H., Kim, M., Eltohamy, M., Won, J.-E., Lee, E.-J., et al.: Capacity of mesoporous bioactive glass nanoparticles to deliver therapeutic molecules. Nanoscale (2012). doi:10.1039/c2nr31775c
60. Shruti, S., Salinas, A.J., Ferrari, E., Malavasi, G., Lusvardi, G., Doadrio, A.L., et al.: Curcumin release from cerium, gallium and zinc containing mesoporous bioactive glasses. Microporous Mesoporous Mater. **180**, 92–101 (2013). doi:10.1016/j.micromeso.2013.06.014
61. Wu, C., Fan, W., Gelinsky, M., Xiao, Y., Simon, P., Schulze, R., et al.: Bioactive SrO-SiO_2 glass with well-ordered mesopores: Characterization, physiochemistry and biological properties. Acta Biomater. **7**, 1797–1806 (2011). doi:10.1016/j.actbio.2010.12.018
62. Jones, J.R.: Review of bioactive glass: From Hench to hybrids. Acta Biomater. **9**, 4457–4486 (2013). doi:10.1016/j.actbio.2012.08.023
63. Lopes, J.H., Mazali, I.O., Landers, R., Bertran, C.A.: Structural investigation of the surface of bioglass 45S5 enriched with calcium ions. J. Am. Ceram. Soc. **96**, 1464–1469 (2013). doi:10.1111/jace.12305
64. Hench, L.L.: Feature 1705. Stress Int. J. Biol. Stress **28**, 1705–1728 (1998)
65. Murphy, S., Boyd, D., Moane, S., Bennett, M.: The effect of composition on ion release from Ca–Sr–Na–Zn–Si glass bone grafts. J. Mater. Sci. Mater. Med. **20**, 2207–2214 (2009). doi:10.1007/s10856-009-3789-y
66. Christodoulou, I., Buttery, L.D.K., Saravanapavan, P., Tai, G., Hench, L.L., Polak, J.M.: Dose- and time-dependent effect of bioactive gel-glass ionic-dissolution products on human fetal osteoblast-specific gene expression. J. Biomed. Mater. Res. B Appl. Biomater. **74**, 529–537 (2005). doi:10.1002/jbm.b.30249
67. Xynos, I.D., Hukkanen, M.V.J., Batten, J.J., Buttery, L.D., Hench, L.L., Polak, J.M.: Bioglass ®45S5 stimulates osteoblast turnover and enhances bone formation in vitro: implications and applications for bone tissue engineering. Calcif. Tissue Int. **67**, 321–329 (2000). doi:10.1007/s002230001134
68. Valerio, P., Pereira, M.M., Goes, A.M., Leite, M.F.: The effect of ionic products from bioactive glass dissolution on osteoblast proliferation and collagen production. Biomaterials **25**, 2941–2948 (2004). doi:10.1016/j.biomaterials.2003.09.086
69. Mourino, V., Cattalini, J.P., Boccaccini, A.R.: Metallic ions as therapeutic agents in tissue engineering scaffolds: an overview of their biological applications and strategies for new developments. J. R. Soc. Interface **9**, 401–419 (2012). doi:10.1098/rsif.2011.0611
70. Hoppe, A., Güldal, N.S., Boccaccini, A.R.: A review of the biological response to ionic dissolution products from bioactive glasses and glass-ceramics. Biomaterials **32**, 2757–2774 (2011). doi:10.1016/j.biomaterials.2011.01.004
71. Maeno, S., Niki, Y., Matsumoto, H., Morioka, H., Yatabe, T., Funayama, A., et al.: The effect of calcium ion concentration on osteoblast viability, proliferation and differentiation in monolayer and 3D culture. Biomaterials **26**, 4847–4855 (2005). doi:10.1016/j.biomaterials.2005.01.006
72. Gentleman, E., Fredholm, Y.C., Jell, G., Lotfibakhshaiesh, N., O'Donnell, M.D., Hill, R.G., et al.: The effects of strontium-substituted bioactive glasses on osteoblasts and osteoclasts in vitro. Biomaterials **31**, 3949–3956 (2010). doi:10.1016/j.biomaterials.2010.01.121

73. Zreiqat, H., Howlett, C.R., Zannettino, A., Evans, P., Schulze-Tanzil, G., Knabe, C., et al.: Mechanisms of magnesium-stimulated adhesion of osteoblastic cells to commonly used orthopaedic implants. J. Biomed. Mater. Res. **62**, 175–184 (2002). doi:10.1002/jbm.10270
74. Diba, M., Tapia, F., Boccaccini, A.R., Strobel, L.A.: Magnesium-containing bioactive glasses for biomedical applications. Int. J. Appl. Glas. Sci. **3**, 221–253 (2012). doi:10.1111/j.2041-1294.2012.00095.x
75. Wu, C., Zhou, Y., Fan, W., Han, P., Chang, J., Yuen, J., et al.: Hypoxia-mimicking mesoporous bioactive glass scaffolds with controllable cobalt ion release for bone tissue engineering. Biomaterials **33**, 2076–2085 (2012). doi:10.1016/j.biomaterials.2011.11.042
76. Gérard, C., Bordeleau, L.J., Barralet, J., Doillon, C.J.: The stimulation of angiogenesis and collagen deposition by copper. Biomaterials **31**, 824–831 (2010). doi:10.1016/j.biomaterials.2009.10.009
77. Balamurugan, A., Balossier, G., Laurent-Maquin, D., Pina, S., Rebelo, A.H.S., Faure, J., et al.: An in vitro biological and anti-bacterial study on a sol–gel derived silver-incorporated bioglass system. Dent. Mater. **4**, 1343–1351 (2008). doi:10.1016/j.dental.2008.02.015
78. Shruti, S., Salinas, A.J., Malavasi, G., Lusvardi, G., Menabue, L., Ferrara, C., et al.: Structural and in vitro study of cerium, gallium and zinc containing sol–gel bioactive glasses. J. Mater. Chem. **22**, 13698 (2012). doi:10.1039/c2jm31767b
79. Marie, P.J.: The calcium-sensing receptor in bone cells: a potential therapeutic target in osteoporosis. Bone **46**, 571–576 (2010). doi:10.1016/j.bone.2009.07.082
80. Zhou, H., Wei, J., Wu, X., Shi, J., Liu, C., Jia, J., et al.: The bio-functional role of calcium in mesoporous silica xerogels on the responses of osteoblasts in vitro. J. Mater. Sci. Mater. Med. **21**, 2175–2185 (2010). doi:10.1007/s10856-010-4083-8
81. Li, H.C., Wang, D.G., Hu, J.H., Chen, C.Z.: Influence of fluoride additions on biological and mechanical properties of Na_2O–CaO–SiO_2–P_2O_5 glass-ceramics. Mater. Sci. Eng. C **35**, 171–178 (2014). doi:10.1016/j.msec.2013.10.028
82. Lusvardi, G., Malavasi, G., Menabue, L., Aina, V., Morterra, C.: Fluoride-containing bioactive glasses: Surface reactivity in simulated body fluids solutions. Acta Biomater. **5**, 3548–3562 (2009). doi:10.1016/j.actbio.2009.06.009
83. Brauer, D.S., Anjum, M.N., Mneimne, M., Wilson, R.M., Doweidar, H., Hill, R.G.: Fluoride-containing bioactive glass-ceramics. J. Non Cryst. Solids **358**, 1438–1442 (2012). doi:10.1016/j.jnoncrysol.2012.03.014
84. Coulombe, J., Faure, H., Robin, B., Ruat, M.: In vitro effects of strontium ranelate on the extracellular calcium-sensing receptor. Biochem Biophys. Res. Commun. **323**, 1184–1190 (2004). doi:10.1016/j.bbrc.2004.08.209
85. Saidak, Z., Marie, P.J.: Strontium signaling: Molecular mechanisms and therapeutic implications in osteoporosis. Pharmacol. Ther. **136**, 216–226 (2012). doi:10.1016/j.pharmthera.2012.07.009
86. Wei, L., Ke, J., Prasadam, I., Miron, R.J., Lin, S., Xiao, Y., et al.: A comparative study of Sr-incorporated mesoporous bioactive glass scaffolds for regeneration of osteopenic bone defects. Osteoporos. Int. **25**, 2089–2096 (2014). doi:10.1007/s00198-014-2735-0
87. Vasile, E., Popescu, L.M., Piticescu, R.M., Burlacu, A., Buruiana, T.: Physico-chemical and biocompatible properties of hydroxyapatite based composites prepared by an innovative synthesis route. Mater. Lett. **79**, 85–88 (2012). doi:10.1016/j.matlet.2012.03.099
88. Yamaguchi, M.: Role of nutritional zinc in the prevention of osteoporosis. Mol. Cell. Biochem. **338**, 241–254 (2010). doi:10.1007/s11010-009-0358-0
89. Kwun, I.S., Cho, Y.E., Lomeda, R.A.R., Shin, H.I., Choi, J.Y., Kang, Y.H., et al.: Zinc deficiency suppresses matrix mineralization and retards osteogenesis transiently with catch-up possibly through Runx 2 modulation. Bone **46**, 732–741 (2010). doi:10.1016/j.bone.2009.11.003
90. Hatakeyama, D., Kozawa, O., Otsuka, T., Shibata, T., Uematsu, T.: Zinc suppresses IL-6 synthesis by prostaglandin F2α in osteoblasts: inhibition of phospholipase C and phospholipase D. J. Cell. Biochem. **85**, 621–628 (2002). doi:10.1002/jcb.10166

91. Castiglioni, S., Cazzaniga, A., Albisetti, W., Maier, J.A.M.: Magnesium and osteoporosis: Current state of knowledge and future research directions. Nutrients **5**, 3022–3033 (2013). doi:10.3390/nu5083022
92. Jahnen-Dechent, W., Ketteler, M.: Magnesium basics. CKJ Clin. Kidney J. (2012). doi:10.1093/ndtplus/sfr163
93. Torres, P.M.C., Vieira, S.I., Cerqueira, A.R., Pina, S., Da Cruz Silva, O.A.B., Abrantes, J.C.C., et al.: Effects of Mn-doping on the structure and biological properties of β-tricalcium phosphate. J. Inorg. Biochem. **136**, 57–66 (2014). doi:10.1016/j.jinorgbio.2014.03.013
94. Rico, H., Gómez-Raso, N., Revilla, M., Hernández, E.R., Seco, C., Páez, E., et al.: Effects on bone loss of manganese alone or with copper supplement in ovariectomized rats a morphometric and densitometric study. Eur. J. Obstet. Gynecol. Reprod. Biol. **90**, 97–101 (2000). doi:10.1016/S0301-2115(99)00223-7
95. Landete-Castillejos, T., Currey, J.D., Ceacero, F., García, A.J., Gallego, L., Gomez, S.: Does nutrition affect bone porosity and mineral tissue distribution in deer antlers? The relationship between histology, mechanical properties and mineral composition. Bone **50**, 245–254 (2012). doi:10.1016/j.bone.2011.10.026
96. Tanaka, T., Kojima, I., Ohse, T., Ingelfinger, J.R., Adler, S., Fujita, T., et al.: Cobalt promotes angiogenesis via hypoxia-inducible factor and protects tubulointerstitium in the remnant kidney model. Lab. Invest. **85**, 1292–1307 (2005). doi:10.1038/labinvest.3700328
97. Azevedo, M., Jell, G., O'Donnell, M., Law, R., Hill, R., Stevens, M.: Synthesis and characterization of hypoxia-mimicking bioactive glasses for skeletal regeneration. J. Mater. Chem. (2010). doi:10.1039/c0jm01111h
98. Wang, Y., Wan, C., Deng, L., Liu, X., Cao, X., Gilbert, S.R., et al.: The hypoxia-inducible factor α pathway couples angiogenesis to osteogenesis during skeletal development. J. Clin. Invest. **117**, 1616–1626 (2007). doi:10.1172/JCI31581
99. Ye, J., He, J., Wang, C., Yao, K., Gou, Z.: Copper-containing mesoporous bioactive glass coatings on orbital implants for improving drug delivery capacity and antibacterial activity. Biotechnol. Lett. **36**, 961–968 (2014). doi:10.1007/s10529-014-1465-x
100. Goh, Y.F., Alshemary, A.Z., Akram, M., Abdul Kadir, M.R., Hussain, R.: Bioactive glass: an in-vitro comparative study of doping with nanoscale copper and silver particles. Int. J. Appl. Glas. Sci. **266**, 255–266 (2014). doi:10.1111/ijag.12061
101. Bejarano, J., Caviedes, P., Palza, H.: Sol–gel synthesis and in vitro bioactivity of copper and zinc-doped silicate bioactive glasses and glass-ceramics. Biomed. Mater. **10**, 025001 (2015). doi:10.1088/1748-6041/10/2/025001
102. Hoppe, A., Meszaros, R., Stähli, C., Romeis, S., Schmidt, J., Peukert, W., et al.: In vitro reactivity of Cu doped 45S5 Bioglass® derived scaffolds for bone tissue engineering. J. Mater. Chem. B **1**, 5659 (2013). doi:10.1039/c3tb21007c
103. Finney, L., Vogt, S., Fukai, T., Glesne, D.: Copper and angiogenesis: unravelling a relationship key to cancer progression. Clin. Exp. Pharmacol. Physiol. **36**, 88–94 (2009). doi:10.1111/j.1440-1681.2008.04969.x
104. Newby, P.J., El-Gendy, R., Kirkham, J., Yang, X.B., Thompson, I.D., Boccaccini, A.R.: Ag-doped 45S5 Bioglass̄-based bone scaffolds by molten salt ion exchange: Processing and characterisation. J. Mater. Sci. Mater. Med. **22**, 557–569 (2011). doi:10.1007/s10856-011-4240-8
105. Ruparelia, J.P., Chatterjee, A.K., Duttagupta, S.P., Mukherji, S.: Strain specificity in antimicrobial activity of silver and copper nanoparticles. Acta Biomater. **4**, 707–716 (2008). doi:10.1016/j.actbio.2007.11.006
106. Deliormanlı, A.M.: Synthesis and characterization of cerium- and gallium-containing borate bioactive glass scaffolds for bone tissue engineering. J. Mater. Sci. Mater. Med. (2015). doi:10.1007/s10856-014-5368-0
107. Mouriño, V., Newby, P., Boccaccini, A.R.: Preparation and characterization of gallium releasing 3-d alginate coated 45s5 bioglass® based scaffolds for bone tissue engineering. Adv. Eng. Mater. **12**, 283–291 (2010). doi:10.1002/adem.200980078

108. Valappil, S.P., Ready, D., Abou Neel, E.A., Pickup, D.M., O'Dell, L.A., Chrzanowski, W., et al.: Controlled delivery of antimicrobial gallium ions from phosphate-based glasses. Acta Biomater. **5**, 1198–1210 (2009). doi:10.1016/j.actbio.2008.09.019
109. Schubert, D., Dargusch, R., Raitano, J., Chan, S.W.: Cerium and yttrium oxide nanoparticles are neuroprotective. Biochem. Biophys. Res. Commun. **342**, 86–91 (2006). doi:10.1016/j.bbrc.2006.01.129
110. Horie, M., Nishio, K., Kato, H., Fujita, K., Endoh, S., Nakamura, A., et al.: Cellular responses induced by cerium oxide nanoparticles: Induction of intracellular calcium level and oxidative stress on culture cells. J. Biochem. **150**, 461–471 (2011). doi:10.1093/jb/mvr081
111. Hu, Y., Du, Y., Jiang, H., Jiang, G.: Cerium promotes bone marrow stromal cells migration and osteogenic differentiation via Smad1/ 5/ 8 signaling pathway. Int. J. Clin. Exp. Pathol. **7**, 5369–5378 (2014)
112. Lin, W., Huang, Y.-W., Zhou, X.-D., Ma, Y.: Toxicity of cerium oxide nanoparticles in human lung cancer cells. Int. J. Toxicol. **25**, 451–457 (2015). doi:10.1080/10915810600959543
113. Karakoti, A.S., Tsigkou, O., Yue, S., Lee, P.D., Stevens, M.M., Jones, J.R., et al.: Rare earth oxides as nanoadditives in 3-D nanocomposite scaffolds for bone regeneration. J. Mater. Chem. **20**, 8912 (2010). doi:10.1039/c0jm01072c
114. Julien, M., Khoshniat, S., Lacreusette, A., Gatius, M., Bozec, A., Wagner, E.F., et al.: Phosphate-dependent regulation of MGP in osteoblasts: role of ERK1/2 and Fra-1. J. Bone Miner. Res. **24**, 1856–1868 (2009). doi:10.1359/jbmr.090508
115. Saravanapavan, P., Jones, J.R., Pryce, R.S., Hench, L.L.: Bioactivity of gel-glass powders in the $CaO–SiO_2$ system: a comparison with ternary ($CaO–P_2O_5–SiO_2$) and quaternary glasses ($SiO_2–CaO–P_2O_5–Na_2O$). J Biomed Mater Res A **66**, 110–119 (2003). doi:10.1002/jbm.a.10532
116. Bolsover, S.R.: Calcium signalling in growth cone migration. Cell Calcium **37**, 395–402 (2005). doi:10.1016/j.ceca.2005.01.007
117. Yu, B., Poologasundarampillai, G., Turdean-Ionescu, C., Smith, M.E., Jones, J.R.: A new calcium source for bioactive sol–gel hybrids. Bioceram. Dev. Appl. **1**, 1–3 (2011). doi:10.4303/bda/D110178
118. Yu, B., Turdean-Ionescu, C.A., Martin, R.A., Newport, R.J., Hanna, J.V., Smith, M.E., et al.: Effect of calcium source on structure and properties of sol–gel derived bioactive glasses. Langmuir **28**, 17465–17476 (2012). doi:10.1021/la303768b
119. Newport, R.J., Skipper, L.J., Carta, D., Pickup, D.M., Sowrey, F.E., Smith, M.E., et al.: The use of advanced diffraction methods in the study of the structure of a bioactive calcia: Silica sol–gel glass. J. Mater. Sci. Mater. Med. **17**, 1003–1010 (2006). doi:10.1007/s10856-006-0436-8
120. Pereira, M.M., Clark, A.E., Hench, L.L.: Homogeneity of bioactive sol–gel-derived glasses in the system $CaO–P_2O_5–SiO_2$.pdf. J. Mater. Synth. Process. **2**, 189–195 (1994)
121. Li, A., Shen, H., Ren, H., Wang, C., Wu, D., Martin, R.A., et al.: Bioactive organic/inorganic hybrids with improved mechanical performance. J. Mater. Chem. B **3**, 1379–1390 (2015). doi:10.1039/C4TB01776E
122. Shah, F.A., Brauer, D.S., Hill, R.G., Hing, K.A.: Apatite formation of bioactive glasses is enhanced by low additions of fluoride but delayed in the presence of serum proteins. Mater. Lett. **153**, 143–147 (2015). doi:10.1016/j.matlet.2015.04.013
123. Fredholm, Y.C., Karpukhina, N., Law, R.V., Hill, R.G.: Strontium containing bioactive glasses: glass structure and physical properties. J. Non Cryst. Solids **356**, 2546–2551 (2010). doi:10.1016/j.jnoncrysol.2010.06.078
124. Goel, A., Rajagopal, R.R., Ferreira, J.M.F.: Influence of strontium on structure, sintering and biodegradation behaviour of $CaO–MgO–SrO–SiO_2-P_2O_5-CaF_2$ glasses. Acta Biomater. **7**, 4071–4080 (2011). doi:10.1016/j.actbio.2011.06.047

125. Isaac, J., Nohra, J., Lao, J., Jallot, E., Nedelec, J.M., Berdal, A., et al.: Effects of strontium-doped bioactive glass on the differentiation of cultured osteogenic cells. Eur. Cells Mater. **21**, 130–143 (2011)
126. O'Donnell, M.D., Hill, R.G.: Influence of strontium and the importance of glass chemistry and structure when designing bioactive glasses for bone regeneration. Acta Biomater. **6**, 2382–2385 (2010). doi:10.1016/j.actbio.2010.01.006
127. Zhang, W., Shen, Y., Pan, H., Lin, K., Liu, X., Darvell, B.W., et al.: Effects of strontium in modified biomaterials. Acta Biomater. **7**, 800–808 (2011). doi:10.1016/j.actbio.2010.08.031
128. Aina, V., Malavasi, G., Fiorio Pla, A., Munaron, L., Morterra, C.: Zinc-containing bioactive glasses: Surface reactivity and behaviour towards endothelial cells. Acta Biomater. **5**, 1211–1222 (2009). doi:10.1016/j.actbio.2008.10.020
129. Zhang, X.F., Kehoe, S., Adhi, S.K., Ajithkumar, T.G., Moane, S., O'Shea, H., et al.: Composition-structure-property (Zn^{2+} and Ca^{2+} ion release) evaluation of Si–Na–Ca–Zn–Ce glasses: potential components for nerve guidance conduits. Mater. Sci. Eng., C **31**, 669–676 (2011). doi:10.1016/j.msec.2010.12.016
130. Anand, V., Singh, K.J., Kaur, K.: Evaluation of zinc and magnesium doped 45S5 mesoporous bioactive glass system for the growth of hydroxyl apatite layer. J. Non Cryst. Solids **406**, 88–94 (2014). doi:10.1016/j.jnoncrysol.2014.09.050
131. Oki, A., Parveen, B., Hossain, S., Adeniji, S., Donahue, H.: Preparation and in vitro bioactivity of zinc containing sol–gel-derived bioglass materials. J. Biomed. Mater. Res. A **69**, 216–221 (2004). doi:10.1002/jbm.a.20070
132. Haimi, S., Gorianc, G., Moimas, L., Lindroos, B., Huhtala, H., Räty, S., et al.: Characterization of zinc-releasing three-dimensional bioactive glass scaffolds and their effect on human adipose stem cell proliferation and osteogenic differentiation. Acta Biomater. **5**, 3122–3131 (2009). doi:10.1016/j.actbio.2009.04.006
133. Rude, R.K., Gruber, H.E., Wei, L.Y., Frausto, A., Mills, B.G.: Magnesium deficiency: Effect on bone and mineral metabolism in the mouse. Calcif. Tissue Int. **72**, 32–41 (2003). doi:10.1007/s00223-001-1091-1
134. Maier, J.A.M., Bernardini, D., Rayssiguier, Y., Mazur, A.: High concentrations of magnesium modulate vascular endothelial cell behaviour in vitro. Biochim. Biophys. Acta Mol. Basis Dis. **1689**, 6–12 (2004). doi:10.1016/j.bbadis.2004.02.004
135. Dietrich, E., Oudadesse, H., Lucas-Girot, A., Mami, M.: In vitro bioactivity of melt-derived glass 46S6 doped with magnesium. J. Biomed. Mater. Res. A **88**, 1087–1096 (2009). doi:10.1002/jbm.a.31901
136. Jallot, E.: Role of magnesium during spontaneous formation of a calcium phosphate layer at the periphery of a bioactive glass coating doped with MgO. Appl. Surf. Sci. **211**, 89–95 (2003). doi:10.1016/S0169-4332(03)00179-X
137. Saboori, A., Rabiee, M., Moztarzadeh, F., Sheikhi, M., Tahriri, M., Karimi, M.: Synthesis, characterization and in vitro bioactivity of sol–gel-derived SiO_2–CaO–P_2O_5–MgO bioglass. Mater. Sci. Eng. C **29**, 335–340 (2009). doi:10.1016/j.msec.2008.07.004
138. Imani Fooladi, A.A., Hosseini, H.M., Hafezi, F., Hosseinnejad, F., Nourani, M.R.: Sol–gel-derived bioactive glass containing SiO_2–MgO–CaO–P_2O_5 as an antibacterial scaffold. J. Biomed. Mater. Res. A **101A**, 1582–1587 (2013). doi:10.1002/jbm.a.34464
139. Landi, E., Logroscino, G., Proietti, L., Tampieri, A., Sandri, M., Sprio, S.: Biomimetic Mg-substituted hydroxyapatite: from synthesis to in vivo behaviour. J. Mater. Sci. Mater. Med. **19**, 239–247 (2008). doi:10.1007/s10856-006-0032-y
140. Miola, M., Brovarone, C.V., Maina, G., Rossi, F., Bergandi, L., Ghigo, D., et al.: In vitro study of manganese-doped bioactive glasses for bone regeneration. Mater. Sci. Eng., C **38**, 107–118 (2014). doi:10.1016/j.msec.2014.01.045
141. Bae, Y.J., Kim, M.H.: Manganese supplementation improves mineral density of the spine and femur and serum osteocalcin in rats. Biol. Trace Elem. Res. **124**, 28–34 (2008). doi:10.1007/s12011-008-8119-6
142. Culotta, V.C., Yang, M., Hall, M.D.: Manganese transport and trafficking: lessons learned from. Society **4**, 1159–1165 (2005). doi:10.1128/EC.4.7.1159

143. Lüthen, F., Bulnheim, U., Müller, P.D., Rychly, J., Jesswein, H., Nebe, J.G.B.: Influence of manganese ions on cellular behavior of human osteoblasts in vitro. Biomol. Eng. **24**, 531–536 (2007). doi:10.1016/j.bioeng.2007.08.003
144. Sopyan, I., Ramesh, S., Nawawi, N.A., Tampieri, A., Sprio, S.: Effects of manganese doping on properties of sol–gel derived biphasic calcium phosphate ceramics. Ceram. Int. **37**, 3703–3715 (2011). doi:10.1016/j.ceramint.2011.06.033
145. Beattie, J.H., Avenell, A.: Trace element nutrition and bone metabolism. Nutr. Res. Rev. **5**, 167–188 (1992). doi:10.1079/NRR19920013
146. Landete-Castillejos, T., Currey, J.D., Estevez, J.A., Fierro, Y., Calatayud, A., Ceacero, F., et al.: Do drastic weather effects on diet influence changes in chemical composition, mechanical properties and structure in deer antlers? Bone **47**, 815–825 (2010). doi:10.1016/j.bone.2010.07.021
147. Pabbruwe, M.B., Standard, O.C., Sorrell, C.C., Howlett, C.R.: Bone formation within alumina tubes: effect of calcium, manganese, and chromium dopants. Biomaterials **25**, 4901–4910 (2004). doi:10.1016/j.biomaterials.2004.01.005
148. Bracci, B., Torricelli, P., Panzavolta, S., Boanini, E., Giardino, R., Bigi, A.: Effect of Mg^{2+}, Sr^{2+}, and Mn2+ on the chemico-physical and in vitro biological properties of calcium phosphate biomimetic coatings. J. Inorg. Biochem. **103**, 1666–1674 (2009). doi:10.1016/j.jinorgbio.2009.09.009
149. Simonsen, L.O., Harbak, H., Bennekou, P.: Cobalt metabolism and toxicology-A brief update. Sci. Total Environ. **432**, 210–215 (2012). doi:10.1016/j.scitotenv.2012.06.009
150. Quinlan, E., Partap, S., Azevedo, M.M., Jell, G., Stevens, M.M., O'Brien, F.J.: Hypoxia-mimicking bioactive glass/collagen glycosaminoglycan composite scaffolds to enhance angiogenesis and bone repair. Biomaterials **52**, 358–366 (2015). doi:10.1016/j.biomaterials.2015.02.006
151. Peters, K., Schmidt, H., Unger, R.E., Kamp, G., Pröls, F., Berger, B.J., et al.: Paradoxical effects of hypoxia-mimicking divalent cobalt ions in human endothelial cells in vitro. Mol. Cell. Biochem. **270**, 157–166 (2005). doi:10.1007/s11010-005-4504-z
152. Buttyan, R., Chichester, P., Stisser, B., Matsumoto, S., Ghafar, M.A., Levin, R.M.: Acute intravesical infusion of a cobalt solution stimulates a hypoxia response, growth and angiogenesis in the rat bladder. J. Urol. **169**, 2402–2406 (2003). doi:10.1097/01.ju.0000058406.16931.93
153. Kramer, E., Itzkowitz, E., Wei, M.: Synthesis and characterization of cobalt-substituted hydroxyapatite powders. Ceram. Int. **40**, 13471–13480 (2014). doi:10.1016/j.ceramint.2014.05.072
154. Srivastava, A.K., Pyare, R.: Characterization of CuO substituted 45S5 bioactive glasses and glass—ceramics. Int. J. Sci. Technol. Res. **1**, 28–41 (2012)
155. Pratten, J., Nazhat, S.N., Blaker, J.J., Boccaccini, A.R.: In vitro attachment of Staphylococcus epidermidis to surgical sutures with and without Ag-containing bioactive glass coating. J. Biomater. Appl. **19**, 47–57 (2004). doi:10.1177/0885328204043200
156. Hu, G., Xiao, L., Tong, P., Bi, D., Wang, H., Ma, H., et al.: Antibacterial hemostatic dressings with nanoporous bioglass containing silver. Int. J. Nanomed. **7**, 2613–2620 (2012). doi:10.2147/IJN.S31081
157. Simon, V.: Addressing the optimal silver content in bioactive glass systems in terms of BSA adsorption. J. Mater. Chem. (2014). doi:10.1039/C4TB00733F
158. Pickup, D.M., Moss, R.M., Qiu, D., Newport, R.J., Valappil, S.P., Knowles, J.C., et al.: Structural characterization by X-ray methods of novel antimicrobial gallium-doped phosphate-based glasses. J. Chem. Phys. (2009). doi:10.1063/1.3076057
159. Salinas, A.J., Shruti, S., Malavasi, G., Menabue, L., Vallet-Regí, M.: Substitutions of cerium, gallium and zinc in ordered mesoporous bioactive glasses. Acta Biomater. **7**, 3452–3458 (2011). doi:10.1016/j.actbio.2011.05.033
160. Zhang, J., Zhu, Y.: Synthesis and characterization of CeO_2-incorporated mesoporous calcium-silicate materials. Microporous Mesoporous Mater. **197**, 244–251 (2014). doi:10.1016/j.micromeso.2014.06.018

161. Das, S., Dowding, J.M., Klump, K.E., McGinnis, J.F., Self, W., Seal, S.: Cerium oxide nanoparticles: applications and prospects in nanomedicine. Nanomedicine **8**, 1483–1508 (2013). doi:10.2217/nnm.13.133
162. Leonelli, C., Lusvardi, G., Malavasi, G., Menabue, L., Tonelli, M.: Synthesis and characterization of cerium-doped glasses and in vitro evaluation of bioactivity. J. Non Cryst. Solids **316**, 198–216 (2003). doi:10.1016/S0022-3093(02)01628-9

What Can We Learn from Atomistic Simulations of Bioactive Glasses?

Alfonso Pedone and Maria Cristina Menziani

Abstract In the last decades, most experimental efforts have been devoted to design bioactive glasses (please consult the Editor's note in order to clarify the usage of the terms bioglass, bioactive glass and biocompatible glasses) with enhanced biological and mechanical properties by adding specific ions to known bioactive compositions. Concurrently, computational research has been focused to the understanding of the relationships between bioactivity and composition by rationalization of the role of the doping ions. Thus, a deep knowledge of the structural organization of the constituent atoms of the bioactive glasses has been gained by the employment of ab initio and classical molecular dynamics simulations techniques. This chapter reviews the recent successes in this field by presenting, in a concise way, the structure–properties relationships of silicate, phospho-silicate and phosphate glasses with potential bioactive properties.

1 Introduction

Bioactive glasses are widely employed for repair and replacement of diseased and damaged bone tissues, as bioactive coatings for bioinert metal/alloy implants, as toothpaste additives, and for several other biomedical applications [1, 2].

Once in contact with body fluids, a rapid sequence of chemical reactions occurs at the surface of the bioactive glasses yielding to the formation of a hydroxycarbonate apatite (HCA) layer similar to bone mineral. HCA interacts with collagen fibrils to integrate with the host bone, giving rise to a strong chemical interface [3].

Since bioactivity strongly depends on the release of ionic species in the physiological environment, a prerequisite for straightforward prediction of the bioactive response of glasses is the correct understanding, at atomic level, of the structural

A. Pedone (✉) · M.C. Menziani
Dipartimento di Scienze Chimiche e Geologiche, Università degli Studi di Modena e Reggio Emilia, Via G. Campi 103, 41125 Modena, Italy
e-mail: alfonso.pedone@unimore.it

J. Marchi (ed.), *Biocompatible Glasses*, Advanced Structured Materials 53,
DOI 10.1007/978-3-319-44249-5_5

organization of the constituting components, and of their modifications occurring over (sub)-nanometer scales, when the glass composition is altered. With this knowledge, new glass compositions for biomaterials with more attention to the application needs of the end users can be rationally designed reducing development costs, and speeding up the time to market.

Understanding the structure of glass is crucial but not trivial. The combination of advanced characterization techniques is required to collect different, complementary information of amorphous structures [4]. The data obtained often depict apparent contradictory structural evidences, and are of difficult interpretation.

Thus, in the last years a fervent computational research activity has been carried out with the aim of supporting in the interpretation of the experimental results. In particular, atomistic computer simulations have shown to provide a detailed picture of the glass structures, and precious information on the structure–properties relationships of complex glasses [5–9]. In fact, the structural and dynamical features that control dissolution and bioactivity cover length and time scales accessible to molecular dynamics (MD) simulations [10–14] Therefore, computational studies have now remarkably advanced the understanding of bioactive glasses, as documented by the numerous reviews and perspective articles published in recent years [9, 10, 12, 13].

This chapter reviews the recent efforts to uncover sound relationships among the structure of crucial components and the physico-chemical properties of silicate, phospho-silicate and phosphate glasses with potential bioactive properties.

The chapter is organized as follows: first computational details for classical and ab initio MD simulations are given with emphasis on critical points for oxide glasses treatment, then some important structural descriptors derived from the computational simulations are described. Section 4 summarizes the key structural features of silicate glasses, and the determinants of glass bioactivity are discussed. Some important computational results that allow significant insight into the effect of dopants such as Mg, Sr, Zn, Ga, Al, Ce, … on glass structure are then reviewed and compared with the available experimental data. The salient features of the glass surface are summarized in Sect. 5. Finally, the computational description of Phosphate glasses is reported.

2 How to Obtain the Glass Structure Models: A Brief Overview of Classical and Ab Initio Molecular Dynamics

2.1 Classical Molecular Dynamics

The melt-and-quench approach commonly used to obtain glasses through MD simulations mimics the experimental process. In this approach, the glass structure is represented by a classical ensemble of particles in a box, interacting through empirical force fields [14].

The Newton's equations of motion for each particle in the ensemble is solved with an iterative process: positions and velocities are updated in small increments of time, known as timesteps. Once equilibration is reached, the structure of the glass is obtained as an average over a large number (thousands or hundred-thousands). Large system sizes, on the order of $\sim 10^4$ atoms, is now accessible with a high level of accuracy, thanks to the accurate force fields now available [15–18]. Moreover, models of length size between 2 and 10 nm yield relevant structural properties for the glass dissolution with high statistical accuracy.

The interatomic pair potential based on the Born model can be written as:

$$U_{ij}(r) = \frac{q_i q_j e^2}{r} + \phi_{ij}(r) \tag{1}$$

where q_i and q_j are the ionic charges, r is the inter-atomic distance, φ_{ij} is the short-range interaction term, which accounts for of the repulsion between electron clouds, van der Waals attraction, polarization effects and, when needed, bond terms.

For ionic or partially ionic materials the rigid ionic model which neglect the ionic polarizability is the most commonly used. However, the atomic polarizability can be explicitly accounted for by modelling polarizable atoms such as the oxide ions with core-shell dipoles, i.e. two opposite charges connected by a harmonic spring [19].

Force fields, spatial (size of the box) and temporal (cooling procedure) dimensions of the MD simulation may have a considerable impact on the final atomic arrangement obtained [11]. Hence, the reliability of the structural model obtained is proved by the comparison with the experimental data.

2.2 *Ab Initio Molecular Dynamics*

In ab initio molecular dynamics (AI MD) the forces acting on the nuclei are computed from electronic structure calculations as the molecular dynamics trajectory is generated. The explicit treatment of electronic structure makes AI MD extremely useful, in terms of accuracy and predictability, for the study of systems difficult to parametrize, such as multi-coordination, and multi-oxidation states of species, reactivity at surfaces or dynamical processes in melts.

However, the increased in computational costs is significant, thus only relatively small system size (100–300 atoms) and time (10–100 ps) are affordable via ab initio MD. Therefore, statistically sound descriptions of medium-range features in glasses containing more than four oxides are still not obtained by these methods.

2.3 Mixed Classical-AI MD Procedure

The computational protocol usually adopted in first-principles simulations of glasses consists in using as a 'starting guess' an initial structure obtained through classical MD with an empirical potential [6, 20, 21]. A partial relaxation of the structure is then carried out at the ab initio level. However, restrictions due to the high computational costs prevent a full relaxation at the medium-range order, which usually remains completely determined by the quality of the empirical potential used to construct the initial structure. Therefore, the scope of these mixed classical/ab initio approaches is limited to the investigation of properties with local character [22–26].

3 Structural Descriptors for Bioactivity Prediction

The short and medium range structure features of the glasses can be extracted from the tree-dimensional models obtained by MD simulations. Besides the bond length, bond angle distributions, and coordination geometries of the constituting ions, other important structural features at length scales beyond the first coordination shell affect the dissolution and the bioactive behaviour of the glass. In particular, the network connectivity, the coordination environment of network formers and network modifier cations, the tendency of cation to cluster and the formation of inhomogeneous regions [7, 8, 22, 27], as well as the occurrence of chain and ring fragments [28], and the diffusion properties of modified cations [29]. Some of these structural descriptors used in almost all the papers reviewed in this chapter, are describe in the following paragraphs.

3.1 The Network Connectivity

The network connectivity (NC) of a glass is the most common structural descriptor used to predict the bioactivity [29]. NC depends critically on composition being defined as average number of bridging oxygen atoms per network former. In general, highly bioactive glasses are characterized by a low network connectivity (≤ 2.5), denoting a fragmented silicate matrix, mainly constituted by linear polymer chains. In this case, the release of $–O–[Si–O–]_n$ chains needed for biodegradation requires breaking a lower number of Si–O bonds compared to highly ramified structure characterized by Q^3 and Q^4 silicate units (Q designates 'quaternary' and *n* the number of bridging oxygens (BO) connected to other network former cations.) (Fig. 1a, c). The presence of hydroxyl groups in sol–gel glasses yields an actual NC lower than that calculated from the nominal composition [30].

NC as calculated from the nominal molecular formula only [29] is an average value and relies on two assumptions: (a) the glass is homogeneous in nature;

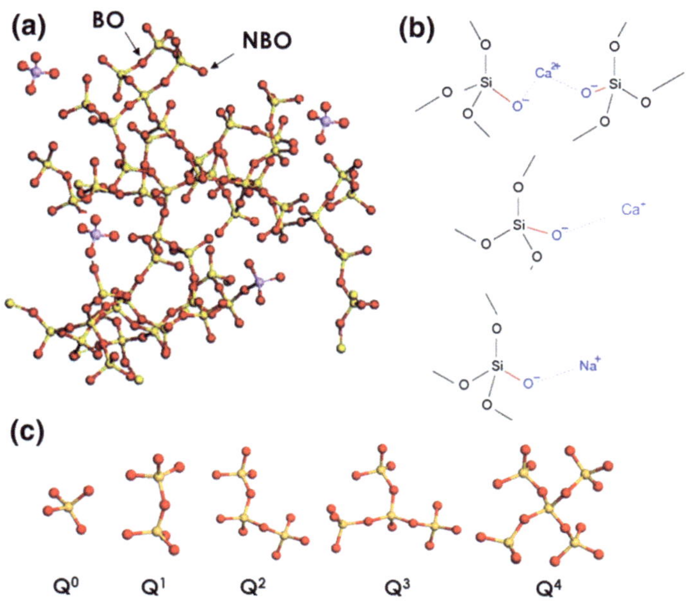

Fig. 1 **a** A fragment of branched network chain in 45S5 (modifiers have been removed for clarity) *yellow ball* silicon; *red ball* oxygen; *purple ball* phosphorus; **b** interaction of Na and Ca ions with the silicate network, and, **c** three dimensional representations of the different Q^n species (*central atom*). **a** Adapted with permission from Ref. [51], copyright 2011 American Chemical Society. **c** Adapted with permission from Ref. [26], copyright 2013 Royal Society of Chemistry

(b) when a bridging oxygen has been replaced by two non-bridging oxygens, the bond is completely broken. However, (a) in multicomponent glasses segregation of ions in specific region gives rise to heterogeneous glasses (for example, fluorinated 45S5 bioglass presents silicate-rich and silicate-poor regions [31–33], and (b) the disrupting effect on the network can vary depending on the type of modifier cation introduced (i.e. Na has a more disrupting effect compared to Ca, which can also assume the intermediate role of charge compensator).

In this respect, NC computed by computer simulations as weighted average of the Q^n distributions of network former ions is more appropriate. It is defined as:

$$NC = \sum_{n=0}^{4} x_n \cdot n \tag{2}$$

where x_n is the percentage of the Q^n species (n = 0, 1, 2, 3, 4). It can be computed over all the three-dimensional model of the glass and/or in specific zones when mesoscale segregation of network occurs, and the real effect of cations with intermediate network-former/modifier character can be taken into account, as shown in the following paragraphs.

3.1.1 Strength of the Glass Network

A theoretical structural descriptor that estimates the degree of connectivity of the network and its overall strength (F_{net}) has been derived to take into account the different energetics of the X–O and X–F bonds in fluorinated bioactive glasses [8, 31]. F_{net} is obtained by using the formula:

$$F_{net} = \frac{1}{N}\left[\sum_{i}^{cations}\sum_{j}^{anions} n_i \cdot CN_{ij} \cdot BE_{ij} \cdot m_{ij}\right] \quad (3)$$

where N is the total number of atoms, n_i is the number of atoms of the ith species; CN_{ij} is the mean coordination number of ij pairs atoms (i = Si, P, Zn, Na, Ca; j = O^{2-}, F^{-}) whereas BE_{ij} are the gas phase bond enthalpies. The multiplicative factor m_{ij} represents the maximum number of SiO_4 and PO_4 units linked to the i–O or i–F bonds, and tunes the contribution of each bond to the overall network strength.

3.1.2 Strength of Modifier-Mediated Cross-Link Interactions

It is generally assumed that the variation in the ion strength depends on the number of O–M–O inter tetrahedral connections.

Thus, an evaluation of the overall strength of modifiers which mediates cross-link interactions in the glass can be obtained from the MD structure, by combining the density of the inter-tetrahedral links T_M formed by each modifier cation M with the corresponding M–O ionic bond strength [34, 35].

In particular, a linear combination of the NC, T_M and $R_{M–M}$ (see next paragraph for definition) descriptors:

$$s = \alpha \cdot NC + \beta \cdot R_{M-M} + \gamma \cdot T_M \quad (4)$$

has been derived and used to understand the behavior of known compositions of yttrium-doped bioactive glasses, and extrapolate this insight to new potentially interesting compositions [36].

3.2 *Clustering of Network and Modifying Cations*

Clustering effects have important consequences on ion mobility, repolymerization of the silica network, and crystallization tendency. Therefore these are key factors in biodegradation since they may inhibit or enhance leaching of the ions in the surrounding environment.

The ratio R_{X-Y} between the number of Y ions found around the coordination sphere of X computed from the MD model and that expected from a homogeneous distribution of the $X - Y$ cations is a statistical measure of the tendency of the X and Y cations to cluster in the glass matrix. The ratio is computed such as $R_{X-Y} = 1$ indicates that the uniform distribution is respected (i.e. no clustering), while $R_{X-Y} > 1$ implies spatial clustering [37, 38] If X = Y self-aggregation is accounted for.

An important issue that involve ion clustering is the pronounced devitrification tendency of bioglasses. The highly disrupted silicate network facilitates the rearrangement of the structural units to form critical size nuclei for crystallization.

Partial crystallization will not necessarily reduce the bioactivity, depending on the crystal phases forming and the composition of the remaining glass phase [2]. A simple descriptor for predicting the crystals that could separate from glasses has been proposed [39, 40]. Based on the assumption that the nucleating tendency depends on the structural similarity between the glass and its isochemical crystals, the algorithm analyzes the stoichiometry of different spherical regions in the bulk glass and compares it with the stoichiometry ratio of compositionally equivalent crystalline phases stored in a database.

4 SiO_2-Based Bioactive Glass Systems

Silicate-based glasses exhibit bioactivity only over a relatively narrow range of compositions.

The 45S5 Bioglass (46.1 % SiO_2, 24.4 % Na_2O, 26.9 % CaO, 2.6 % P_2O_5, in mol%), was the first material able to form an interfacial bond with host tissue, when implanted in rats [41]. Kokubo and co-workers [42] demonstrated that also P_2O_5-free Na_2O–CaO–SiO_2 glasses are bioactive with the rate of formation of the biologically active apatite layer similar to that of 45S5 Bioglass.

However, numerous recent investigations conducted both in vitro and in vivo reveal that the presence of P enhance the bioactivity [1]. The rate at which Ca, P, Si ions enter the fluid surrounding the glass [43], which is crucial for triggering the osteoblast activity, strongly depends on the amount of phosphate units into the glass. Moreover, the ion release also controls the local pH and the presence of P avoids excessive acidity that inhibits bone bonding [44].

4.1 Structure of Bioglass 45S5

The atomic structure of silica glasses is determined by the silica tetrahedra connected by –Si–O–Si– bridging oxygen bonds (Fig. 1a). Silicon is therefore the glass network-forming atom. Network-modifying cations (e.g. alkali and alkaline-earth metal oxides) can disrupt the network by forming non-bridging oxygen (NBO) bonds such as $Si–O^- \ Na^+$ (Fig. 1b).

The medium-range order around the network-forming cation is expressed as Q^n species distribution where Q designates 'quaternary' and *n* the number of BO oxygens connected to other network former cations ranges from 0 to 4 (Fig. 1c). Q^n therefore provides a direct link to the polymerization degree of the structure. Thus, Q^4 describes a three-dimensional network, Q^3—two-dimensional sheets, Q^2—chains and rings, Q^1 and Q^0 correspond to isolated dimers and tetrahedra, respectively.

The results of a pioneering MD-GIPAW [26] study on 45S5 bioactive glass clearly showed and confirmed that the host silica network is described by a tri-nomial Q^n distribution consisting of chains and rings of Q^2 Si (67.2 %) SiO_4 tetrahedra cross-linked with Q^3 Si (22.3 %) species and terminated by a low quantity of Q^1 Si (10.1 %) species [25].

The structural role of phosphorus in bioglass has been debated for long and only recently been clarified. The controversy regarded its presence as orthophosphate units (Q^0), with charge balanced by sodium and/or calcium, (^{31}P and ^{17}O NMR) or in mixed silicate/phosphate network containing Si–O–P bonds, and originated both by the results of NMR experiments [45–47] and theoretical studies [12, 25, 27, 48, 49]. It is now recognized that while the majority of phosphorus atoms are present as isolated orthophosphate tetrahedra, small amounts of Si–O–P bonds ($\sim$8 %) are also present at high P_2O_5 content [50].

These orthophosphate groups are surrounded by modifier cations for charge-balancing purposes, and it has recently be shown that the P atoms in short-range scale phosphosilicate glasses are randomly distributed in the glass. In particular, across a short-range scale inferior of 450 pm. The dispersion of the phosphate-ions is independent on the degree of polymerization of silicate network and nearly independent of the P content of the glass in the range of 1–6 mol% P_2O_5 [52].

While early MD simulation experiments [53, 54] have reported different Ca and Na distributions in series of glasses with increased P_2O_5 content, a random distribution between the silicate rich regions and the phosphate rich regions of the glass structure seems to be preferred in the bioglass 45S5 [2, 23, 48, 54].

A recent study carried out with a mixed computational (MD) and experimental (NMR) approach [55] has investigated the intermixing of network modifying Na^+/Ca^{2+} ions around the silicate and phosphate tetrahedra in a wide series of soda lime phosphosilicate glasses, whose P content and silicate network connectivity were varied independently. The extent of Na^+/Ca^{2+} ordering around a given Q^n of Si or P computed by MD simulations indicates that Na and Ca ions intermixed nearly randomly. The overall weak preferences are essentially independent of the Si and P contents of the glass, but depend of the total amount of network modifiers. The most negatively charged P Q^0, and Si Q^1, and Q^2 groups present in 45S5 bioactive silicate glass, show the strongest preferences for the divalent Ca^{2+} cations, but this preference becomes less pronounced by increasing the total amount of network modifiers, whereas the preference of the lower-charged P Q^1 and Si Q^3 species for Na^+ cations increases.

Very recently, the structural features of a series of 45S5 bioactive silicate glass derivatives spanning a wide range of Na, Ca, Si, and P compositions has been reported [56]. The results from MD and NMR studies shown that it is possible to obtain both a rapid degradation of the glass network and fast dissolution of biologically active ions by a fine tuning of network connectivity and of the amounts of readily released orthophosphate ions. On this process, the propensity of P to be arranged in orthophosphate groups detached from the glass network is the key factor.

4.2 *The Structure–Property Relationships of Substituted Bioactive Glasses*

Over the last decade, research activity has been focused on adding modifier ions in bioactive glasses to increase their potential therapeutic benefit. A certain degree of flexibility in glass composition allows for addition of several elements in different concentrations [57], thus improving their physical-chemical properties for specific applications. For example, the strength, toughness, and elastic properties, which are a major bottleneck for the resistance of an implant against mechanic loads; high solubility may be the major disadvantage of bioglasses when used for long-term implants, since most of the released ions may be transported away from the region near the implant from the biological fluid prior to the formation of new bone.

However, the same property, high solubility, can be exploit to release specific ions with therapeutic action in the human body exactly at the site where they are needed, with minimized side effects. Furthermore, by controlling the rate of bioactive glasses dissolution through variation of the glass network connectivity and the type of modifier or intermediate ion, long term sustained therapeutic effects can be obtained [2].

In the following, we review the contribution of molecular simulations studies to the understanding of the composition–structure–property relationships obtained by several additive ions, such as magnesium (Mg), strontium (Sr), zinc (Zn), aluminum (Al), gallium (Ga), cerium (Ce) and fluoride (F).

4.2.1 Magnesium-Bioactive Glasses

The replacement of CaO for MgO in glasses derived from the parent 45S5 Bioglass ($46.2SiO_2{\cdot}24.3Na_2O{\cdot}(26.9 - x)CaO{\cdot}2.6P_2O_5{\cdot}x MgO$ where $x = 0$, 5, 10, 15, 20, and 26.9 mol%) produces significant changes on the structure, chemical durability, and elastic properties as detected by means of molecular dynamics simulations [35].

The results show that the Mg ions are mainly fivefold coordinated; however, non-negligible amount of 4- and a small amount of sixfold coordinated species are also observed as a function of the MgO content.

The total number of NBOs in the glass is unchanged with respect to the 45S5 Bioglass, therefore the overall network connectivity (NC) with an open structure dominated by Si Q^2 species is also similar. Differences are instead observed in the small number of shared edges between MgO_5 and SiO_4 polyhedra with respect to the CaO_6–SiO_4 ones. In fact, the higher field strength of Mg allows the coordination from NBOs belonging to different tetrahedra only. Thus, the larger rings formed improving the solubility and the melt viscosities of Mg-containing silicate glasses.

Segregation of modifying cations is observed: Na and Ca are found in the phosphate rich regions, whereas Na, Ca, and Mg ions are homogeneously distributed in the silicate matrix. Ca and Mg manifest a clear preference for low-n Q silicate sites whereas the Na ions are preferably found around high-n sites. Therefore, an increasing of the Na leaching is expected because weaker interactions of sodium ions with bridging oxygens of high-n Si Q^n sites facilitate Na diffusion as reported for soda-lime glasses [58].

On these basis, the authors suggest that MgO content below 10 mol% would improve the mechanical properties of bioglass 45S5, preserving good bioactivity.

The insertion of higher field strength Mg ions in alkali-free bioactive glasses also results in a decreasing in network connectivity. In this case, the expected increase in bioactivity was indeed confirmed by in vitro bio-mineralization activity [59].

4.2.2 Strontium-Bioative Glasses

The effect of the SrO/CaO substitution on the glass structure and diffusion of a series of bioactive glasses was studied by Du and Xiang [51, 60] using MD simulations. Although in biomedical applications the SrO concentration is usually below 5 mol%, a wide range of Sr concentrations was used to understand the strontium substitution effect: $46.1SiO_2{\cdot}24.4Na_2O{\cdot}(26.9-x)CaO{\cdot}2.6P_2O_5{\cdot}xSrO$ with x = 0, 1, 5, 10, 15, 20 and 26.9 mol%. It was shown that the substitution does not considerably change the medium range structure although a linear increase of glass density and decrease of molar volume as a function of Sr addition was found. Ca and Sr ions were preferentially distributed around phosphorus ions. Therefore, the authors concluded that the enhanced dissolution rate in Sr containing glasses is mainly due to the increase of free volume and the non-local effect that weakens the silicon-oxygen network of these systems.

Ionic diffusion MD studies on three bioactive glass compositions (from 46 to 65 mol% SiO_2 and 5 mol% SrO/CaO) [60] showed higher diffusion coefficient and lower diffusion energy barrier for sodium with respect to calcium and strontium (see Fig. 2); the diffusion coefficient of modifier cations decreases significantly with the increasing of silica content. This phenomenon explains the observed decreased solubility and bioactivity in SrO/CaO substituted bioactive glasses.

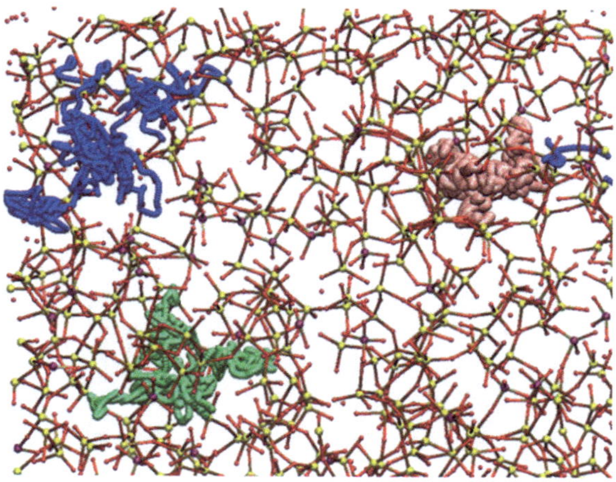

Fig. 2 Diffusion pathways of three atoms: Na, Ca and Sr. Trajectories from MD simulations for 45S5-5Sr glass at 2000 K in the duration of 20 pico-seconds. *Pink ball* Sr; *blue ball* Ca; *green ball* Na; *small yellow ball* Si; *small purple ball* P; *small red ball* O. Figure is reprinted with permission from Ref. [60], copyright 2012 Elsevier

4.2.3 Zinc-Bioactive Glasses

Several MD studies devoted to the optimization of the Zn content on glasses based on the Bioglass 45S5 have been carried out in order to obtain glasses with preserved bioactivity and an optimal zinc oxide releasing rate [40, 49, 61–63]. These represent the first example of a complete cycle in rational glass design reported in the literature obtained by means of the Quantitative Structure–Property Relationships (QSPR) approach [8].

Two series of glasses, prepared by enriching the parent 45S5 bioglass with different percentages of P and/or Zn were analyzed.

$(2\text{-}y)SiO_2 \cdot 1Na_2O \cdot 1.1CaO \cdot yP_2O_5 \cdot xZnO$, (x = 0, 0.13, 0.62, 0.78; y = 0.10, 0.20, 0,36 mol%). The salient feature that emerged is that Zn is always fourfold coordinated and copolymerized with the Si; producing a reinforced network with respect to the parent glass. Moreover, Zn favors the insertion of phosphorous into the network, progressively incorporating it into the network as zinc concentration increases. A highly ramified Si–Zn–P network is thus formed (see Fig. 3) with a uniformly distribution of Na ions and segregation zones for the Ca ions in close proximity to Si and P.

These emerging picture explains the slow rate of Zn dissolution into the contacting media and the decrease in the overall reaction rate of the Zn containing glasses. In fact, the rapid exchange of Na^+ with H_3O^+ ions present in the solution (first step of glass degradation), is hindered by the progressive reduction of suitable percolation channels for Na ions diffusion as a function of Zn addition. In addition, the Na ions mobility is also reduced by the strong electrostatic attraction of the

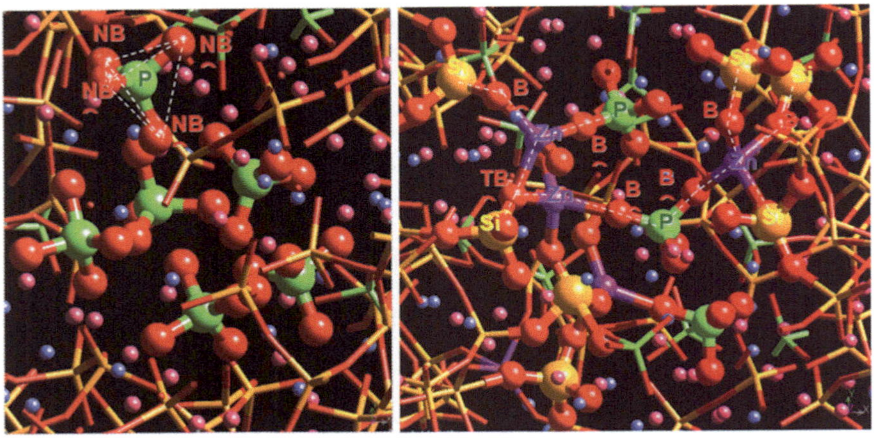

Fig. 3 Snapshot of the simulated 45S5 (*left*) and HP5Z5 (*right*) glasses showing the zone rich in isolated P tetrahedra characteristic of the 45S5 bioglass and the –Si–Zn–P–Zn– stings formed in HP5Z5. Si is represented in *yellow*, Zn in *violet*, P in *green*, O in *red*, Na in *pink*, and Ca in *blue*. Figure is reprinted with permission from Ref. [49], copyright 2005 American Chemical Society

$(ZnO_4)^{2-}$ tetrahedra. Therefore, high concentrations of Zn seem to be responsible for the drastic reduction in the overall leaching activity of the glass and of its inability to form HA. To compensate these effects higher percentages of P_2O_5 with respect to the parent 45S5 bioglass can be added.

HZ5 (x = 0.16, y = 0.0) and HP5Z5 (x = 0.16, y = 0.20) were chosen for further experimental studies on the basis of the results of the QSPR study. Chemical durability tests in water and in vitro observations in a cellular medium [64, 65] confirmed that the HP5Z5, but also the HP5Z10 (x = 0.32, y = 0.20) glasses manifest the pre-requisite for bioactivity, since they are able to form a HA layer on their surface after soaking in SBF solution. Moreover, the HZ5 and HP5Z5 glasses (not HP5Z10) were selected from cell culture tests with MC-3T3 osteoblast cells and related cytotoxicity tests as optimal compositions for cell adhesion and cell growth. Finally, in vivo experiments performed on HZ5 [66] showed glass degradation processes and rates comparable to 45S5.

Alkali-Free Zinc Bioactive Glasses

Insights on the structure of alkali-free bioactive glasses co-doped with strontium, magnesium and zinc have been gained by combining molecular dynamics simulations with solid-state nuclear magnetic resonance spectroscopy [67–69].

The results showed that the silicate network connectivity of Zn^{2+}/Mg^{2+} and Ca^{2+}/Sr^{2+} substituted glasses remains typical of highly bioactive compositions. This phenomenon is due to a similarity in coordination propensity of Zn/Mg and Ca/Sr: both Zn and Mg show a preference to be coordinated to ~5 NBOs form SiO_4

tetrahedra, whereas Ca and Sr are always coordinated to ~6 NBOs form SiO_4 tetrahedra. Although an increase in the Zn^{2+}/Mg^{2+} and Ca^{2+}/Sr^{2+} ratios does not affect the network connectivity, the chemical degradation of the resulting glasses decreases, but no negative effect on the apatite-forming ability is observed.

The authors justified the lack of a straightforward correlation between the network connectivity and the dissolution behaviour by invoking a strategic role of the specific chemistry of ionic species in the glass, including valence and ionic radii.

4.2.4 Fluoride-Bioactive Glasses

Fluoride doped 45S5 bioactive glasses are used as dental biomaterials with enhanced biocompatibility, acidic resistance of enamel, and inhibition of alveolar cavities. Moreover, in these glasses flourapatite (FAp) production is preferred over the HCA, since FAp is chemically more stable and less dissolvable at low pH condition [70].

The release of ionic species (fluoride in particular) in the physiological environment is critical for the suitability of these glasses for biomedical applications, therefore a very accurate picture of the structural organization around fluorine is needed. The results obtained by several studies focused on the effect of fluorine addition to bioactive and other silicate glasses, are often contradictory. In particular, two questions have been deeply debated: what is the affinity of fluorine to silicon, and in the presence of more than one modifier species, how does fluorine prefer to bond to them?

Computational simulations carried out both by ab initio and classical MD [31–33] and mixed computational simulations and NMR measurements [48] agree in depicting the same scenario of F almost exclusively coordinated to modifier cations (Ca and Na) with no clear preference for either ion, and with coordination number close to 4. Figure 4 reports the most common coordination environments found in Car-Parrinello MD simulation [48]. No appreciable amount of Si–F bonds is detected, with only very few (<2 %) of such bonds observed in the glasses with the highest fluorine content. The most important characteristic of these systems is the marked affinity of fluoride to sodium and calcium which leads to the absence of Si–F bonds.

The segregation of ions into two separate regions (alkali-fluoride-rich and phospho-silicate-rich) leads to a network more polymerized with respect to the F-free bioglass, with important consequences on the dissolution of F anions from the glass (Fig. 5).

Since ion clustering in low-silica regions is associated with higher durability and lower bioactivity of glasses [71] this phenomenon can prevent or reduce the formation of the silica gel layer in fluorinated bioglass with significant differences in surface reactivity with respect to F-free 45S5 bioactive silicate glass [31, 72].

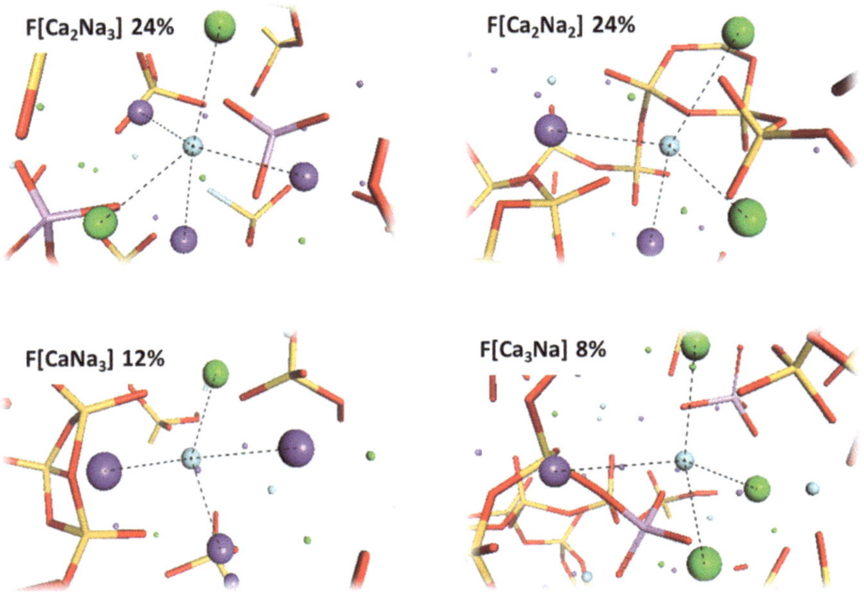

Fig. 4 The most common fluorine environments found in fluorinated 45S5 bioglass. F, Na and Ca atoms are represented as *cyan*, *violet* and *green spheres*, respectively. Si and O atoms are represented as *yellow* and *red sticks*, respectively. Figure is adapted with permission from Ref. [48], copyright 2012 Royal Society of Chemistry

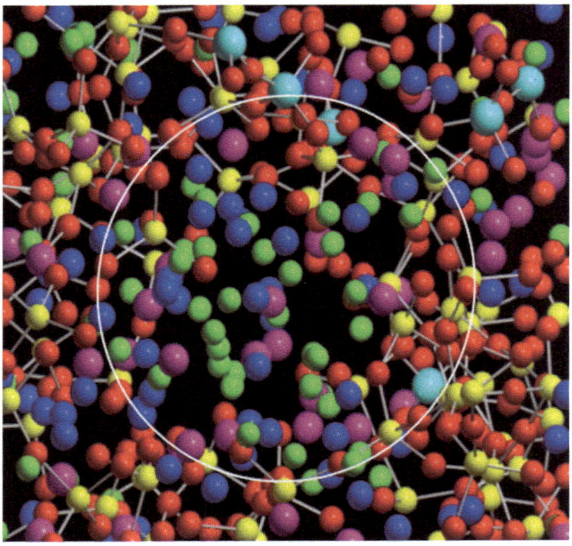

Fig. 5 Snapshot of glass structure $HCaCaF_2$ 15 %. In the *white circle*, is seen the microsegregation zone of Ca, Na and fluorine ions. *Green*, *blue*, *violet*, *cyan*, *yellow* and *red spheres* represent F, Na, Ca, P, Si and O ions, respectively. Figure is reprinted with permission from Ref. [33], copyright 2008 American Chemical Society

4.2.5 Gallium/Alluminum Co-Doped Bioactive Glasses

Gallium is used for the cure of hypercalcemia associated with bone tumour metastasis. Moreover, Ga^{3+} can be introduced in biodegradable materials to prevent bacterial colonization after surgery, avoiding the systematic administration of antibiotics [1].

The structural features of bioactive glasses co-doped with Gallium and Aluminum have been investigate by MD and compared with those of the original 45S5 Bioglass [38]. The three-dimensional model obtained for these glasses supports the interpretation of the experimental data and provides new insights into the different biological behaviours of Ga- and Al-containing phosphosilicate glasses. The fourfold coordination is predominant for Ga whatever interatomic potential model is employed, but small amounts of fivefold and sixfold coordinated atoms have also been detected.

Therefore, the intermediate role of Ga in phosphosilicate glasses is supported, the network of Ga-containing glasses is less polymerized and more degradable than the corresponding ones doped with Al which, on the contrary, plays a network former role.

Small quantities of Ga or Al ions do not change drastically the medium range order characteristic of the 45S5 Bioglass. However, the clustering of Ca ions around phosphorus is more pronounced in Ga-doped to the Al-doped glasses. The formation of insoluble calcium phosphate domains (see Fig. 6) leads to more durable glasses and together with the enhanced clustering of Ca ions observed for Ga and Al-doped bioactive glasses seems to emerge as a marker of non-bioactive behaviour.

In other words, the formation of inhomogeneous regions due to self-aggregation of the Al ions (phenomenon not observed for Ga ions) seems to inhibit the bioactivity; the authors furnished as a possible explanation a reduced mobility of phosphate groups associated with calcium ions in these segregation domains; as a consequence, the kinetics of dissolution is slower than that of the bioactive compositions in which isolated phosphates are embedded in a uniform environment.

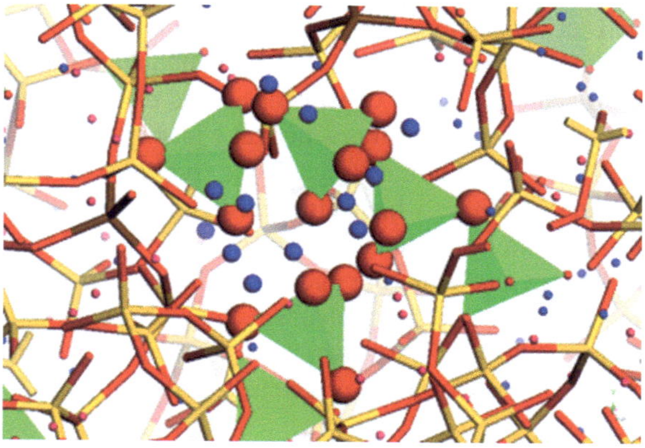

Fig. 6 Example of calcium phosphate domain found in the Al-containing 45S5 bioglass. Phosphorous and oxygen atoms are represented in *green tetrahedral* and *red balls*, while calcium ions in *blue spheres*. Figure is reprinted with permission from Ref. [38], copyright 2013 American Chemical Society

4.2.6 Cerium-Bioactive Glasses

Recently, it has been reported that Ce-containing bioactive glasses are able to inhibit oxidative stress in terms of reduction of hydrogen peroxide by mimicking the catalase enzyme activity [73], and the relationship between structure and antioxidant and bioactivity properties has been investigated by means of MD simulations [73–75]. In fact, it is known that increasing of CeO_2 content in the glass compositions enhances antioxidant ability at the expenses of bioactivity, since CeO_2 delays the formation of the hydroxyapatite layer [76].

The results of computational simulations suggest that this behavior can be related to the medium-range order of the glass matrix. The preference of Ce ions to allocate close to phosphate domains could trigger several phenomena responsible of the retard in the release of phosphate ions from the glass network: (a) entrap the phosphate ions in the glass network reducing the ion release, (b) involve the phosphate ions in the formation of a stable, insoluble $CePO_4$ crystalline phase observed by XRD analysis after thermal treatment of the glass samples, [76] and (c) push the Ca ions in the silicate domains thus preventing the formation of calcium phosphate domains that can act as crystallization nuclei able to speed up the crystallization of $Ca_3(PO_4)_2$ on the glass surface.

Therefore, a good compromise between a high bioactivity level and an efficient catalase mimetic activity requires a proper adjustment of cerium oxide content in the glasses which results in 3.6 and 5.3 mol% of CeO_2 added to 45S5 bioglass.

5 Bioglass Nanoparticles and Surface Reactivity

5.1 Glass Surface

The open silicate network of bioactive glasses allows water molecules to penetrate the glass network much more easily than in more polymerized glasses.

Ab initio or reactive force-field based studies are needed to describe the degradation behavior of a bioactive glass because of the formation of new bonds, defects and surface reconstruction that follows exposure of a glass surface. The size and time limits of these techniques due to computational costs prompted the researchers to verify carefully if the conclusions based on the bulk structure can be used to explain the phenomena that in practice take place predominantly on the surface.

The main findings regard the presence at the surface of relatively stable 2-member rings, which are absent in the bulk of bioactive glasses, whose ring distribution is dominated by 4- and 5-membered sites [71, 77]. Small rings form by linking two neighboring undercoordinated Si atoms with Si–O dangling bonds, and represents one of the mechanisms by which unstable units are healed. Indeed, small rings on the 45S5 surface have been suggested as stable surface sites which are able to guide the nucleation of calcium phosphate on the surface [78, 79].

The high stability of these rings on the surface of the 45S5 Bioglass was confirmed by AIMD simulations [80–82]. These simulations showed that some of these strained surface sites resist hydrolysis long enough to nucleate calcium phosphate precursors, which will then protect them from further reactions [71]. The simulations also suggested that the higher stability of small rings on the bioactive than the pure silica surface is also due to the presence of more favorable absorption sites for water like modifier cations (Na and Ca) and non-bridging oxygens [9].

5.2 *Bioglass Nanparticles*

Nanosized bioactive glass particles represent an attractive alternative to glass micro-sized particles for hard tissue regeneration. Their small size and large surface area lead to higher bioactivity, rapid remineralization, enhanced interaction with fibrinogen and cell proliferation, improved mechanical properties and dentin remineralisation rate.

Classical MD simulations have shown to be useful to investigate the causes of the enhanced activity of nanosized samples of bioglasses [75, 83]. The number of atoms contained, for instance, in an isolated 45S5 bioglass nanoparticle of 5–15 nm is of the order of 10^4–10^5, a manageable size for classical MD simulations.

A comparison of the surface structure of a dry 45S5 nanoparticle to that of a bulk sample exposing a flat surface has been reported recently [83].

The results show a key feature of bioactive glasses most beneficial for their bioactive behaviour such as high fragmentation of the silicate network is further enhanced on the surface of a 45S5 nanoparticle, compared to the bulk glass and to the virtually flat surface of a corresponding larger glass substrate. Moreover, the mobility of modifier cations and the density of small silicate rings—key features to support rapid dissolution and bone bonding processes at the surface—are also enhanced at the nanoparticle surface compared to samples of larger size.

Recently, classical MD simulations have been also used to investigate the different antioxidant properties of Ce-containing bioactive glass nanoparticles with composition based on the Kokubo's and 45S5 glasses [75]. This investigation revealed that the different catalase mimetic activity of the two glass nanoparticles is related to the different Ce^{3+}/Ce^{4+} ratio exposed at the glass surface. In particular, nanoparticles with a similar amount of cerium cations at the surface possess better antioxidant properties.

6 P_2O_2-Based Bioglass Systems

Ternary phosphate glasses in the $CaO–Na_2O–P_2O_5$ system represent another class of biodegradable glasses with a specific bioactivity controllable by varying the composition [84]. In fact, their degradation rates in aqueous solutions can vary from hours to several weeks. Furthermore, specific biological functions and enhanced biocompatibility can be induced by including specific dopants during the synthesis [85–87].

As a result, phosphate glasses find a lot of applications in biomedicine [84], such as in neural repair, tissue engineering [88] and bone fracture fixation [89] or as delivery systems for drugs, nutrients or antimicrobial agents [90].

Compared to phospho-silicate bioactive glasses, there have been only few molecular dynamics simulations of phosphate based glasses in the CaO–Na_2O–P_2O_5 system. One of the first investigation was reported by Tang et al. [91] who employed AIMD simulations to generate structural models of phosphate bioactive glasses with compositions $(CaO)_x(Na_2O)_{0.55-x}$ $(P_2O_5)_{0.45}$ where x = 0.30, 0.35, and 0.40.

The structure of these glasses was dominated by Q^2 and Q^1 species, whereas the number of Q^3 units, constituting the 3D phosphate network, significantly decreased with the calcium oxide content. The calculations revealed that the phosphate tetrahedral becomes more rigid with the concentration of calcium, which tend to be a stronger coordinator than sodium. Both modifiers were found to assume a pseudo-octahedral environment with a coordination number of 6.6 and 6.9, respectively, independently on the composition.

These structural models were then used to validate a new shell model classical force-field by Ainsworth et al. [92] that was later exploited to study the factors affecting the increased durability observed when CaO substitutes Na_2O in larger models by the same authors [93]. They observed that Q^n distribution and network connectivity of the investigated glasses did not change with the composition. The enhanced durability of these glasses when Ca substitutes Na were interpreted by the tendency of calcium atoms to cross-link more phosphate chain and orthophosphate fragments with respect to sodium atoms. Figure 7 shows the binding of a sodium ion with three phosphate chains observed in their simulations.

Further, they showed that this increased cross-linking is a consequence of calcium's higher field strength than sodium that make it more prone to bind NBOs atoms than Na (6.2 vs 5.4). Because of these differences among the two modifier ions when the Ca content increases at the expense of the Na one the structure get more compact and the strengthening of the glass leads to the lower dissolution rates observed experimentally.

6.1 *Fluoride-Bioactive Glasses*

After having disclosed at the molecular level the relationships between the calcium and sodium content and the solubility of such glasses the same authors focused their attention on the investigation of the structural changes caused by the addition of fluorine [94] and silver ions [95, 96]. Fluorinated phosphate glasses are interesting systems because they combine the bioactivity of phosphate glasses with the anti-cariogenic properties of fluoride.

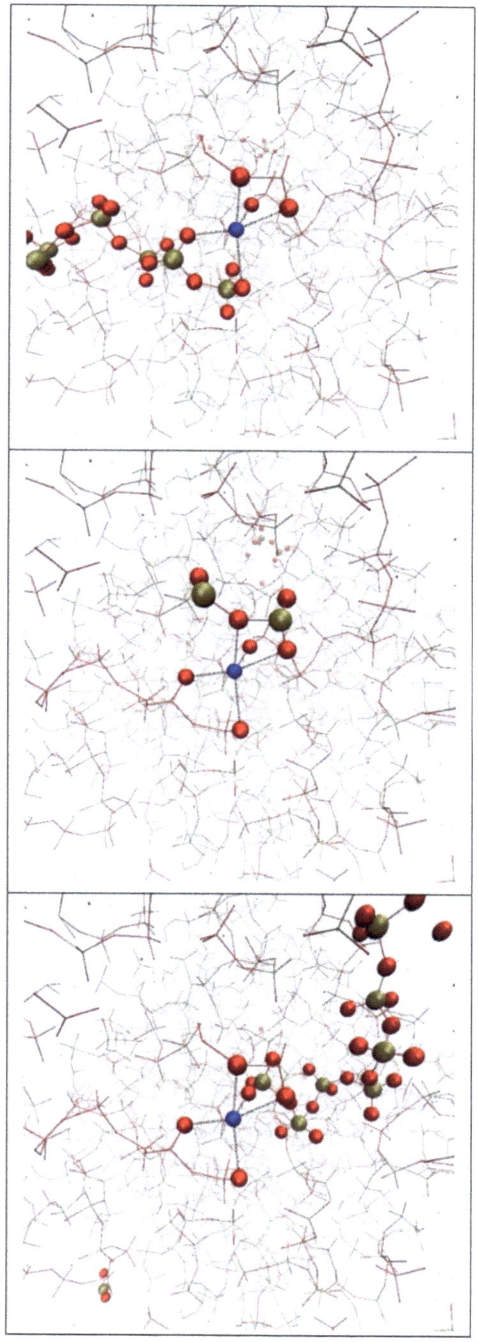

Fig. 7 The picture shows a Na atom (*blue sphere*) bound to three phosphate fragments. *Each picture* shows a different phosphate chain bounded to the Na central ion. Figure is reprinted with permission from Ref. [93], copyright 2013 American Chemical Society

The incorporation of fluorine in phospho-silicate glasses has deleterious effects on the bioactivity because the silica rich layer formed at the glass surface that trigger the precipitation of calcium phosphate is less homogeneous on F-containing phosphosilicate glasses than on F-free phosphosilicate glasses, and in certain conditions is very thin or even absent [72]. This inhomogeneity was associated to the negligible amount of Si–F bonds in such glasses and to the separation of phosphosilicate-rich and Na/Ca/F-rich regions on medium range scales [31, 33]. Christie et al. [94] showed that in phosphate glasses there is a substantial amount of P–F bonds with respect to the amount of Si–F bonds in phosphosilicate glasses. Moreover, since the F–P coordination numbers is similar to the F–Na and F–Ca coordination numbers the mesoscale segregation observed in fluorinated phosphosilicate bioactive glasses is much less important in phosphate glasses. Since clustering of modifier atoms is associated with more durable and less bioactive glasses [37], fluorinated phosphate glasses should be more bioactive than the phosphosilicate counterparts. Christie et al. showed that when fluorine bonds to phosphorous the tetrahedral structure of the latter is preserved since F replaces one of the oxygen atoms in a P–O bond. Moreover, since bridging oxygens are replaced by non-bridging F ions with fluoride addition a slight decrease in the network connectivity with F content was also observed.

Finally, based on their AIMD simulations, they concluded that fluorinated phosphate glasses are a better alternative to Fluorinated phosphosilicate glasses since the incorporation of fluorine does not cause structural changes that would affect their bioactivity.

6.2 *Silver-Bioactive Glasses*

Another ion incorporated in phosphate-based bioactive glasses is silver that is known to have biocidal effects and thus can be incorporated to prevent or cure infections that can occur at the prosthesis interface once implanted in the body [97]. Ag-doped phosphate glasses has a wide range of bactericidal activity against a lot of bacteria [98] thanks to the involvement of the Ag^+ ions on the respiratory chain processes of bacteria and since it reduces the integrity of bacterial membranes [99].

Experimentally, it was observed that the enhancement of Ag concentration in glasses of composition $(P_2O_5)_{0.5}(CaO)_{0.30}(Na_2O)_{0.20-x}(Ag)_x$ (x = 0.00–0.05) reduces the glass dissolution, silver ion release and the bactericidal activity [100]. Therefore, this activity leans on a continuous provision of silver in solution, which in turn depends on the bulk and surface structure as well as ionic diffusion and kinetic of dissolution.

A first attempt to understanding the dissolution phenomena in silver-doped phosphate glasses, from first-principles and classical MD simulations, was done by

Ainsworth et al. [95] They investigated the short- and medium-range structure of phosphate glasses with varying amount of Na and Ca ions and from 0 to 20 mol% of Ag_2O, and tried to correlate the structural changes caused by the incorporation of silver into the glass.

They found that Ag ions have negligible effect on short range order of phosphorous. In these glasses Ag plays a network modifier role and was found to assume a distorted octahedral and trigonal bipyramidal geometry with about 5.5 oxygens and bond lengths of 2.5 Å. A disproportionation reaction ($2Q^2 - Q^1 + Q^3$) was observed when silver ions replaced CaO, but not on silver-doping via Na_2O substitution. Since the network connectivity and the number of phosphate chains bounded to silver and sodium was roughly the same [96], they associated the increased durability of glasses in which silver replaces sodium to the differences between the local bonding of the two ions.

7 Final Remarks

In the last decade, both classical and ab initio MD simulations have been successfully employed to shed light on the structure and properties of silicate, phosphosilicate and phosphate glasses. In this brief overview, we have showed how such techniques have been applied to investigate the structure-bioactivity relationships and to rationalize the effect of the inclusion of several doping ions on the structure and properties of bioactive glasses.

Albeit a lot of progresses have been achieved in the last years to better understand key steps related to the dissolution processes and to design new active compositions with specific properties some improvements in the computational procedures have to be reached. Some challenges remain especially for the production of reliable surface structures of bioactive glasses with different compositions and these must be coupled with a proper investigation of the surface-water interactions as a function of simulation time. The investigation of the affinity between bioactive nanoparticles and blood plasma proteins will be of primary importance to have information on the fate of glass nanoparticles with specific medical properties once injected in the blood stream. However, because of the prohibitive space and time scales that must be spanned the possibility of using coarse grain MD simulations must be exploited. Moreover, since in the dentistry field glass ceramics are mixed with polymeric materials to produce hybrid matrices known as glass ionomer cements future promising directions will be to simulate such systems and their mechanical properties.

Despite these challenges, MD simulations is (and will be) certainly a powerful tool for scientists engaged in the research of new bioactive glass compositions.

References

1. Jones, J.R.: Review of bioactive glass: from Hench to hybrids. Acta Biomater. **9**, 4457–4486 (2013)
2. Brauer, D.S.: Bioactive glasses—structure and properties. Angew. Chem. Int. Ed. **54**, 4160–4181 (2015)
3. Hench, L.L.: Bioceramics. J. Am. Ceram. Soc. **81**, 1705–1728 (1998)
4. Martin, R.A., Yue, S., Hanna, J.V., Lee, P.D., Newport, R.J., Smith, M.E., et al.: Characterizing the hierarchical structures of bioactive sol–gel silicate glass and hybrid scaffolds for bone regeneration. Philos. Transact. A Math. Phys. Eng. Sci. **370**, 1422–1443 (2012)
5. Pedone, A.: Properties calculations of silica-based glasses by atomistic simulations techniques: a review. J. Phys. Chem. C **113**, 20773–20784 (2009)
6. Malavasi, G., Menziani, M.C., Pedone, A., Civalleri, B., Corno, M., Ugliengo, P.: A computational multiscale strategy to the study of amorphous materials. Theor. Chem. Acc. **117**, 933–942 (2007)
7. Malavasi, G., Pedone, A., Menziani, M.C.: Towards a quantitative rationalization of multicomponent glass properties by means of molecular dynamics simulations. Mol. Simul. **32**, 1045–1055 (2006)
8. Pedone, A., Menziani, M.C.: Computational modeling of silicate glasses: a quantitative structure–property relationship perspective. In: Massobrio, C., Du, J., Bernasconi, M., Salmon, P.S. (eds.) Molecular Dynamic Simulation of Disordered Materials [Internet], pp. 113–35. Springer, New York (2015) [cited 2015 Aug 24]. http://link.springer.com/chapter/10.1007/978-3-319-15675-0_5
9. Tilocca, A.: Rationalizing the biodegradation of glasses for biomedical applications through classical and ab-initio simulations. In: Massobrio, C., Du, J., Bernasconi, M., Salmon, P.S. (eds.) Molecular Dynamic Simulation of Disordered Materials [Internet]. Springer, New York, pp. 255–273 (2015) [cited 2015 Aug 24]. http://link.springer.com/chapter/10.1007/978-3-319-15675-0_10
10. Tilocca, A.: Current challenges in atomistic simulations of glasses for biomedical applications. Phys. Chem. Chem. Phys. **16**, 3874–3880 (2014)
11. Du, J.: Challenges in molecular dynamics simulations of multicomponent oxide glasses. In: Massobrio, C., Du, J., Bernasconi, M., Salmon, P.S. (eds.) Molecular Dynamic Simulation of Disordered Materials [Internet]. Springer, New York, pp. 157–180 (2015) [cited 2015 Aug 24]. http://link.springer.com/chapter/10.1007/978-3-319-15675-0_7
12. Tilocca, A.: Structural models of bioactive glasses from molecular dynamics simulations. In: Proceeding of the Royal Society of London A Mathematical, Physical and Engineering Sciences (2009). rspa.2008.0462
13. Cormack, A.N., Tilocca, A.: Structure and biological activity of glasses and ceramics. Philos. Transact. A Math. Phys. Eng. Sci. **370**, 1271–1280 (2012)
14. Allen, M.P., Tildesley, D.J.: Computer Simulation of Liquids. Clarendon Press, Oxford (1987)
15. Pedone, A., Corno, M., Civalleri, B., Malavasi, G., Menziani, M.C., Segre, U., et al.: An ab initio parameterized interatomic force field for hydroxyapatite. J. Mater. Chem. **17**, 2061–2068 (2007)
16. Pedone, A., Malavasi, G., Menziani, M.C., Cormack, A.N., Segre, U.: A new self-consistent empirical interatomic potential model for oxides, silicates, and silica-based glasses. J. Phys. Chem. B **110**, 11780–11795 (2006)
17. Tilocca, A., de Leeuw, N.H., Cormack, A.N.: Shell-model molecular dynamics calculations of modified silicate glasses. Phys. Rev. B. **73**, 104209 (2006)
18. Tilocca, A.: Short- and medium-range structure of multicomponent bioactive glasses and melts: an assessment of the performances of shell-model and rigid-ion potentials. J. Chem. Phys. **129**, 084504 (2008)

19. Yu, H., van Gunsteren, W.F.: Accounting for polarization in molecular simulation. Comput. Phys. Commun. **172**, 69–85 (2005)
20. Ispas, S., Benoit, M., Jund, P., Jullien, R.: Structural and electronic properties of the sodium tetrasilicate glass $Na_2Si_4O_9$ from classical and ab initio molecular dynamics simulations. Phys. Rev. B **64**, 214206 (2001)
21. Tilocca, A., de Leeuw, N.H.: Structural and electronic properties of modified sodium and soda-lime silicate glasses by Car-Parrinello molecular dynamics. J. Mater. Chem. **16**, 1950–1955 (2006)
22. Tilocca, A., de Leeuw, N.H.: Ab initio molecular dynamics study of 45S5 bioactive silicate glass. J. Phys. Chem. B **110**, 25810–25816 (2006)
23. Corno, M., Pedone, A., Dovesi, R., Ugliengo, P.: B3LYP simulation of the full vibrational spectrum of 45S5 bioactive silicate glass compared to nu-silica. Chem. Mater. **20**, 5610–5621 (2008)
24. Corno, M., Pedone, A.: Vibrational features of phospho-silicate glasses: Periodic B3LYP simulations. Chem. Phys. Lett. **476**, 218–222 (2009)
25. Pedone, A., Charpentier, T., Malavasi, G., Menziani, M.C.: New insights into the atomic structure of 45S5 bioglass by means of solid-state NMR spectroscopy and accurate first-principles simulations. Chem. Mater. **22**, 5644–5652 (2010)
26. Charpentier, T., Menziani, M.C., Pedone, A.: Computational simulations of solid state NMR spectra: a new era in structure determination of oxide glasses. Rsc Adv. **3**, 10550–10578 (2013)
27. Tilocca, A., Cormack, A.N., de Leeuw, N.H.: The structure of bioactive silicate glasses: new insight from molecular dynamics simulations. Chem. Mater. **19**, 95–103 (2007)
28. Tilocca, A., Cormack, A.N., de Leeuw, N.H.: The formation of nanoscale structures in soluble phosphosilicate glasses for biomedical applications: MD simulations. Faraday Discuss. **136**, 45–55 (2007)
29. Hill, R.G., Brauer, D.S.: Predicting the bioactivity of glasses using the network connectivity or split network models. J. Non Cryst. Solids **357**, 3884–3887 (2011)
30. Malavasi, G., Menabue, L., Menziani, M.C., Pedone, A., Salinas, A.J., Vallet-Regi, M.: New insights into the bioactivity of SiO_2–CaO and SiO_2–CaO–P_2O_5 sol–gel glasses by molecular dynamics simulations. J. Sol–Gel. Sci. Technol. **67**, 208–219 (2013)
31. Lusvardi, G., Malavasi, G., Tarsitano, F., Menabue, L., Menziani, M.C., Pedone, A.: Quantitative structure–property relationships of potentially bioactive fluoro phospho-silicate glasses. J. Phys. Chem. B **113**, 10331–10338 (2009)
32. Christie, J.K., Pedone, A., Menziani, M.C., Tilocca, A.: Fluorine environment in bioactive glasses: ab initio molecular dynamics simulations. J. Phys. Chem. B **115**, 2038–2045 (2011)
33. Lusvardi, G., Malavasi, G., Cortada, M., Menabue, L., Menziani, M.C., Pedone, A., et al.: Elucidation of the structural role of fluorine in potentially bioactive glasses by experimental and computational investigation. J. Phys. Chem. B **112**, 12730–12739 (2008)
34. Christie, J.K., Tilocca, A.: Integrating biological activity into radioisotope vectors: molecular dynamics models of yttrium-doped bioactive glasses. J. Mater. Chem. **22**, 12023–12031 (2012)
35. Pedone, A., Malavasi, G., Menziani, M.C.: Computational insight into the effect of CaO/MgO substitution on the structural properties of phospho-silicate bioactive glasses. J. Phys. Chem. C **113**, 15723–15730 (2009)
36. Christie, J.K., Tilocca, A.: Molecular dynamics simulations and structural descriptors of radioisotope glass vectors for in situ radiotherapy. J. Phys. Chem. B **116**, 12614–12620 (2012)
37. Christie, J.K., Tilocca, A.: Aluminosilicate glasses as yttrium vectors for in situ radiotherapy: understanding composition-durability effects through molecular dynamics simulations. Chem. Mater. **22**, 3725–3734 (2010)
38. Malavasi, G., Pedone, A., Menziani, M.C.: Study of the structural role of gallium and aluminum in 45S5 bioactive glasses by molecular dynamics simulations. J. Phys. Chem. B **117**, 4142–4150 (2013)

39. Lusvardi, G., Malavasi, G., Menabue, L., Menziani, M.C., Pedone, A., Segre, U.: A computational tool for the prediction of crystalline phases obtained from controlled crystallization of glasses. J. Phys. Chem. B **109**, 21586–21592 (2005)
40. Malavasi, G., Lusvardi, G., Pedone, A., Menziani, M.C., Dappiaggi, M., Gualtieri, A., et al.: Crystallization kinetics of bioactive glasses in the ZnO–Na_2O–CaO–SiO_2 system. J. Phys. Chem. A **111**, 8401–8408 (2007)
41. Hench, L.L., Splinter, R.J., Allen, W.C., Greenlee, T.K.: Bonding mechanisms at the interface of ceramic prosthetic materials. J. Biomed. Mater. Res. **5**, 117–141 (1971)
42. Kokubo, T.: Surface chemistry of bioactive glass-ceramics. J. Non Cryst. Solids **120**, 138–151 (1990)
43. Xynos, I.D., Edgar, A.J., Buttery, L.D., Hench, L.L., Polak, J.M.: Gene-expression profiling of human osteoblasts following treatment with the ionic products of Bioglass 45S5 dissolution. J. Biomed. Mater. Res. **55**, 151–157 (2001)
44. Karlsson, K.H., Fröberg, K., Ringbom, T.: A structural approach to bone adhering of bioactive glasses. J. Non Cryst. Solids **112**, 69–72 (1989)
45. Hill, R.: An alternative view of the degradation of bioglass. J. Mater. Sci. Lett. **15**, 1122–1125 (1996)
46. Lockyer, M.W.G., Holland, D., Dupree, R.: NMR investigation of the structure of some bioactive and related glasses. J. Non Cryst. Solids **188**, 207–219 (1995)
47. Elgayar, I., Aliev, A.E., Boccaccini, A.R., Hill, R.G.: Structural analysis of bioactive glasses. J. Non Cryst. Solids **351**, 173–183 (2005)
48. Pedone, A., Charpentier, T., Menziani, M.C.: The structure of fluoride-containing bioactive glasses: new insights from first-principles calculations and solid state NMR spectroscopy. J. Mater. Chem. **22**, 12599–12608 (2012)
49. Linati, L., Lusvardi, G., Malavasi, G., Menabue, L., Menziani, M.C., Mustarelli, P., et al.: Qualitative and quantitative structure–property relationships analysis of multicomponent potential bioglasses. J. Phys. Chem. B **109**, 4989–4998 (2005)
50. Fayon, F., Duée, C., Poumeyrol, T., Allix, M., Massiot, D.: Evidence of Nanometric-sized phosphate clusters in bioactive glasses as revealed by solid-state 31P NMR. J. Phys. Chem. C **117**, 2283–2288 (2013)
51. Xiang, Y., Du, J.: Effect of strontium substitution on the structure of 45S5 bioglasses. Chem. Mater. **23**, 2703–2717 (2011)
52. Stevensson, B., Mathew, R., Edén, M.: Assessing the phosphate distribution in bioactive phosphosilicate glasses by 31P solid-state NMR and molecular dynamics simulations. J. Phys. Chem. B **118**, 8863–8876 (2014)
53. Tilocca, A., Cormack, A.N.: Structural effects of phosphorus inclusion in bioactive silicate glasses. J. Phys. Chem. B **111**, 14256–14264 (2007)
54. Linati, L., Lusvardi, G., Malavasi, G., Menabue, L., Menziani, M.C., Mustarelli, P., et al.: Medium-range order in phospho-silicate bioactive glasses: insights from MAS–NMR spectra, chemical durability experiments and molecular dynamics simulations. J. Non Cryst. Solids **354**, 84–89 (2008)
55. Mathew, R., Stevensson, B., Edén, M.: Na/ca intermixing around silicate and phosphate groups in bioactive phosphosilicate glasses revealed by heteronuclear solid-state NMR and molecular dynamics simulations. J. Phys. Chem. B **119**, 5701–5715 (2015)
56. Mathew, R., Stevensson, B., Tilocca, A., Edén, M.: Toward a rational design of bioactive glasses with optimal structural features: composition-structure correlations unveiled by solid-state NMR and MD simulations. J. Phys. Chem. B **118**, 833–844 (2014)
57. Hoppe, A., Güldal, N.S., Boccaccini, A.R.: A review of the biological response to ionic dissolution products from bioactive glasses and glass-ceramics. Biomaterials **32**, 2757–2774 (2011)
58. Pedone, A., Malavasi, G., Menziani, M.C., Segre, U., Cormack, A.N.: Role of magnesium in soda-lime glasses: insight into structural, transport, and mechanical properties through computer simulations. J. Phys. Chem. C **112**, 11034–11041 (2008)

59. Kapoor, S., Semitela, Â., Goel, A., Xiang, Y., Du, J., Lourenço, A.H., et al.: Understanding the composition-structure-bioactivity relationships in diopside ($CaO \cdot MgO \cdot 2SiO_2$)-tricalcium phosphate ($3CaO \cdot P_2O_5$) glass system. Acta Biomater. **15**, 210–226 (2015)
60. Du, J., Xiang, Y.: Effect of strontium substitution on the structure, ionic diffusion and dynamic properties of 45S5 Bioactive glasses. J. Non Cryst. Solids **358**, 1059–1071 (2012)
61. Lusvardi, G., Malavasi, G., Menabue, L., Menziani, M.C.: Synthesis, characterization, and molecular dynamics simulation of Na_2O–CaO–SiO_2–ZnO glasses. J. Phys. Chem. B **106**, 9753–9760 (2002)
62. Lusvardi, G., Malavasi, G., Menabue, L., Menziani, M.C.: A combined experimental-computational strategy for the design, synthesis and characterization of bioactive zinc-silicate glasses. Key Eng. Mater. **377**, 211–224 (2008)
63. Lusvardi, G., Malavasi, G., Menabue, L., Menziani, M.C., Pedone, A., Segre, U.: Density of multicomponent silica-based potential bioglasses: quantitative structure–property relationships (QSPR) analysis. J. Eur. Ceram. Soc. **27**, 499–504 (2007)
64. Lusvardi, G., Malavasi, G., Menabue, L., Menziani, M.C., Segre, U., Carnasciali, M.M., et al.: A combined experimental and computational approach to $(Na_2O)1 - x \cdot CaO \cdot (ZnO) x \cdot 2SiO_2$ glasses characterization. J. Non Cryst. Solids **345–346**, 710–714 (2004)
65. Lusvardi, G., Malavasi, G., Menabue, L., Menziani, M.C., Pedone, A., Segre, U., et al.: Properties of zinc releasing surfaces for clinical applications. J. Biomater. Appl. **22**, 505–526 (2008)
66. Lusvardi, G., Zaffe, D., Menabue, L., Bertoldi, C., Malavasi, G., Consolo, U.: In vitro and in vivo behaviour of zinc-doped phosphosilicate glasses. Acta Biomater. **5**, 419–428 (2009)
67. Goel, A., Kapoor, S., Tilocca, A., Rajagopal, R.R., Ferreira, J.M.F.: Structural role of zinc in biodegradation of alkali-free bioactive glasses. J. Mater. Chem. B **1**, 3073–3082 (2013)
68. Xiang, Y., Du, J., Skinner, L.B., Benmore, C.J., Wren, A.W., Boyd, D.J., et al.: Structure and diffusion of ZnO–SrO–CaO–Na_2O–SiO_2 bioactive glasses: a combined high energy X-ray diffraction and molecular dynamics simulations study. RSC Adv. **3**, 5966–5978 (2013)
69. Kapoor, S., Goel, A., Tilocca, A., Dhuna, V., Bhatia, G., Dhuna, K., et al.: Role of glass structure in defining the chemical dissolution behavior, bioactivity and antioxidant properties of zinc and strontium co-doped alkali-free phosphosilicate glasses. Acta Biomater. **10**, 3264–3278 (2014)
70. Rabiee, S.M., Nazparvar, N., Azizian, M., Vashaee, D., Tayebi, L.: Effect of ion substitution on properties of bioactive glasses: a review. Ceram. Int. **41**, 7241–7251 (2015)
71. Tilocca, A.: Models of structure, dynamics and reactivity of bioglasses: a review. J. Mater. Chem. **20**, 6848–6858 (2010)
72. Lusvardi, G., Malavasi, G., Menabue, L., Aina, V., Morterra, C.: Fluoride-containing bioactive glasses: surface reactivity in simulated body fluids solutions. Acta Biomater. **5**, 3548–3562 (2009)
73. Nicolini, V., Gambuzzi, E., Malavasi, G., Menabue, L., Menziani, M.C., Lusvardi, G., et al.: Evidence of catalase mimetic activity in Ce^{3+}/Ce^{4+} doped bioactive glasses. J. Phys. Chem. B **119**, 4009–4019 (2015)
74. Nicolini, V., Varini, E., Malavasi, G., Menabue, L., Menziani, M.C., Lusvardi, G., et al.: The effect of composition on structural, thermal, redox and bioactive properties of ce-containing glasses. Mater. Des. **97**, 73–85 (2016)
75. Pedone, A., Muniz-Miranda, F., Tilocca, A., Menziani, M.C.: The antioxidant properties of Ce-containing bioactive glass nanoparticles explained by molecular dynamics simulations. Biomed. Glas. **2**, 19–28 (2016)
76. Leonelli, C., Lusvardi, G., Malavasi, G., Menabue, L., Tonelli, M.: Synthesis and characterization of cerium-doped glasses and in vitro evaluation of bioactivity. J. Non Cryst. Solids **316**, 198–216 (2003)
77. Berardo, E., Pedone, A., Ugliengo, P., Corno, M.: DFT modeling of 45S5 and 77S Soda-lime phospho-silicate glass surfaces: clues on different bioactivity mechanism. Langmuir **29**, 5749–5759 (2013)

78. Sahai, N., Anseau, M.: Cyclic silicate active site and stereochemical match for apatite nucleation on pseudowollastonite bioceramic-bone interfaces. Biomaterials **26**, 5763–5770 (2005)
79. Bolis, V., Busco, C., Aina, V., Morterra, C., Ugliengo, P.: Surface properties of silica-based biomaterials: ca species at the surface of amorphous silica as model sites. J. Phys. Chem. C **112**, 16879–16892 (2008)
80. Tilocca, A., Cormack, A.N.: Exploring the surface of bioactive glasses: water adsorption and reactivity. J. Phys. Chem. C **112**, 11936–11945 (2008)
81. Tilocca, A., Cormack, A.N.: Modeling the water–bioglass interface by ab initio molecular dynamics simulations. ACS Appl. Mater. Interfaces. **1**, 1324–1333 (2009)
82. Pedone, A., Malavasi, G., Menziani, M.C., Segre, U., Musso, F., Corno, M., et al.: FFSiOH: a new force field for silica polymorphs and their hydroxylated surfaces based on periodic B3LYP calculations. Chem. Mater. **20**, 2522–2531 (2008)
83. Tilocca, A.: Molecular dynamics simulations of a bioactive glass nanoparticle. J. Mater. Chem. **21**, 12660–12667 (2011)
84. Neel, E.A.A., Pickup, D.M., Valappil, S.P., Newport, R.J., Knowles, J.C.: Bioactive functional materials: a perspective on phosphate-based glasses. J. Mater. Chem. **19**, 690–701 (2009)
85. Knowles, J.C.: Phosphate based glasses for biomedical applications. J. Mater. Chem. **13**, 2395–2401 (2003)
86. Ahmed, I., Collins, C.A., Lewis, M.P., Olsen, I., Knowles, J.C.: Processing, characterisation and biocompatibility of iron-phosphate glass fibres for tissue engineering. Biomaterials **25**, 3223–3232 (2004)
87. Neel, E.A.A., Ahmed, I., Pratten, J., Nazhat, S.N., Knowles, J.C.: Characterisation of antibacterial copper releasing degradable phosphate glass fibres. Biomaterials **26**, 2247–2254 (2005)
88. Ahmed, I., Lewis, M., Olsen, I., Knowles, J.C.: Phosphate glasses for tissue engineering: part 1. Processing and characterisation of a ternary-based P_2O_5–CaO–Na_2O glass system. Biomaterials **25**, 491–499 (2004)
89. Uo, M., Mizuno, M., Kuboki, Y., Makishima, A., Watari, F.: Properties and cytotoxicity of water soluble Na_2O–CaO–P_2O_5 glasses. Biomaterials **19**, 2277–2284 (1998)
90. Valappil, S.P., Ready, D., Abou Neel, E.A., Pickup, D.M., O'Dell, L.A., Chrzanowski, W., et al.: Controlled delivery of antimicrobial gallium ions from phosphate-based glasses. Acta Biomater. **5**, 1198–1210 (2009)
91. Tang, E., Di Tommaso, D., de Leeuw, N.H.: An ab initio molecular dynamics study of bioactive phosphate glasses. Adv. Eng. Mater. **12**, B331–B338 (2010)
92. Ainsworth, R.I., Tommaso, D.D., Christie, J.K., de Leeuw, N.H.: Polarizable force field development and molecular dynamics study of phosphate-based glasses. J. Chem. Phys. **137**, 234502 (2012)
93. Christie, J.K., Ainsworth, R.I., Di Tommaso, D., de Leeuw, N.H.: Nanoscale chains control the solubility of phosphate glasses for biomedical applications. J. Phys. Chem. B **117**, 10652–10657 (2013)
94. Christie, J.K., Ainsworth, R.I., de Leeuw, N.H.: Ab initio molecular dynamics simulations of structural changes associated with the incorporation of fluorine in bioactive phosphate glasses. Biomaterials **35**, 6164–6171 (2014)
95. Ainsworth, R.I., Christie, J.K., de Leeuw, N.H.: On the structure of biomedical silver-doped phosphate-based glasses from molecular dynamics simulations. Phys. Chem. Chem. Phys. **16**, 21135–21143 (2014)
96. Christie, J.K., Ainsworth, R.I., de Leeuw, N.H.: Investigating structural features which control the dissolution of bioactive phosphate glasses: beyond the network connectivity. J. Non-Cryst. Solids [Internet]. [cited 2015 Jul 30]. http://www.sciencedirect.com/science/article/pii/S0022309315000332
97. Sheridan, R., Doherty, P.J., Gilchrist, T., Healy, D.: The effect of antibacterial agents on the behaviour of cultured mammalian fibroblasts. J. Mater. Sci. Mater. Med. **6**, 853–856 (1995)

98. Ahmed, I., Ready, D., Wilson, M., Knowles, J.C.: Antimicrobial effect of silver-doped phosphate-based glasses. J. Biomed. Mater. Res. A **79A**, 618–626 (2006)
99. Randall, C.P., Oyama, L.B., Bostock, J.M., Chopra, I., O'Neill, A.J.: The silver cation (Ag +): antistaphylococcal activity, mode of action and resistance studies. J. Antimicrob. Chemother. **68**, 131–138 (2013)
100. Valappil, S.P., Pickup, D.M., Carroll, D.L., Hope, C.K., Pratten, J., Newport, R.J., et al.: Effect of silver content on the structure and antibacterial activity of silver-doped phosphate-based glasses. Antimicrob. Agents Chemother. **51**, 4453–4461 (2007)

Bioactive Glasses: Advancing from Micro to Nano and Its Potential Application

Mengchao Shi, Jiang Chang and Chengtie Wu

Abstract Bioactive glasses or bioglasses in short (please consult the Editor's note in order to clarify the usage of the terms bioglass, bioactive glass and biocompatible glasses) have attracted much attention in application for bone regeneration since 1970s. With the development of the preparation strategies from conventional quenching to modified sol–gel methods, bioglasses of different structures and varied compositions have been reported as their physicochemical and biological properties being well-studied. Mesoporous bioglasses, which possessed unique mesopore channels for drug delivery, has become a hotspot in the last decade. In this chapter, the fabrication of bioglasses including porous scaffolds, coatings, fibers and particles especially the development of its nanoscale form, and several bioglasses involved composite materials are discussed. Recent studies on therapeutic ion substitution (e.g. Sr, Co) of bioglasses and their biological properties both in vivo and in vitro are mentioned. The potential application of bioglasses in different forms for the hard tissue engineering (e.g. dental implantation, bone regeneration), and some recent reports on soft tissue engineering (e.g. would healing) are also referred to. As one of the most promising candidate for bone/soft tissue regeneration application, both the great chances and challenges, and the potential direction of bioglasses for its development are summarized.

M. Shi · J. Chang (✉) · C. Wu (✉)
State Key Laboratory of High Performance Ceramics and Superfine Microstructure, Shanghai Institute of Ceramics, Chinese Academy of Sciences, Shanghai 200050, People's Republic of China
e-mail: jchang@mail.sic.ac.cn

C. Wu
e-mail: chengtiewu@mail.sic.ac.cn

J. Marchi (ed.), *Biocompatible Glasses*, Advanced Structured Materials 53,
DOI 10.1007/978-3-319-44249-5_6

1 Introduction

1.1 Origin of Conventional Bioactive Glasses (BG)

Invented by Professor Larry Hench at the University of Florida in 1969, bioglasses (later termed 45S5 Bioglass®) were the first man-made biomaterials that can bond closely with the host bone tissue. The "grandfather" composition (46.1 mol% SiO_2, 24.4 mol%, Na_2O, 26.9% mol% CaO and 2.6 mol% P_2O_5) of Bioglass® made it possible to form a strong bond with bone which could not be removed unless breaking the bone [1, 2]. This launched the field of bioactive ceramics, including variation of 45S5 Bioglass, glass-ceramics, hydroxyapatite, calcium phosphates and so on. It has also been the milestone of the third-generation of biomedical materials, or the bioactive material, which was defined as to stimulate a beneficial response from the body, particularly bonding to host tissue [3]. In the past 45 years, bioglasses, taking 45S5 as a golden standard, with its generally excellent bioactivity, osteoconductivity, osteostimulation and potential to enhance angiogenesis, have been widely studied by researchers and applied as bone filling materials and bioactive coatings for dentistry, orthopedics and small bone implants in hard/soft tissue regeneration application [4, 5].

The mechanism behind new bone formation on bioglasses is attributed to a hydroxycarbonate apatite (HCA) layer on the surface, which is associated with the release of Na and Ca ions [6, 7]. The HCA is similar to bone mineral and could interact with collagen fibrils to integrate with the host bone. Further studies have revealed that the dissolution products, including Ca and Si ions from 45S5 could stimulate osteoblast proliferation and differentiation [8].

Apart from the silicate based bioglasses borate based bioglasses were developed in 1990 by replacing partial silica with boron to gain more desirable bioactivity [9]. The glasses possess lower chemical durability and could convert more rapidly and thoroughly to apatite. The sintering behavior is more controlled than 45S5 Bioglass®. As a trace element required for bone health, the biosafety of boron is concentration dependent and the excessive amount could be toxicity [10, 11]. Potential application of borate glasses and the composites have recently been reported in some literatures [12, 13]. Another bioglass is phosphate based glasses that proposed in 1980 [14]. With P_2O_5 being the network former oxide, the asymmetric structure of P–O–P bonds hydrated easily and lead to the good biodegradability. It has been studied as controlled release vehicles of antibacterial ions including zinc, gallium, silver and copper in recent years [4]. In this chapter, we mainly focused on the most widely investigated silicate based bioglasses, from the conventional 45S5 Bioglass® prepared by melting quenching approach to the developed ones synthesized by the chemistry-based sol–gel methods.

45S5 Bioglass® was first synthesized by mixing all the powder containing silicon, calcium, sodium salts/oxides and phosphate and melting them at high temperature (1300–1500 °C). It is essential for the temperature to be at the sintering window (the temperature difference between T_g and $T_{c,\ onset}$) [9, 15, 16]. Being effected by the particle sizes, structure of silica network and the whole composition, the sintering window is too small to avoid crystallization, which could have negative impact on the bioactivity of bioglasses. Bioglasses cannot induce the HCA layer formation if the content of SiO_2 exceeds 60 % since the network is too stable to release Na or Ca, leading to insufficient OH groups on the glass surface. Besides, another disadvantage is the lack of microporous structure and low specific surface area of melt glasses, let alone the high energy consuming during the sintering process [17, 18]. Later after that, a new approach named sol–gel method was applied in bioglasses preparation, through which larger surface area, porosity, higher SiO_2 content and varied compositions could be attained. Details will be discussed in Sect. 1.2.

1.2 Development of Mesoporous Bioactive Glasses (MBG)

In 1990s, the discovery of ordered mesoporous silica sieves known as MCM41 by Mobil Oil Company launched the field of unique mesoporous materials [19]. The material possesses higher surface area, tunable pore volume and size, possibility of surface modification and has been widely studied the field of catalysis, adsorption/separation, electronics and biomedical applications [20, 21]. Years after that, studies on mesoporous materials were expended into the bone regeneration since the investigation of in vitro apatite formation found that HCA layers could be deposited on the surfaces of several types of mesoporous materials (e.g. phosphorous-doped MCM-41, SBA-15) [22]. Interestingly, the mesoporous silica materials present a similar chemical surface to bioglasses, which may led to its application as bone regenerators. However, scientists have noticed that the compared with pure silica content, bioglasses with a combined composition of SiO_2–CaO–P_2O_5 showed more active apatite formation ability [23, 24]. It is of great interests to introduce mesoporous structure to bioactive glasses to improve the bioactivity.

Meanwhile, problems such as bacterial infection in bone reconstruction process have caused great pain of patients. Conventional treatments including systemic antibiotic administration, surgical debridement and wound drainage are not always efficient, which may lead to extra surgeries. One of the best solution is to introduce a proper local drug release system into the implant site [25, 26]. Under this circumstance, the in situ introduction of mesoporous structure, which could endow the bioactive glasses with drug/growth factor loading capacity stood out as a wise candidate. Apart from the antibacterial drugs, growth factors enhancing the osteogenesis and angiogenesis could also be delivered [27, 28]. In the year 2004, mesoporous bioactive glass (MBG) was first synthesized by Yan et al. using non-ionic block copolymers as template via the evaporation-induced self-assembly process [29]. The prepared MBG possessed highly ordered mesoporous channels and large specific surface area, pore volume and pore size (351 $m^2\ g^{-1}$, 0.49 $cm^3\ g^{-1}$ and 4.6 nm by BET, respectively), showing a significant improvement compared to BG with some composition. The mineralization property of MBG tested in simulated body fluid (SBF) was also greatly enhanced. After that, different types of MBG such as particles, fibers and scaffolds were synthesized.

2 Preparation and Properties of Different Forms of Bioactive Glasses

2.1 Synthesis of Bioglasses: From Melt Quenching to Sol–Gel Methods

Conventional route to prepare bioglasses is the well-known melt quenching method, which was similar to the preparation of glasses. Typically, stoichiometric amounts of different constituent oxides or carbonates of high purity are mixed by ball mill and the obtained powders are sintered at high temperature (1300–1500 °C) [30] depending on the varied compositions (Fig. 1). However, it is worth noting that bioglasses containing less than 10 % alkali oxide are difficult to melt due to the high viscosities, while their silica contents exceeding 60 % could fail the formation of HCA layers, thus the effective bond to host bone [9].

Despite the excellent bioactivity of bioglasses, the narrow compositions with regulatory approval as particulate synthetic bone filling/grafting materials are not suitable to be fabricated into fibers, coatings or scaffolds [31]. In order to obtain bioglasses with adjustable compositions with higher silica content, the sol–gel methods, which could be manipulated at room temperature, become a popular approach to prepare bioglasses [32]. Typical process of this chemistry-based synthesis route is as follows: the compositional precursors are mixed in a solution, and then the precursors undergo a polymer-type reaction to form a gel, in which a wet inorganic network of covalently bonded silica is generated. The gel is then dried

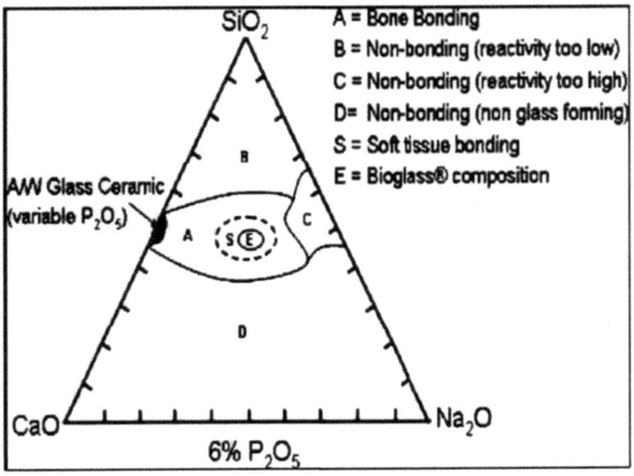

Fig. 1 Ternary compositional diagram given for 45 % SiO_2-24.5 % Na_2O-24.5 % CaO-6 % P_2O_5 (wt%) glass by Hench for bone-bonding [30]

Table 1 Compositions of several bioactive glasses [6]

Compositions (wt%)	45S5	13-93	13-93B1	13-93B3	6P53B	58S	70S30C
Na_2O	24.5	6.0	5.8	5.5	10.3	0	0
K_2O	0	12.0	11.7	11.1	2.8	0	0
MgO	0	5.0	4.9	4.6	10.2	0	0
CaO	24.5	20.0	19.5	18.5	18.0	32.6	28.6
SiO_2	45.0	53.0	34.4	0	52.7	58.2	71.4
P_2O_5	6.0	4.0	3.8	3.7	6.0	9.2	0
B_2O_3	0	0	19.9	56.6	0	0	0

and heated to 550–650 °C to become a glass [33]. Compared to the dense melt-quenching glasses with similar compositions, bioglasses prepared by this approach possess an inherent nanoporosity that can result in increased specific surface area, larger pore volume, thus the higher dissolution rates and improved cellular response. Moreover, the improved concentration of silanol groups (Si–OH) on the surface tend to induce better bioactive behaviors [34]. As the role of Na_2O in melt- quenched bioglasses is to lower the melting point and improve the processability, which is useless in sol–gel methods, the sol–gel glasses tend to have fewer components than the conventional ones. Various compositions of bioglasses (e.g. 58S SiO_2 58.2 wt%, CaO 32.6 wt%, P_2O_5 9.2 wt%) are shown in Table 1 [6].

In order to prepare bioglasses with mesoporous structures, surfactants including cationic surfactant (e.g. CTAB) and nonionic block copolymer (e.g. P123) are added into the precursors to act as structure-directing agents. Mesopores can be formed by calcination at a relatively low temperature (<700 °C) to remove the surfactant [35].

2.2 *Fabrication of Bioglasses: From Micro to Nano*

2.2.1 Bioglasses Particulates for Clinical Use

Being the second most commonly transplanted tissues in body, bone plays an essential role in health. Bone defects caused by trauma, diseases such as osteoporosis or tumour removal, especially those large ones beyond the self-healing ability of human, can only be regenerated by grafts. With the limitation of autografts and the underlying risks of allografts, the demand for bioactive bone repair materials has become an emergency [36–38]. It is exactly the original and most important application for bioglasses. First synthesized in 1969 and used in clinical trials, bioglasses were used in the form of particles or granules since they can be pressed easily into a defect. The granules have a size range of 90–710 μm. They were used to save tooth in the root or to repair bone in the jaw. Figure 2 showed a typical image of the bioglass product calle Novabone [31].

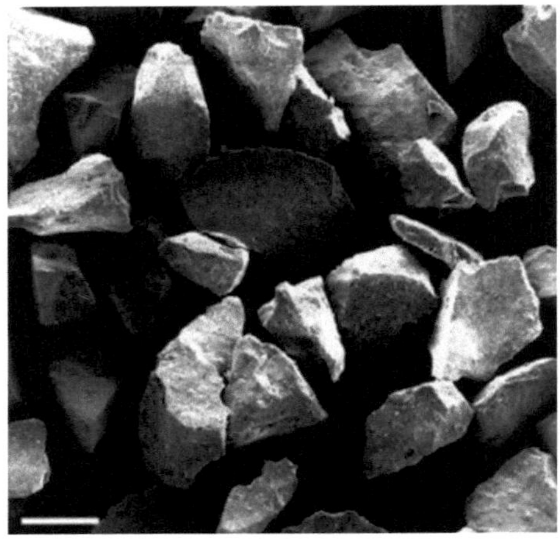

Fig. 2 SEM image of the bioglass particles for clinical use. *Scale bar* is 200 μm [31]

2.2.2 Bioglasses Scaffolds for Bone Regeneration

While the particulates of several to hundreds of micrometers were used in defect filling to help the bone/teeth repair in orthopedic/oral operations, the concept of bone regeneration put forward the use of porous scaffolds to guide bone repair, mimicking the natural bone (Fig. 3). It is proposed that the scaffolds should not only provide the mechanical support at the defect site, but also allow the cells (e.g. bone marrow stem cells) to attach, proliferate and differentiate, stimulate them to form new bone, and, offer space for the neovascularization [39, 40]. Moreover, the scaffolds should be degradable to let the new bone remodel naturally.

Scaffolds formed by bioglasses particulates undergoes a thermally bond of loose packing of particles/short fibers in a designed geometry. But the low porosity of 40–50 % and the insufficient interconnection of the porous structure occurred as the main disadvantages [6].On an early stage, fugitive phase (e.g. NaCl, starch), which could be removed by dissolution or decomposition before sintering, was introduced in the forming of scaffolds (Fig. 4). However, the problem of connectivity still remained.

Later after that polymer foam was used to serve as template for microstructure. The porosity of silicate, borosilicate and borate bioglass scaffolds was increased to the range 60–90 % by the methods [39, 40]. The solution/suspension freezing approach has also been carried out in a controlled manner to make bioglass scaffolds with oriented microstructure. Compared to the randomly oriented ones, mechanical strength of these scaffolds were significantly improved. By varying the composition and mixture of the suspensions, the pore diameter and structure could be adjusted. For instance, scaffolds of bioglass (13-93) showed pore diameters of 100–150 μm (Fig. 4d, e).

The developing technology of three dimensional (3D) printing, the rapid prototyping methods, or the solid freeform fabrication (SFF) have brought new options for scaffolds preparation [41–43]. Both the external shape and internal structure

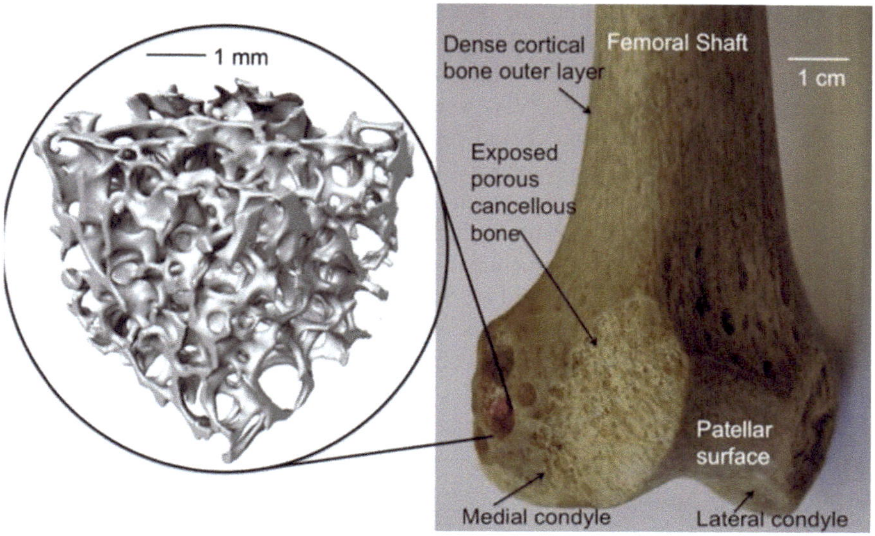

Fig. 3 Photograph of a human femur with a core-drilled piece removed. *Inset* X-ray microtomography (micro-CT) image of the cancellous bone removed from the femur proximal to the knee joint [31]

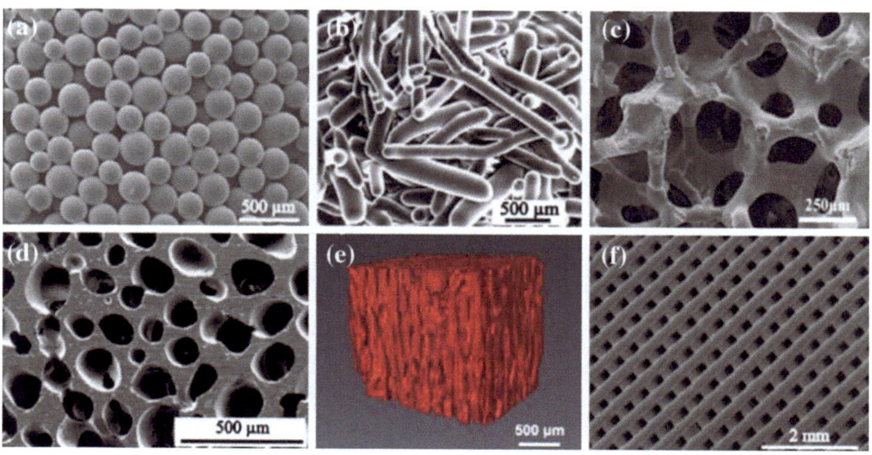

Fig. 4 Microstructures of bioglass scaffolds created by a variety of processing methods: **a** thermal bonding (sintering) of particles (microspheres); **b** thermal bonding of short fibers; **c** "trabecular" microstructure prepared by a polymer foam replication technique; **d** oriented microstructure prepared by unidirectional freezing of suspensions (plane perpendicular to the orientation direction); **e** X-ray micro-CT image of the oriented scaffold shown in (**d**); **f** grid-like microstructure prepared by robocasting. Glass composition: **a** 16CaO-21Li_2O-63B_2O_3; **b–e** 13-93; **f** 6P53B [31]

could be defined by controlling the pore size and distribution. A typical process of 3D printing involve the building of objects layer by layer form a computer-generated model with the assistance of proper software (e.g. CAD). Binder (e.g. polyvinylalcohol, PVA) were mixed with the sieved bioglasses powders to get the paste-like suspension for printing. A narrow-diameter syringe or nozzle was used to print the suspension onto a substrate with a robotic deposition device. The formed scaffolds were then transferred to a muffle furnace and heated slowly to remove the binder or further bond the powders. By controlling the geometric and interconnected structure of scaffolds, the mechanical properties could also be manipulated. As shown in Fig. 5, a 3-D printed MBG scaffolds under mild conditions using PVA as a binder possessed 200 times higher compressive strength than the PS-templated ones while maintaining the apatite-formation ability and drug delivery property [44].

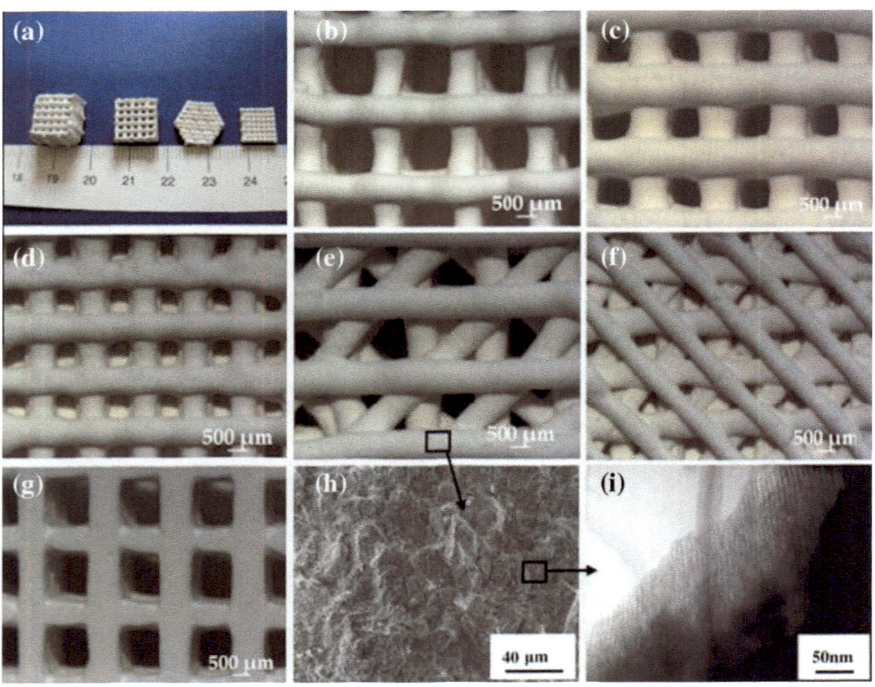

Fig. 5 Pore morphology and microstructure of MBG scaffolds. **a** MBG scaffolds produced by 3-D printing of different sizes, shapes and morphologies. **b–d** MBG scaffolds with different pore sizes varying from **b** 1307 ± 40, to **c** 1001 ± 48, to **d** 624 ± 40 μm. **d–f** MBG scaffolds with different pore morphologies. **g** Pore morphology of the bottom side of the MBG scaffolds. The pores on the bottom side remain open. **h** SEM image of the microstructure of pore walls. **i** TEM micrographs demonstrating the well-ordered mesopore channel structure of the pore walls in the scaffolds. The size of the mesopore channel is about 5 nm. The 3-D printed scaffolds obtained have controllable large pores (from several hundred micrometers to more than a millimeter) for cell seeding and tissue in-growth and nanopores (5 nm) suitable for drug loading and delivery [44]

Sol–gel process is also involved in porous scaffolds preparation. With tolerance of wider range of bioglass compositions, scaffolds as 58S (60 mol% SiO_2, 36 mol% CaO, 4 mol%. P_2O_5) could be fabricated. The whole process includes the hydrolysis, polymerization, gelation, drying and dehydration. A conventional acid-catalysed preparation of sol initiates the formation of the silica network [45, 46]. Nanoparticles of silica form and coalesce before the formation of Si–O–Si bonds between them. The gelation time could be accelerated from days to minutes by adding hydrofluoric acid (HF) in the system. Proper surfactant is then added by vigorous agitation. The surfactant-involved process produces interconnected macropores and maintain the inherent nanoporous texture [47]. To obtain ordered mesopores by this method at the same time, nonionic block copolymer (P123) and polyurethane sponges as co-template are usually applied in the system. Figure 6 shows the macroporous structure with ordered mesoporous channels on the scaffolds [48].

2.2.3 Bioglasses Coatings

Despite the excellent bioactivity and controllable biodegradability of bioglasses, the inherent brittleness of scaffolds fully constituted by bioglasses severely affected its further application. While biomaterials such as magnesium and its alloys, which possessed good mechanical properties, have the problems as high reactivity and insufficient corrosion resistance in physiological fluids [49]. It is a wise choice to coat suitable inorganic/organic materials on the surface of these implants. Distinct modification of the surface could not only break the limitations as corrosion, but also improve the biological properties and lead to better bone-to-implant interfaces [50]. Therefore, the distinguished osteoconductivity of bioglasses, especially the large surface area and pore volume of mesoporous bioglasses that could load and

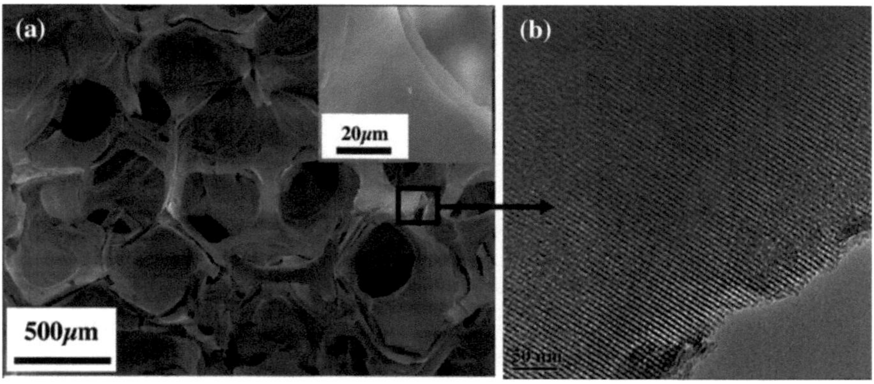

Fig. 6 SEM **a** image of macroporous structure and TEM **b** image of ordered-mesopore channels on MBG scaffolds [48]

release drugs make it an outstanding option. With the aid of heat treatment, spinning coating, electrophoretic deposition (EPD) or simply immersing in sol–gel solution of bioglasses, a coating with adjustable thickness could be acquired [51]. Typical SEM images of bioglasses coating on surface of Mg substrate is shown in Fig. 7. The thickness of both coatings were similar at around 1.5 μm while the MBG coating was observed crack free [52]. Apart from modification of metallic substrate, bioglasses are also used on the surface of glass-ceramic scaffolds [53] and Ti–6Al–4V substrate [54].

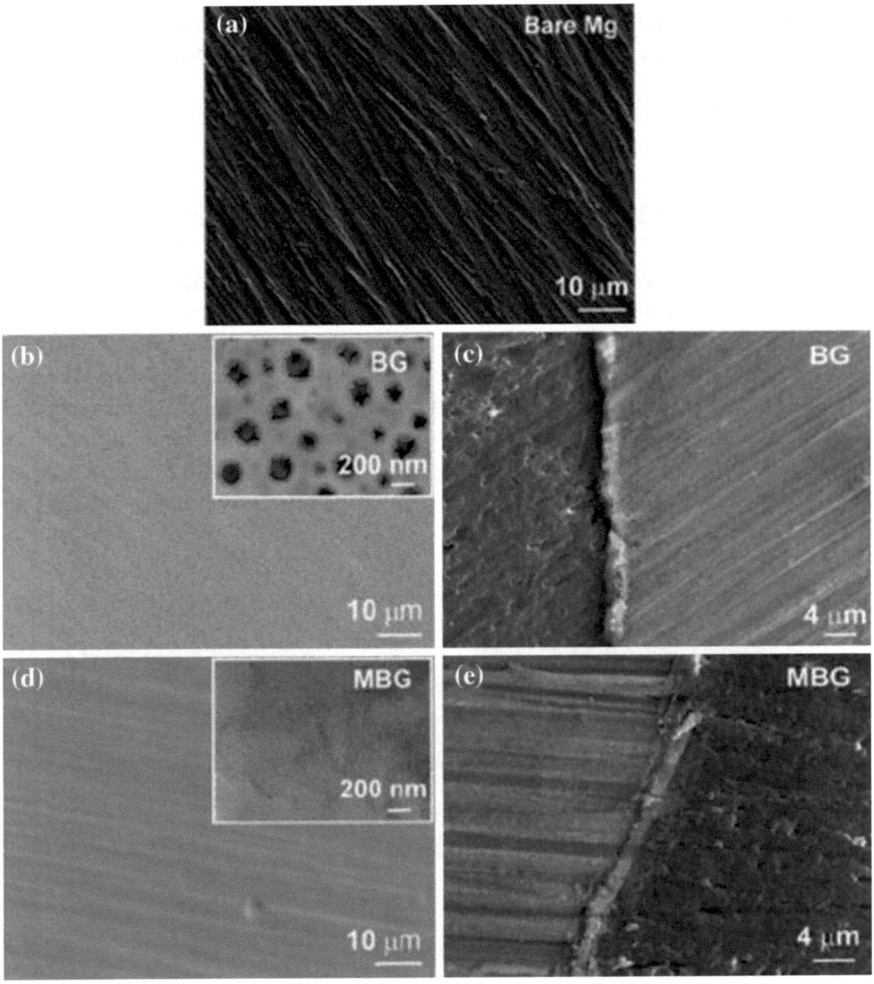

Fig. 7 Surface morphology of **a** the uncoated Mg, **b** the BG coated Mg substrate, *inset* is enlarged view of (**b**), **c** cross-section of the BG coated Mg substrate, **d** the MBG coated Mg substrate, *inset* is the enlarged view of (**d**), and **e** cross-section of the MBG coated Mg substrate [52]

2.2.4 Bioglasses Fibers

Fabricated matrix composed of fibers can mimic the three-dimensional structure of natural extracellular matrix and it is of high possibility to enhance the cellular responses [55, 56]. In the past decades, along with the development of various compositions of bioglasses by sol–gel methods, many studies on bioglasses fibers fabrication have been conducted. The most widely used technique is electrospinning, of which an electric field that sends fine streams of solution to a collector was used. In most cases, some polymer will be added and the diameter of fibers could be controlled by varying the viscosity of solution and the value of voltage. Glass fiber meshes are gained after burning out the polymer during stabilization. Fibers with a diameter from hundreds of nanometers to tens of micrometers could be obtained [57]. Figure 8 shows fibers with a highly ordered, two-dimensional hexagonal structure. Bioglass 45S5 fibers could also be produced by a novel laser spinning approach [58]. A small pool of molten bioglasses was created using a high-velocity gas jet from a supersonic nozzle. The fibers possess a rapid degradation rate in SBF

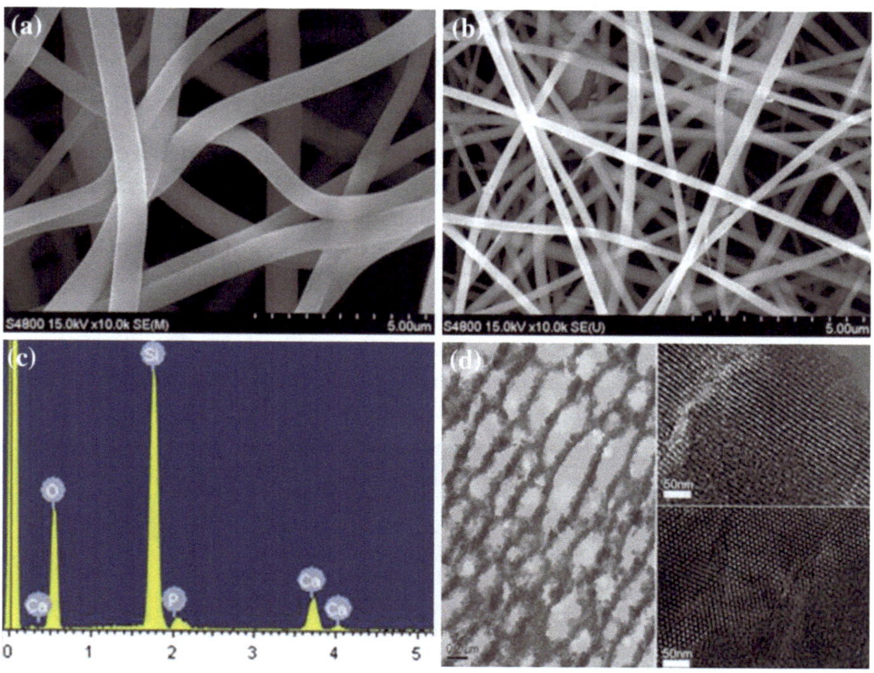

Fig. 8 SEM images of mesoporous bioactive glass nanofiber (MBGNF) matrices **a** after electrospinning and **b** after heat treatment at 600 °C. **c** SEM-EDS pattern of calcined MBGNFs and **d** TEM micrograph of ultramicrotomed MBGNFs embedded in resin. The MBGNF matrix showed characteristics typical of highly ordered, one-dimensional channels in a hexagonally packed mesostructure. *Left* nanofibrous structure. *Bottom right* highly ordered, two-dimensional hexagonal structure. *Top right* long, one-dimensional channels. *Left* magnification of 50 k, *scale bar* 0.2 mm. *Right* magnification of 250 k, *scale bar* 50 nm [57]

owning to its small diameters and highly bioactive composition. Besides the pure bioglass fibers, those composite ones with certain polymer are prepared in some recent studies. Details of them will be discussed in Sect. 2.4.

2.2.5 Bioglasses Nanoparticles

Nanostructured biomaterials are playing an important role in bone regeneration due to their unique nanostructure and functions [59, 60]. Although microparticles of bioglasses (diameter 1–1000 μm) have been investigated for many years, the preparation and application of nanoparticles (10–1000 nm) have only been looked into in the past decade [61, 62]. Nanoparticles possess specific advantages as follows: firstly, they can be directly endocytosed to affect the cellular behavior; secondly, rapid clearance by phagocytes can be avoided due to their inherent small size; thirdly, nanoparticles with porous channels can serve as drug delivery system in situ and work as therapeutic agent [63, 64]. Finally, they can be used as building blocks for bottom-up preparation of injectable gels and composite scaffolds.

Similar to the preparation of mesoporous silica nanoparticles, supramolecular chemistry and sol–gel process with proper structure-directing agents (CTAB, F127, P123, etc.) and hydrolysis catalyst (acid or alkali) were applied in the synthesis of MBG nanoparticles. Under proper synthesis conditions such as hydrothermal treatment, the template molecular self-organized to micelles which then linked with the silicate precursors, hydrolysed and assembled to form ordered mesoporous structure. High surface area and porosity were obtained after the removal of the template. MBG particles ranging from hundred nanometers to a few micrometers were prepared in the past 20 years. Via a facile hydrothermal method using CTAB and PVP as co-templates with an original molar ration of Ca/P/Si being 15/5/80, MBG nanospheres (size of 50–100 nm), which possessed typical mesoporous channels inside the particles, was successfully synthesized (Fig. 9). Excellent apatite-mineralization ability and high loading efficiency of anti-cancer drug was

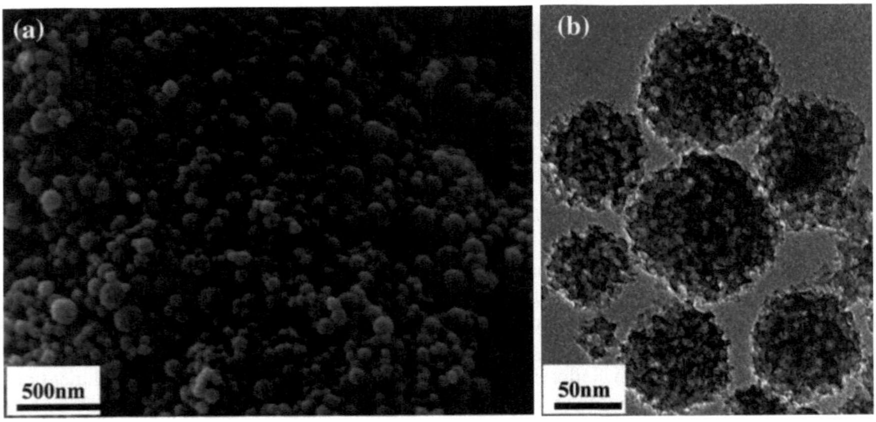

Fig. 9 SEM (**a**) and TEM (**b**) images of MBG nanoparticles [65]

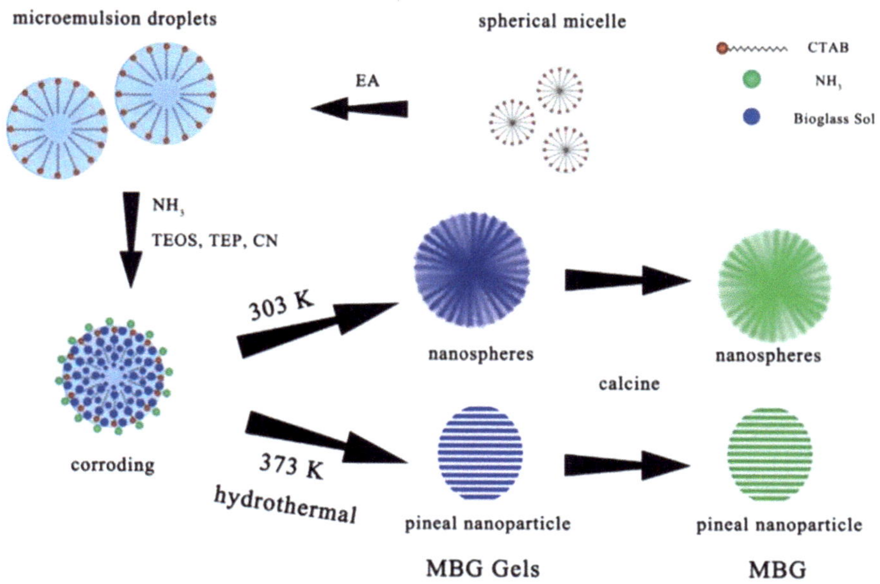

Fig. 10 Schematic illustration of the formation of MBG particles [66]

shown by the MBG nanospheres while the release behavior could be controlled by varying the pH microenvironment [65].

As illustrated in a latest report (Fig. 10), CTAB micelle self-assembled with the hydrophobic molecule ethyl acetate in water to form oil/water micro-emulsion droplets which served as template [66]. The bioglass sol then hydrolyzed and condensed at the interface by ammonia molecules. Under different temperature and pressure conditions, the size and shape of nanoparticles were obtained (Fig. 11).

2.3 *Ion Substitution of Bioglasses*

As mentioned above, bioglasses based on SiO_2–CaO–P_2O_5 system are beneficial for repair and replacement of bone tissue defects. The essential HCA layer on its surface forms as a result of a sequence of chemical reactions in the body fluid [7, 67]. It is proposed that three main stages are involved in the HCA formation [1, 68].

Stage 1. Rapid exchange of Na^+ and Ca^{2+} with H_3O^+ from the fluid, resulting in the hydrolysis of the silica groups and formation of silanols (Si–OH). With the consumption of H^+, the pH of the solution increased.

$$\mathrm{Si{-}O{-}Na^+ + H^+ + OH^- \rightarrow Si{-}OH^+ + Na^+(aq) + OH^-}$$

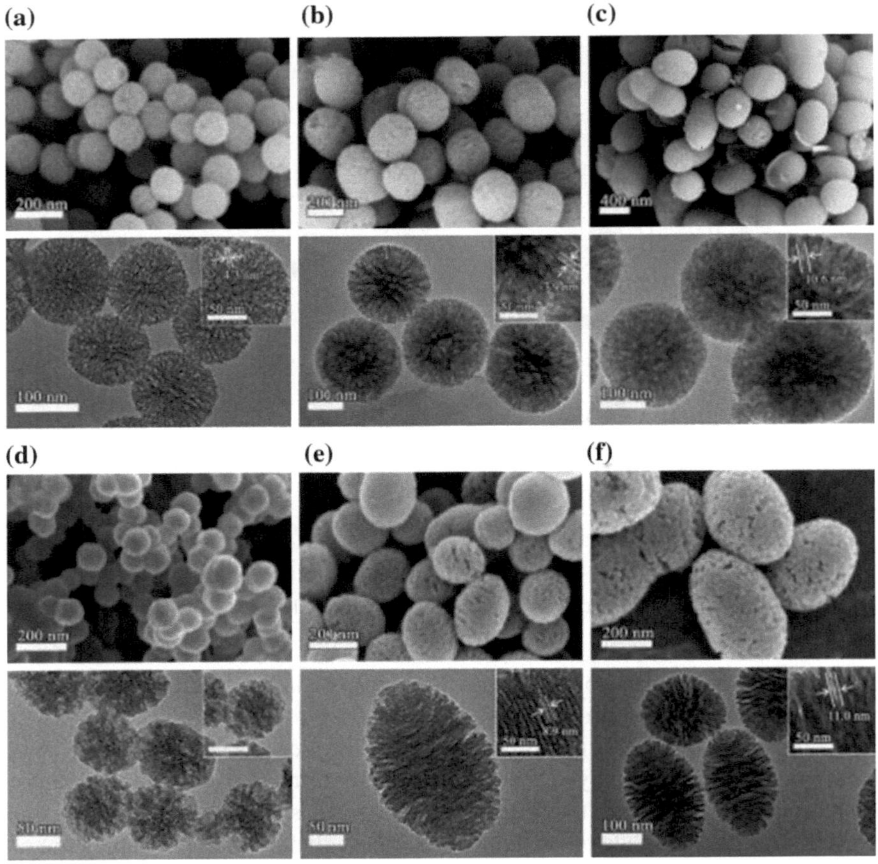

Fig. 11 Morphology of MBG particles prepared in different concentrations of the aqueous ammonia (1 mol L^{-1} for **a** and **d**, 3 mol L^{-1} for **b** and **e**, 5 mol L^{-1} for **c** and **f**), under different temperature (303 K for **a**–**c**, 373 K for **d**–**f**) [66]

Stage 2. The increasing concentration of hydroxyl in solution leads to the attack of silica glass network. The breaking Si–O–Si bonds and forming silanol groups at the interface result in the increasing Si $(OH)_4$ (dissolved silica) to the solution.

$$\mathrm{Si{-}O{-}Si} + \mathrm{H_2O} \rightarrow \mathrm{Si{-}OH} + \mathrm{HO{-}Si}$$

Stage 3. The condensation and repolymerization of the silanol groups on the surface leads to a silica-rich layer, after which Ca^{2+} and PO_4^{3+} groups migrate to the surface to form a CaO–P_2O_5 rich film on top. Then with the incorporation of OH^- and CO_3^{2-} anions from the solution, the CaO–P_2O_5 film crystallizes to make a mixed carbonated hydroxyl apatite HCA layer.

However, a major disadvantage is the high solubility of bioglasses. Resulting from the low fracture toughness, most of the released ions might be transported away from the surrounding of the implantation site by body fluid before new bone formation [46, 69, 70]. Moreover, with the advanced studies on cellular response, approaches to prevent bacterial infection with different therapeutic ions (mostly trace element of human being), the original composition of Ca, Si and P seems insufficient for the biomedical applications [71]. The trend of incorporation of various elements into bioglasses to modulate their physical, chemical and biological properties has become a hot spot in the last two decades [4].

In order to incorporate foreign ions in bioglasses, mostly by the sol–gel method, the structure-directing agent (e.g. P123) is firstly dissolved in ethanol solution and then certain ionic salts together with the basic compositions of bioglasses are all dissolved in the system. After an evaporation-induced self-assembly process and completely drying of the samples, calcination process should be conducted to remove P123 and obtain the therapeutic ion-doped bioglasses materials [72, 73]. The ion release kinetics could be modulated by tailoring the content of several precursors. Significant stimulation on anti-bacterial activity, osteogenesis, angiogenesis and cementogenesis is obtained by the ion substituted bioglasses.

Strontium (Sr) ions have been reported to inhibit osteoclast activity, therefore be beneficial for patients suffering from osteoporosis [74]. The amount of Sr in the skeleton is 0.335 % [75] of Calcium (Ca) content, its biological feature relating to the chemical correspondence to Ca. A high concentration of Sr can accumulate in bone and displace Ca in hard tissue metabolic process. 5 wt% Sr substituted sol–gel bioglasses have showed positive effect on fetal mouse calvarial bone cells [76]. Lithium ($Li+$) has been widely used as a long-term mood stabilizer in the treatment of bipolar and depressive disorders [77]. 5 % Li-doped MBG scaffolds with hierarchically large pores of 300–500 μm and well-ordered mesopores of 5 nm have been reported to enhance the proliferation and osteogenic/cementogenic differentiation of hPDLCs via the activation of Wnt/β-catenin signaling pathway.

Hypoxia (low oxygen pressure) plays a vital role in coupling angiogenesis with osteogenesis and the inducing of hypoxia on the defect site has been recognized as an important part for new bone tissue regeneration. Ions as copper (Cu) and cobalt (Co) incorporated in bioglasses have been proved to activate the expression of hypoxia inducing factor-1α (HIF-1α) transcription factor, which initiates the expression of a number of genes associated with neovascularization. BMSCs cultured on Cu/Co doped MBG scaffolds showed an improved HIF and VEGF expression, but it was reported the Co doped ones tend to be cytotoxic [72, 73]. Boron (B), possessing the biological effects such as stimulation of bone healing in vivo and angiogenesis in vitro, has been incorporated into bioglasses. A similar report by Haro et al. assessed the pro-angiogenic capacity of B-doped bioglass on embryonic quail chorioallantoic membrane (CAM) and found that the introduction of B significantly increase angiogenesis [12].

Bacterial infection is the main reason that cause failure of the implant in defect sites, which may results in revision surgery and prolonging time of hospitalization.

Typical bacteria including *Pseudomonas aeruginosa, Escherichia coli* and *Staphylococcu aureus* are usually found in the implant site [78]. Therefore, the anti-bacterial property is essential for biomaterials in bone regeneration. Silver (Ag), one of the most well-known precious metal, has been used to test the toxicity of food since ancient times [79]. Its ionic products, Ag ions, being doped in the network of bioglasses, could endow the materials with anti-bacterial activity. However, the addition of Ag in bioglasses structure can trigger the enhancement of quartz and metallic silver crystallization, and excessive Ag ions in bioglasses would cause toxicity to cells. It has been shown that bioglass containing 2 wt% Ag had negative effect on cell viability while that containing 0.75 and 1 wt% were safe.

Apart from these, therapeutic ions such as Zn, Fe, Mg, and Al were all applied in bioglasses composition modification [80]. The effects of these ions have been included in Table 2. Further details of ion substituted bioglasses properties will be discussed in Sect. 3.

2.4 Bioglasses Composites

In recent years, composite materials made of inorganic bioactive glasses combined with bioactive polymers have attracted much attention for bone tissue engineering application. As mentioned above, bioglasses possess excellent apatite-formation ability and osteoinduction ability. However, the inherent brittleness, generally low mechanical strength impede its clinical use. Meanwhile, another promising biomaterial, bioactive polymer (e.g. PCL, PLLA), which showed good handling characteristics for various fabrication, favorable mechanical properties, lacks sufficient bioactivity to build close bond to bone tissue [81–83]. Moreover, drug delivery capacity and controllable release profile could be obtained via the combination of these two materials [84]. Three-dimensional highly porous composite scaffolds of bioglass/PDLLA were successfully prepared by the foam replication technique (Fig. 12, W and B represented two types of foams used in scaffold preparation, 45 ppi and 60 ppi, respectively.). Highly porous structure with interconnected porosity was shown, the polymeric coating showing no negative affect on the interconnectivity. The mechanical stress test has revealed that the PDLLA-coated samples have significantly improved value compared to the non-polymer ones (Fig. 13) [85].

On the other side, polymer scaffolds (e.g. PHBV) with poor hydrophilicity could be modulated via the addition of bioglasses in the system [86]. PHBV/BG scaffolds were prepared by a solvent casting-particulate leaching method (Fig. 14). Open pores with a size from 30 to 300 μm were maintained with 20 wt% of bioglasses while the compressive strength and water absorptivity of the scaffolds increased from 0.11 to 0.34 MPa, 52–91%, respectively (the water absorptivity shown in Fig. 15). Other property modification including the degradation rate and drug release kinetics by the composite of polymer/bioglasses materials has also been conducted by researchers [87]. Some of the results are displayed in Figs. 16 and 17.

Table 2 Some therapeutic ions and their biological roles

Element	Role
K	Principal cation in extracellular fluid, regulation of osmotic pressure, glycogenesis, muscle contraction of cardiac muscles
Na	Principal cation of extracellular fluid, regulates plasma volume, maintains osmotic pressure, transmission of nerve impulses, absorptive processes for bile salts and amino acids
Ca	Constituent of bones and teeth, regulation of nerves, enzyme activation, neuromuscular excitability
Mg	Component of enzyme system with thymine pyrophosphate cofactor. Constituent of bones and teeth, activator for phosphate transferring enzymes
Zn	Cofactor for many enzymes, cell replication, metabolism of vitamin A and E, tissue repair and wound healing
Sr	Helpful in calcification of bones and teeth, bone healing, bone resorption
Cr	Maintains the configuration of RNA molecule, active ingredient in glucose tolerant factor
Co	Constituent of vitamin B12, cofactor of enzymes involved in DNA biosynthesis
Cu	Essential for hematologic and neurologic systems, formation of myelin sheaths in nervous systems, constituent of many enzymes, helps in iron absorption
Fe	Required for hemoglobin, component of enzymes for cellular respiration, myelination of spinal cord, synthesis and packaging of neurotransmitters
Mn	Cofactor of hydrolase, decarboxylase, involved in glycoprotein, part of enzymes required for urea formation and pyruvate metabolism
Se	Constituent of glutathione peroxidase, part of defense system protecting organisms from harmful free radicals, oxidant with vitamin E
Al	Decreasing the bioactivity Stabilizing the glass structure Decreasing the expansion coefficient
Si	Calcification of bone, component of mucopolysaccharides, component of connective tissues, cross linking agent, helps in resiliency of connective tissues
B	Helps in both osteogenesis and angiogenesis
P	Constituent of teeth, bones, adenosine triphosphate and nucleic acids
F	Increases hardness of bones, increases enamel remineralization, prevents dental caries
S	Required for amino acid, connective tissue, skin, nails and hair
Cl	Fluid and electrolyte balance, principal anion in extracellular fluid and gastric juice
I	Component of thyroid hormones Iron Required for hemoglobin, component of enzymes for cellular respiration, myelination of spinal cord, synthesis and packaging of neurotransmitters

Apart from biodegradable organic polymers, studies on bioglass/inorganic composites have been widely reported [53, 88]. Implants manufactured using titanium, cobalt alloys and stainless steel possess high mechanical property but have sever shortcomings as limited corrosion resistance in biological fluid and lack of bioactivity. A strategy to decrease these undesired effects is the superficial modifications by bioceramics (e.g. Bioglasses, HA) via the technique of atmospheric plasma spraying or flame spraying process. Figure 18 gives the image of the section

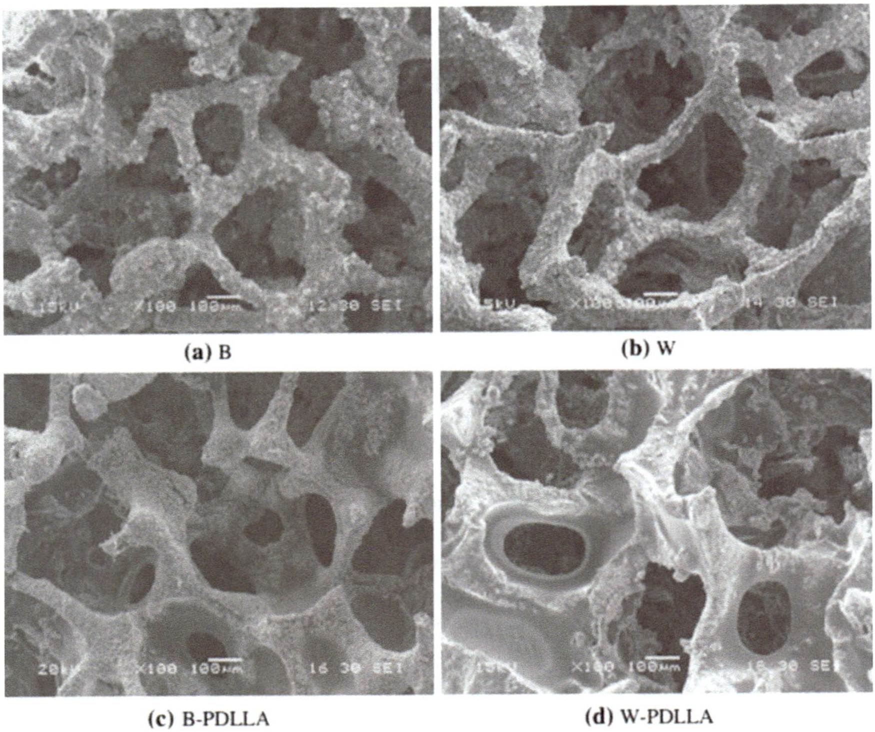

Fig. 12 SEM micrographs of B-type BioglassR-based scaffolds **a** before and **c** after PDLLA coating, and of W-type scaffolds **b** before and **d** after PDLLA coating [85]

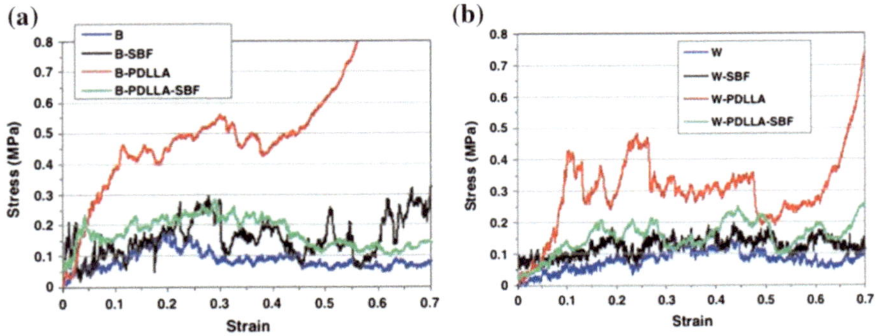

Fig. 13 Compressive stress–strain diagrams of **a** uncoated and PDLLA-coated B-type scaffolds, before and after 28 days in SBF and **b** uncoated and PDLLA-coated W-type scaffolds, before and after 28 days in SBF [85]

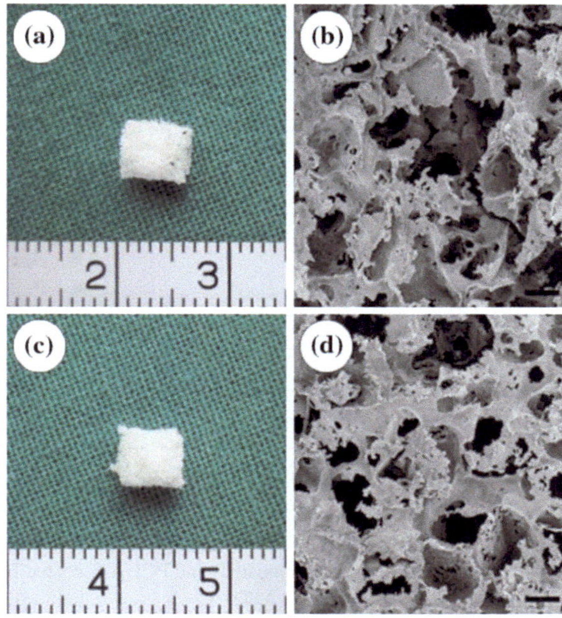

Fig. 14 Optical and SEM micrographs of the PHBV and PHBV/BG scaffolds. The PHBV and PHBV/BG scaffolds prepared using the compression molding, thermal processing and salt particulate leaching method had a regular shape, and some pores on the surface of the scaffolds can be observed. The SEM images show that the PHBV and PHBV/BG scaffolds exhibited a macroporous structure with interconnected open pores, and the pore size varied from 30 to 300 mm. *Scale bar* 100 mm [86]

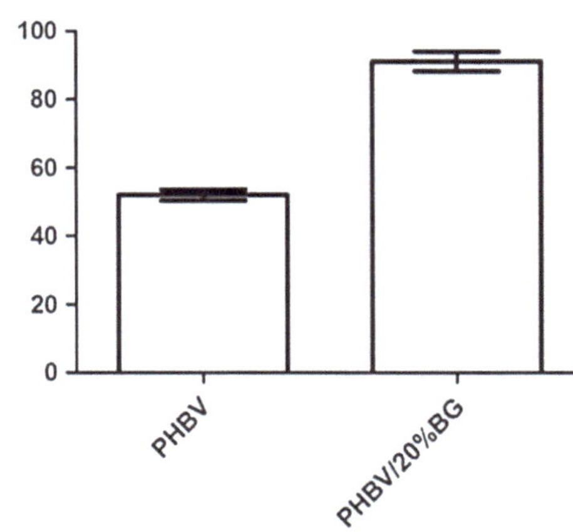

Fig. 15 Water absorptivity before and after BG addition [86]

between bioglasses and the metallic substrate [51]. Further studies have revealed that the apatite formation ability was significantly improved by the surface modification. Similar experiments were conducted on the Mg alloy surface in other reports (Fig. 19) and the water contact angle was significantly decreased, showing a greatly improved hydrophilcity (Fig. 20) [49].

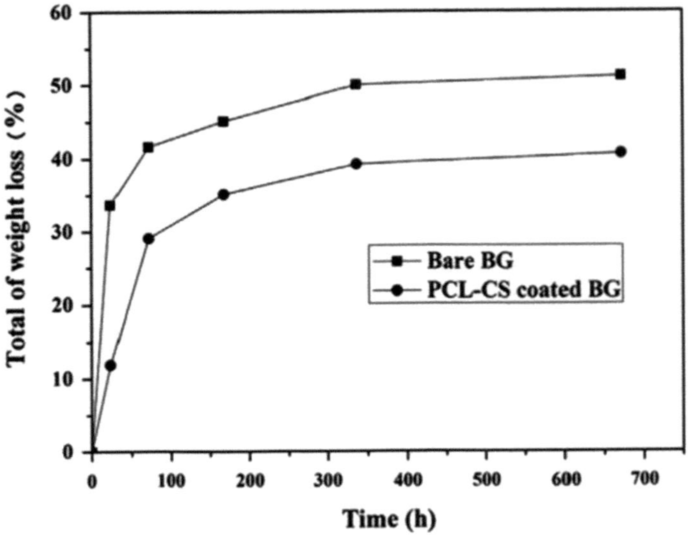

Fig. 16 Weight loss of bare (uncoated) and PCL–CS coated BG scaffolds after immersion in PBS solution for 28 days

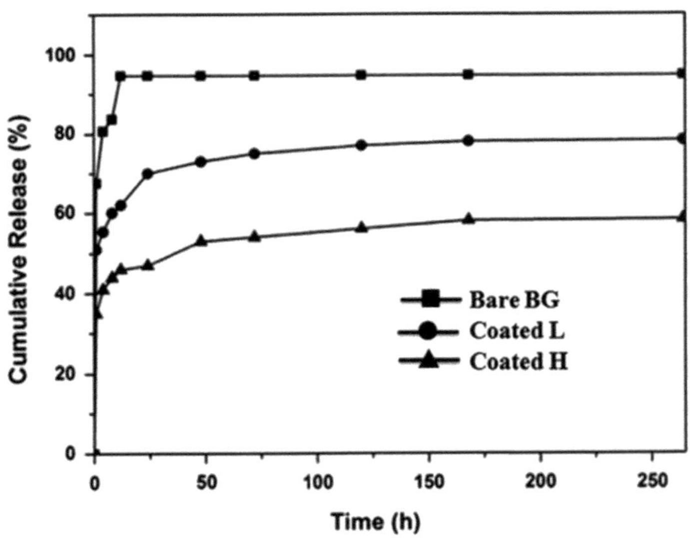

Fig. 17 In vitro vancomycin released from bare and coated BG scaffolds. Coated BG scaffolds were loaded with the drug at two different concentrations (vancomycin/solvent: 25 mg/ml (L) and 50 mg/ml (H))

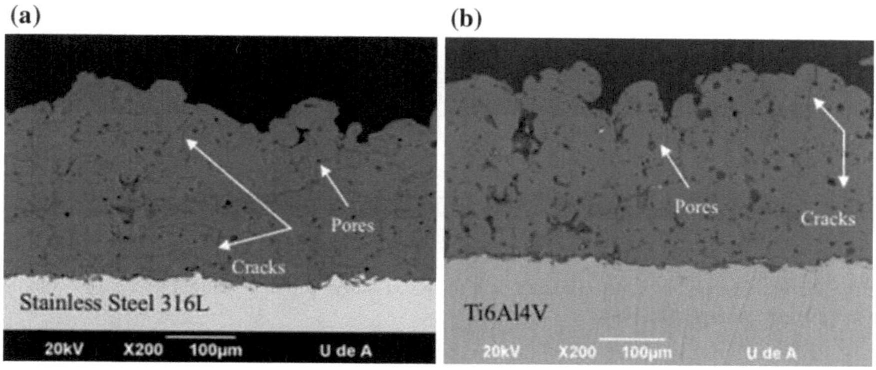

Fig. 18 SEM cross-section of different metallic surface covered with bioglassess [51]. **a** bioglasses on Stainless Steel 316L, **b** bioglasses on Ti6Al4V

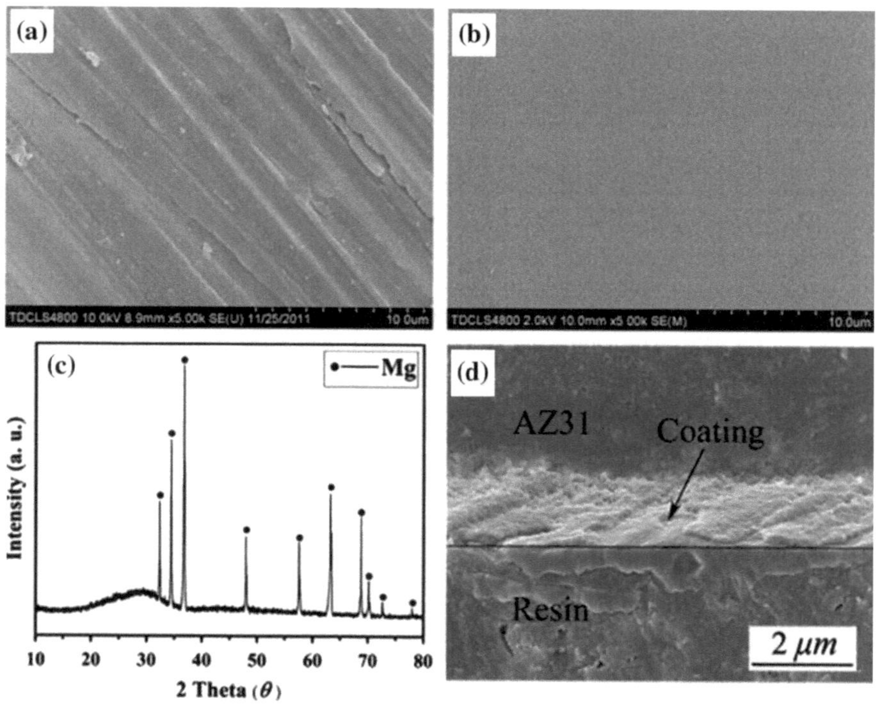

Fig. 19 Surface morphologies of AZ31 alloy without (**a**) and with (**b**) 58S MBG coatings. The XRD pattern (**c**) and cross-section micrograph (**d**) of 58S MBG coated samples [49]

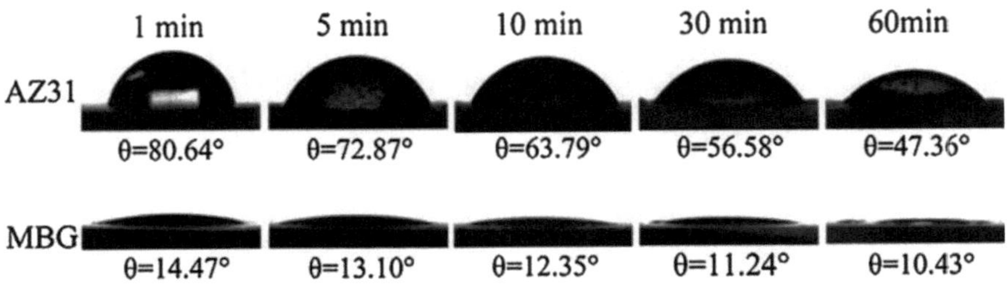

Fig. 20 Photographs of water contact angle on AZ31 alloy with and without 58S MBG coatings for different contact time [49]

3 Application Potential of Bioglasses in Tissue Engineering

3.1 Drug/Growth Factor Delivery by Bioglasses

One of the most important issues in biomedical application is the controlled release of drugs/growth factors by the drug delivery systems (DDSs) [89]. Multifunctional therapeutic effects can be maintained via the controlled release rate and enough release period of certain drug delivery [90–92]. To intensify the positive effect of bioglasses for bone tissue applications and to endow the material with anti-bacterial capacity, considerable researches have been conducted to use bioglasses as platforms to encapsulate and carry drugs, growth factors, hormones and peptides. With the development of their mesoporous forms, the drug delivery ability of bioglasses has been largely improved for the easy loading and prolonged release of various biomolecules [77]. The abundant Si–OH groups inside the MBG channels might play a key role in interacting with drugs and factors by hydrogen bond and Van der Waals force while Fickian diffusion mechanism is usually involved in the release behavior [93].

One of the approaches to load drugs in bioglasses is to add drugs into the sol–gel solution for glass preparation [26]. As the reaction of sol–gel process was usually conducted at room temperature, the activity of drugs (e.g. antibiotic Tetracyline) could be preserved. The samples were obtained after freeze-drying. The antibiotic was incorporated into the bioglass structure by the chemical connection between the phosphate group and the tetracycline acid moiety. Drug release in SBF showed that 12 % of the drug were burstly released at the first 8 h while a sustained release behavior lasted for the next 80 days of 22–25 % of the drug.

Improved drug loading and release behavior becomes possible by the application of bioglasses with mesoporous channels. Previous studies used MBG scaffolds to deliver DMOG, a small molecular drug that could induce hypoxia via counteract the effect of HIF-PH ad stabilize HIF-1α expression [94, 95]. To modulate the

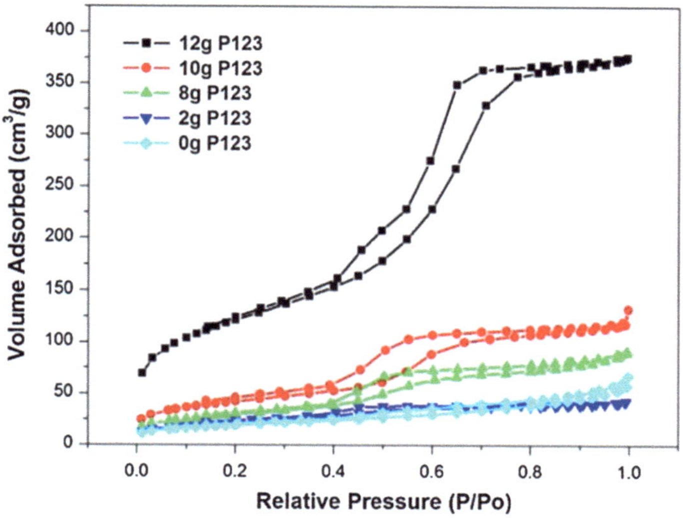

Fig. 21 Nitrogen adsorption–desorption isotherm analysis for bioactive glass scaffolds prepared using different contents of P123 template [48]

loading capacity of scaffolds, different amounts of the mesopore template P123 were added in the preparation and scaffolds with different specific surface were obtained (Fig. 21). The 12 g-P123@ MBG scaffolds showed a maximum loading efficiency of 23 % DMOG and possessed the lowest burst release kinetics of the drug (Fig. 22) [48].

Bioglass/polymer composite materials have been designed to serve as drug carriers. As reported in a recent study, osteogenic enhancer fibroblast growth factor-18 (FGF-18) loaded mesporous bioglass nanospheres were combined with FGF-2 loaded biopolymer fibers (Fig. 23). The obtained composite nanofibrous scaffolds showed increased apatite-formation ability and mechanical property. In vitro study revealed the stimulatory effect on the activity of MSCs while the in vivo study carried out on rat calvarium defects showed significantly enhanced proliferation of osteocytes, bone lining cells and vessel forming cells. PLGA scaffolds coated with MBG possessed favored BMCs proliferation and osteogeic differentiation while the MBG surface improved the BMP-2 delivery of the scaffolds [96].

3.2 *Application in Bone/Teeth Regeneration*

Started with the discovery of 45S5, numerous investigations have been conducted on the important properties of bioglasses on bone and tooth repair and regeneration for orthopedic and dental applications [97–99]. The outstanding osteoconduction

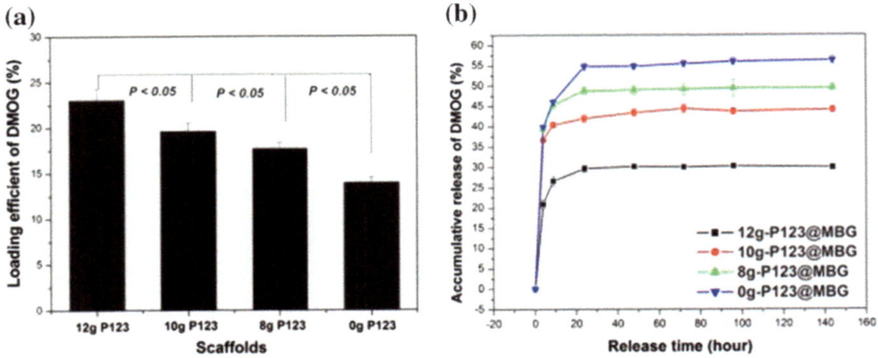

Fig. 22 **a** Drug loading and **b** release of DMOG in MBG scaffolds prepared using different contents of P123 template [48]

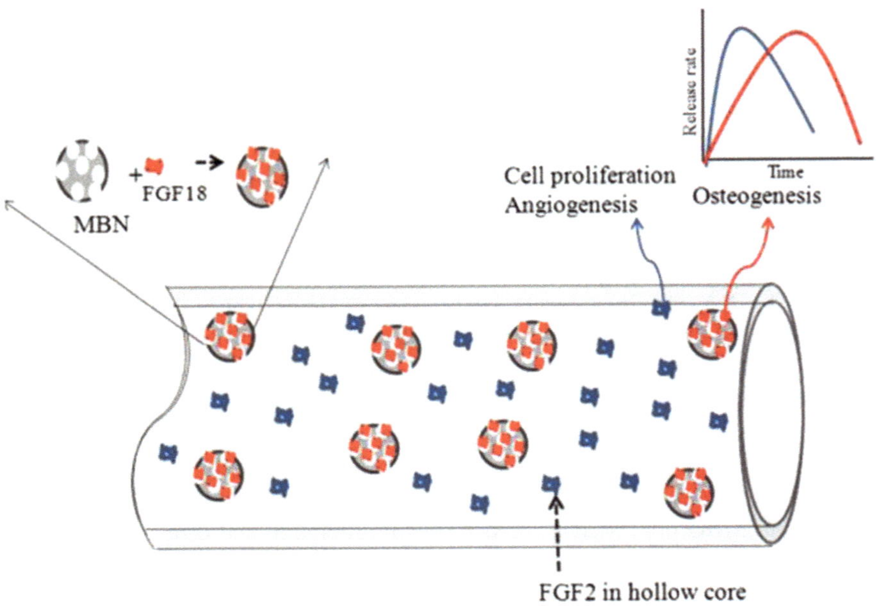

Fig. 23 Schematic design of the present study and the development of a novel therapeutic bone scaffold where FGF18 preloaded within MBG nanoparticles were incorporated within an FGF2-loaded core–shell electrospun polymeric fiber. FGF2 is released initially to stimulate cellular mitosis and possible angiogenesis, while FGF18 is released more slowly to promote osteogenesis [96]

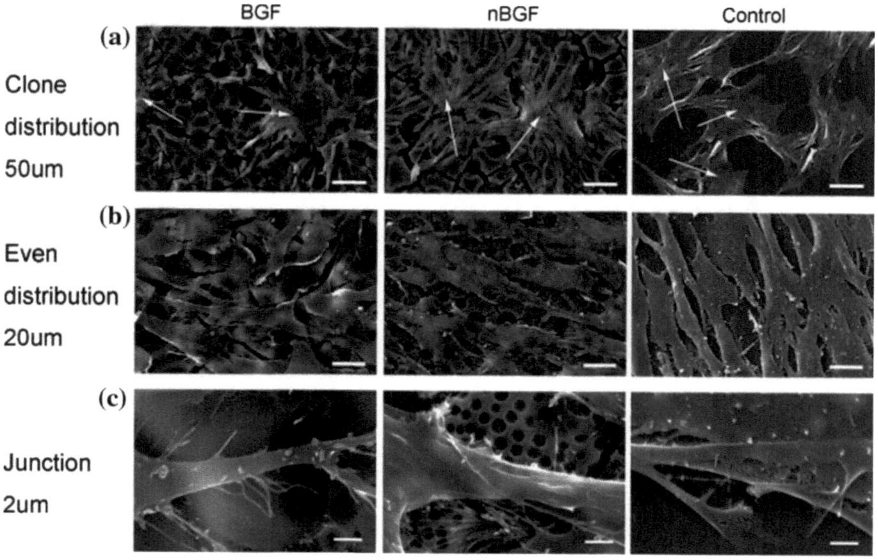

Fig. 24 SEM images of BMSCs attached on BGF (1), nBGF (2) and control glass slide (3). **a** The colony-like distribution of BMSCs after attachment for 6 h, *bar* 50 m. **b** The ordering distribution of BMSCs grew and filled the gaps between colonies after attachment for 3 days, *bar* 20 m. **c** The junctions connecting BMSCs and films. *White arrows* point to BMSCs [102]

and osteostimulation capacities of bioglasses have been studied in depth both in vitro and in vivo. Studies on the interaction between bioglasses and typical bone-related cells, mesenchymal stem cells, osteoblasts and osteoclasts have been looked into [100, 101]. The effect of dissolved ion concentrations, surface morphology on the cellular behavior (adhesion, proliferation, differentiation, gene/protein expressions) was further investigated. In previous report, nanoporous bioglasses film on commercial glass slide prepared by sol–gel method could be attached by BMSCs tightly. While the control group of commercial glass surface appeared a relatively oblate polygons of cells rather than obvious community-like structure, the cells on bioglasses and nanoporous bioglass film presented in a gyrate configuration with order, fulfilled with proliferated BMSCs (Fig. 24). It was clearly indicated that rougher surface with nanoporous structure was more beneficial in promoting the attachment of cells and therefore the combination with bone tissues [102].

The apatite formation ability, which is essential for the close bond to host bone or teeth, has been widely examined in many previous studies on bioglasses. Nanofibers (diameter: 240–470 nm according to the ratio of water/TEOS) of bioglass 70S were fabricated by electrospinning [103]. After immersion in SBF solution, cauliflower-like structure could be seen on the fiber surface, the porous lamella-like mineral deposition being a typical feature of bone-like apatite formed (Fig. 25). The SADE pattern also showed obvious diffraction rings, suggesting the polucrystalline nature of apatite coverage wrapping the amorphous bioglass fibers.

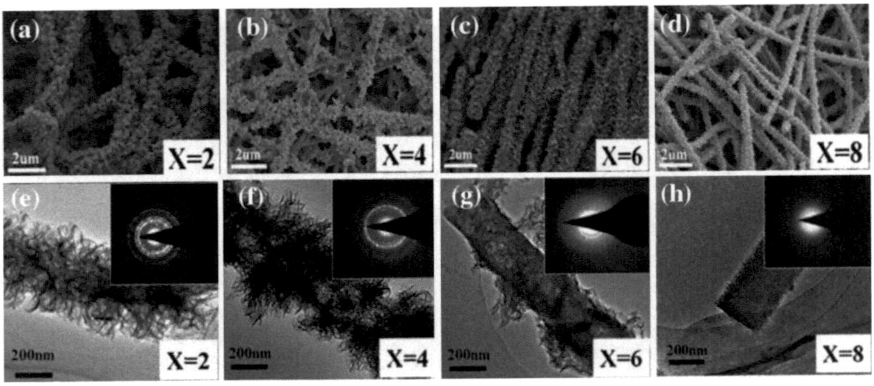

Fig. 25 **a–d** SEM images and **e–h** TEM images of BG fibers prepared with different X ratio after soaking in SBF for 30 h. The *insets* show SAED patterns of the corresponding samples [103]

Porous scaffolds made of 13-93 bioglass implanted in a non-healing rodent calvaria defect model for up to 12 weeks have successfully induced the apatite formation in the defect site. Analysis by von-Kossa and hematocylin and eosin (H&E) staining method revealed the large amount of newly formed bones [104].

As mentioned in Sect. 2.3, the biological property of ion-substituted bioglasses has also attracted much attention. For instance, Sr-incorporated MBG scaffolds was prepared in order to combine the therapeutic effects of Sr ions on osteoporosis with the bioactivity of MBG to regenerate osteoporotic-related fractures [105]. Experiments on critical sized femur defects created in ovariectomised rats showed a stimulatory effect of Sr ions on osteogenesis (Fig. 26).

3.3 Application in Soft Tissue Engineering

Not surprisingly, given the inorganic nature and mechanical rigidity of bioglasses, more attention has been paid on the application in hard tissue engineering. Yet, noticing that quite a lot of characteristics that is key to hard tissue regeneration are also important for soft tissue engineering, lots of studies on the application potential of bioglasses in this area have emerged in recent years [106].

Neovascularization, a key role in both new bone and soft tissue (e.g. wound healing) regeneration process, has been one of the most hotspot in biological researches. Suitable transport of nutrient and growth factors, as well as removal of waste products from the new tissue formation site are largely depended on the formed blood vessels [107]. To be more specific, strategies to improve the angiogenic stimulation of biomaterials should be taken into consideration. Years ago, fibroblasts cultured on 45S5 has be found to have a significantly increased secretion

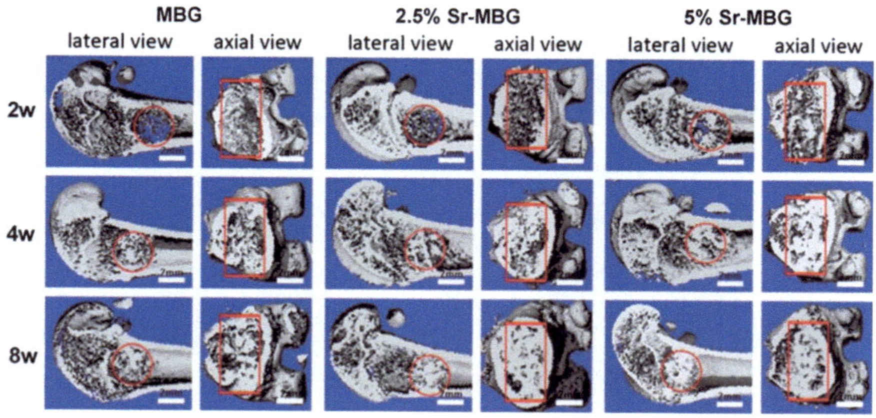

Fig. 26 3D reconstruction of longitudinal section and cross-section images by micro-CT at 2, 4 and 8 weeks post-operation of the critical femoral defect. The *circle* and *rectangle* describe the boundary of the defects. Only a little new bone was present in defects at 2 weeks, while abundant new bone regenerated at 4 and 8 weeks which depicted visible difference among the three groups. *Scale bar* 2 mm

of both VEGF and bFGF, which were representative markers for angiogenesis [108]. Besides, ion-doped bioglass (e.g. Cu) has been applied to accelerate the new vessel formation. In a previous report, Cu-doped (3 wt% in CuO) bioglass scaffolds were implanted in the rat calvarial defect for 8 weeks. Analysis by micro-CT tests have shown that a much higher number density of blood vessels on the defects were obtained in the group of BG-3Cu scaffolds compared to that of the pure BG scaffolds and blank control.

Bioactive glass microspheres have been applied as hemostatic agents for wound healing. It is proposed that the increased Ca ions, as well as the surface area of the bioglass, may accelerate the blood coagulation [109, 110]. A following study using mesoporous silver-exchanged silica spheres enriched with Ca (diameter 600 μm to 1.2 mm) showed that the additional ions into the silica network increased the degradability, therefore increased the blood clotting rates. With the aim of improving the healing of full thickness skin wounds, both 58S nanoscale bioactive glass (NBG-58S) by sol–gel method and melt-derived 45S5 bioglass powders were applied to the superficial injuries in healthy and diabetic rats [111]. Wound healing was compared by calculating the healed area as a percentage of the total wound every 2 days up to 16 days (Fig. 27). The sol–gel derived glasses led to quicker and more effective wound healing than the melt-derived glasses, which was attributed to the larger surface area and surface nanoscale topography of the sol–gel bioglasses. Importantly, both the groups showed better healing than the control group, which indicated the potential of bioglasses for soft tissue engineering.

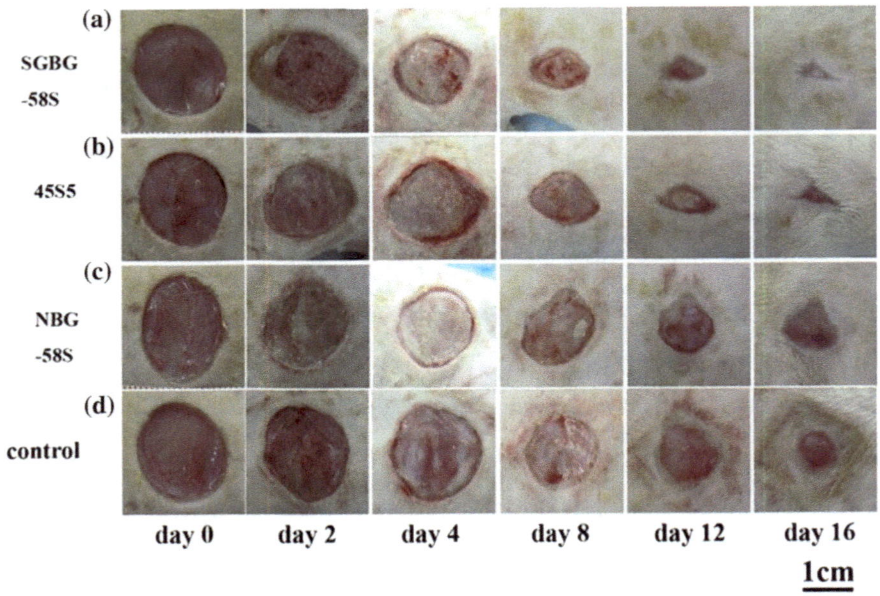

Fig. 27 BG treated and untreated wounds from days 0–16 according to Lin et al. Wounds were treated with different types of BGs, as indicated. It can be seen that SGBG-58S led to the fastest healing rates [111]

4 Conclusion and Perspective

Since the discovery of melt-derived 45S5 Bioglass by Larry Hench in 1970s, great progress has been achieved in the preparation of bioactive glasses in the past 40 years. Apart from the tunable compositions, both on the adjustment of the orginal calcium, silicate, sodium and phosphate contents and the incorporation of foreign ions including copper, zinc, strontium, sliver, etc., as well as mesoporous structure has been successfully introduced to bioglasses. With the modification of sol–gel methods and other developed fabrication techniques, different forms of micro-powders, bulks, scaffolds, films, fibers and nanoparticles of bioglasses could be obtained with specific morphology and surface characteristics. Moreover, their combination with other bioceramics, bioactive polymers and alloys in various forms has provided vast choice to satisfy the multi-requirements for potential application. As the outstanding biological property being the stimulatory effect on osteoblastic differentiation of stem cells without addition of osteogenic induction, bioglasses have been widely studied in bone tissue engineering. In the past several years, their positive effect on soft tissue regeneration (e.g. wound healing) has emerged and growing attentions have be attracted. Studies on cellular effect of bioglasses on different types of cells concerning the stem cells, osteoblasts, endothelial cells and even immune cells (skeleton system is closely connected with immune system) have been pushed forward and there are still much left to be done. Several products have been put into clinical use while many of the newly synthesized samples are undergoing fundamental researches in laboratory by biomaterial scientists. Bioglasses, being the promising candidate for bone/soft tissue regeneration application, are facing with both great chances and challenges.

There are several important issues that suggested to be the potential directions for the study of bioglasses. First, more trials need to be conducted on the preparation of bioglasses with nanoscale architecture, including chemistry-based methods to the synthesis of nanoparticles and the construction of meso/nanoporous structures on both surface and inside the main body. For one thing, cell adhesion and new tissue growth stimulation could be achieved by nanostructured materials. For another, the incorporation of nanoscale particles into two or three dimensional coatings or scaffolds may show improvements of properties such as mechanical strength and surface roughness, being crucial to following effects on its biological properties. Second, the better delivery of drugs/growth factors, as well as the dissolution of therapeutic ions (both original and substituted) should be further studied. The possible synergistic mechanism of ions and biomolecules on the multifunctional properties, together with the release kinetics should be focused on, of which some relevant co-culture of different cells, more appropriate animal models may be involved. Last but not least, researches in the fabrication of both pure bioglasses materials and their hybrids with proper polymers, metals, other inorganic materials via additive manufacturing technologies need to move beyond current progress. By combining certain chemical process with the advanced techniques, bioglasses in various forms with optimized properties for clinical trials will not be far.

References

1. Hench, L.L.: Bioceramics—from concept to clinic. Am. Ceram. Soc. Bull. **72**, 93–98 (1993)
2. Hench, L.L., Splinter, R.J., Allen, W.C., Greenlee, T.K.: Bonding mechanisms at the interface of ceramic prosthetic materials. J. Biomed. Mater. Res. **5**, 117–141 (1971)
3. Hench, L.L., Polak, J.M.: Third-generation biomedical materials. Science **295**, 1014–1017 (2002)
4. Kaur, G., Pandey, O.P., Singh, K., Homa, D., Scott, B., Pickrell, G.: A review of bioactive glasses: their structure, properties, fabrication and apatite formation. J. Biomed. Mater. Res. Part A **102**, 254–274 (2014)
5. Hench, L., Hench, J.W., Greenspan, D.: Bioglass: a short history and bibliography. J. Australas. Ceram. Soc. **40**, 1–42 (2004)
6. Rahaman, M.N., Day, D.E., Bal, B.S., Fu, Q., Jung, S.B., Bonewald, L.F., Tomsia, A.P.: Bioactive glass in tissue engineering. Acta Biomater. **7**, 2355–2373 (2011)
7. Pantano, C.G., Clark, A.E., Hench, L.L.: Multilayer corrosion films on bioglass surfaces. J. Am. Ceram. Soc. **57**, 412–413 (1974)
8. Wu, C.T., Chang, J.: Silicate bioceramics for bone tissue regeneration. J. Inorg. Mater. **28**, 29–39 (2013)

9. Brink, M.: The influence of alkali and alkaline earths on the working range for bioactive glasses. J. Biomed. Mater. Res. **36**, 109–117 (1997)
10. Liang, W., Rahaman, M.N., Day, D.E., Marion, N.W., Riley, G.C., Mao, J.J.: Bioactive borate glass scaffold for bone tissue engineering. J. Non-Cryst. Solids **354**, 1690–1696 (2008)
11. Fu, H., Fu, Q., Zhou, N., Huang, W., Rahaman, M.N., Wang, D., Liu, X.: In vitro evaluation of borate-based bioactive glass scaffolds prepared by a polymer foam replication method. Mater. Sci. Eng. C Mater. Biol. Appl. **29**, 2275–2281 (2009)
12. Haro Durand, L.A., Vargas, G.E., Romero, N.M., Vera-Mesones, R., Porto-Lopez, J.M., Boccaccini, A.R., Zago, M.P., Baldi, A., Gorustovich, A.: Angiogenic effects of ionic dissolution products released from a boron-doped 45S5 bioactive glass. J. Mater. Chem. B **3**, 1142–1148 (2015)
13. Zhao, S., Wang, H., Zhang, Y., Huang, W., Rahaman, M.N., Liu, Z., Wang, D., Zhang, C.: Copper-doped borosilicate bioactive glass scaffolds with improved angiogenic and osteogenic capacity for repairing osseous defects. Acta Biomater. **14**, 185–196 (2015)
14. Gao, H.S., Tan, T.N., Wang, D.H.: Dissolution mechanism and release kinetics of phosphate controlled release glasses in aqueous medium. J. Control. Release **96**, 29–36 (2004)
15. Brink, M., Turunen, T., Happonen, R.P., YliUrpo, A.: Compositional dependence of bioactivity of glasses in the system Na_2O–K_2O–MgO–CaO–B_2O_3–P_2O_5–SiO_2. J. Biomed. Mater. Res. **37**, 114–121 (1997)
16. Lin, S., Ionescu, C., Pike, K.J., Smith, M.E., Jones, J.R.: Nanostructure evolution and calcium distribution in sol–gel derived bioactive glass. J. Mater. Chem. **19**, 1276–1282 (2009)
17. Vedel, E., Arstila, H., Ylanen, H., Hupa, L., Hupa, M.: Predicting physical and chemical properties of bioactive glasses from chemical composition. Part 1: viscosity characteristics. Glass Technol. Eur. J. Glass Sci. Technol. Part A **49**, 251–259 (2008)
18. O'Donnell, M.D.: Predicting bioactive glass properties from the molecular chemical composition: glass transition temperature. Acta Biomater. **7**, 2264–2269 (2011)
19. Zhao, D.Y., Feng, J.L., Huo, Q.S., Melosh, N., Fredrickson, G.H., Chmelka, B.F., Stucky, G.D.: Triblock copolymer syntheses of mesoporous silica with periodic 50 to 300 angstrom pores. Science **279**, 548–552 (1998)
20. Mamaeva, V., Sahlgren, C., Linden, M.: Mesoporous silica nanoparticles in medicine—recent advances. Adv. Drug Deliv. Rev. **65**, 689–702 (2013)
21. Slowing, I., Viveroescoto, J., Wu, C., Lin, V.: Mesoporous silica nanoparticles as controlled release drug delivery and gene transfection carriers. Adv. Drug Deliv. Rev. **60**, 1278–1288 (2008)
22. Henstock, J.R., Canham, L.T., Anderson, S.I.: Silicon: the evolution of its use in biomaterials. Acta Biomater. **11**, 17–26 (2015)
23. Groh, D., Doehler, F., Brauer, D.S.: Bioactive glasses with improved processing. Part 1. Thermal properties, ion release and apatite formation. Acta Biomater. **10**, 4465–4473 (2014)
24. Beck Jr., G.R., Ha, S.-W., Camalier, C.E., Yamaguchi, M., Li, Y., Lee, J.-K., Weitzmann, M.N.: Bioactive silica-based nanoparticles stimulate bone-forming osteoblasts, suppress bone-resorbing osteoclasts, and enhance bone mineral density in vivo. Nanomed. Nanotechnol. Biol. Med. **8**, 793–803 (2012)
25. Vallet-Regi, M., Colilla, M., Izquierdo-Barba, I.: Bioactive mesoporous silicas as controlled delivery systems: application in bone tissue regeneration. J. Biomed. Nanotechnol. **4**, 1–15 (2008)
26. Hum, J., Boccaccini, A.: Bioactive glasses as carriers for bioactive molecules and therapeutic drugs: a review. J. Mater. Sci. Mater. Med. **23**, 2317–2333 (2012)
27. Vallet-Regi, M., Ramila, A., Del Real, R., Pérez-Pariente, J.: A new property of MCM-41: drug delivery system. Chem. Mater. **13**, 308–311 (2001)
28. Vallet-Regi, M., Izquierdo-Barba, I., Colilla, M.: Structure and functionalization of mesoporous bioceramics for bone tissue regeneration and local drug delivery. Philos. Trans. R. Soc. A Math. Phys. Eng. Sci. **370**, 1400–1421 (2012)

29. Yan, X., Yu, C., Zhou, X., Tang, J., Zhao, D.: Highly ordered mesoporous bioactive glasses with superior in vitro bone-forming bioactivities. Angew. Chem. Int. Ed. **43**, 5980–5984 (2004)
30. Hench, L.L.: The story of bioglass (R). J. Mater. Sci. Mater. Med. **17**, 967–978 (2006)
31. Jones, J.R.: Review of bioactive glass: from Hench to hybrids. Acta Biomater. **9**, 4457–4486 (2013)
32. Sepulveda, P., Jones, J.R., Hench, L.L.: Characterization of melt-derived 45S5 and sol–gel-derived 58S bioactive glasses. J. Biomed. Mater. Res. **58**, 734–740 (2001)
33. Siqueira, R.L., Peitl, O., Zanotto, E.D.: Gel-derived SiO_2–CaO–Na_2O–P_2O_5 bioactive powders: synthesis and in vitro bioactivity. Mater. Sci. Eng. C Mater. Biol. Appl. **31**, 983–991 (2011)
34. Letaief, N., Lucas-Girot, A., Oudadesse, H., Dorbez-Sridi, R.: New 92S6 mesoporous glass: influence of surfactant carbon chain length on the structure, pore morphology and bioactivity. Mater. Res. Bull. **60**, 882–889 (2014)
35. Yan, X.X., Yu, C.Z., Zhou, X.F., Tang, J.W., Zhao, D.Y.: Highly ordered mesoporous bioactive glasses with superior in vitro bone-forming bioactivities. Angew. Chem. Int. Ed. **43**, 5980–5984 (2004)
36. Lovelace, T.B., Mellonig, J.T., Meffert, R.M., Jones, A.A., Nummikoski, P.V., Cochran, D. L.: Clinical evaluation of bioactive glass in the treatment of periodontal osseous defects in humans. J. Periodontol. **69**, 1027–1035 (1998)
37. Mengel, R., Soffner, M., Flores-De-Jacoby, L.: Bioabsorbable membrane and bioactive glass in the treatment of intrabony defects in patients with generalized aggressive periodontitis: Results of a 12-month clinical and radiological study. J. Periodontol. **74**, 899–908 (2003)
38. Low, S.B., King, C.J., Krieger, J.: An evaluation of bioactive ceramic in the treatment of periodontal osseous defects. Int. J. Periodontics Restor. Dent. **17**, 358–367 (1997)
39. Schopper, C., Ziya-Ghazvini, F., Goriwoda, W., Moser, D., Wanschitz, F., Spassova, E., Lagogiannis, G., Auterith, A., Ewers, R.: HA/TCP compounding of a porous CaP biomaterial improves bone formation and scaffold degradation—a long-term histological study. J. Biomed. Mater. Res. Part B Appl. Biomater. **74B**, 458–467 (2005)
40. Peters, F., Reif, D.: Functional materials for bone regeneration from beta-tricalcium phosphate. Materialwiss. Werkstofftech. **35**, 203–207 (2004)
41. Leong, K.F., Cheah, C.M., Chua, C.K.: Solid freeform fabrication of three-dimensional scaffolds for engineering replacement tissues and organs. Biomaterials **24**, 2363–2378 (2003)
42. Sachlos, E., Czernuszka, J.T.: Making tissue engineering scaffolds work. Review: the application of solid freeform fabrication technology to the production of tissue engineering scaffolds. Eur. Cells Mater. **5**, 29–39 (2003). (discussion 39–40)
43. Liu, C.Z., Czernuszka, J.T.: Development of biodegradable scaffolds for tissue engineering: a perspective on emerging technology. Mater. Sci. Technol. **23**, 379–391 (2007)
44. Wu, C., Luo, Y., Cuniberti, G., Xiao, Y., Gelinsky, M.: Three-dimensional printing of hierarchical and tough mesoporous bioactive glass scaffolds with a controllable pore architecture, excellent mechanical strength and mineralization ability. Acta Biomater. **7**, 2644–2650 (2011)
45. Sepulveda, P., Jones, J.R., Hench, L.L.: Bioactive sol–gel foams for tissue repair. J. Biomed. Mater. Res. **59**, 340–348 (2002)
46. Jones, J.R., Lin, S., Yue, S., Lee, P.D., Hanna, J.V., Smith, M.E., Newport, R.J.: Bioactive glass scaffolds for bone regeneration and their hierarchical characterisation. Proc. Inst. Mech. Eng. Part H J. Eng. Med. **224**, 1373–1387 (2010)
47. Yun, H.-S., Kim, S.-E., Hyun, Y.-T., Heo, S.-J., Shin, J.-W.: Hierarchically mesoporous–macroporous bioactive glasses scaffolds for bone tissue regeneration. J. Biomed. Mater. Res. Part B Appl. Biomater. **87B**, 374–380 (2008)
48. Wu, C., Zhou, Y., Chang, J., Xiao, Y.: Delivery of dimethyloxallyl glycine in mesoporous bioactive glass scaffolds to improve angiogenesis and osteogenesis of human bone marrow stromal cells. Acta Biomater. **9**, 9159–9168 (2013)

49. Huang, K., Cai, S., Xu, G., Ren, M., Wang, X., Zhang, R., Niu, S., Zhao, H.: Sol–gel derived mesoporous 58S bioactive glass coatings on AZ31 magnesium alloy and in vitro degradation behavior. Surf. Coat. Technol. **240**, 137–144 (2014)
50. Li, H., Chen, S., Wu, Y., Jiang, J., Ge, Y., Gao, K., Zhang, P., Wu, L.: Enhancement of the osseointegration of a polyethylene terephthalate artificial ligament graft in a bone tunnel using 58S bioglass. Int. Orthop. **36**, 191–197 (2012)
51. Monsalve, M., Lopez, E., Ageorges, H., Vargas, F.: Bioactivity and mechanical properties of bioactive glass coatings fabricated by flame spraying. Surf. Coat. Technol. **268**, 142–146 (2015)
52. Wang, X., Wen, C.: Corrosion protection of mesoporous bioactive glass coating on biodegradable magnesium. Appl. Surf. Sci. **303**, 196–204 (2014)
53. Fiorilli, S., Baino, F., Cauda, V., Crepaldi, M., Vitale-Brovarone, C., Demarchi, D., Onida, B.: Electrophoretic deposition of mesoporous bioactive glass on glass-ceramic foam scaffolds for bone tissue engineering. J. Mater. Sci. Mater. Med. **26**, 1–2 (2015)
54. Tan, F., Naciri, M., Al-Rubeai, M.: Osteoconductivity and growth factor production by MG63 osteoblastic cells on bioglass-coated orthopedic implants. Biotechnol. Bioeng. **108**, 454–464 (2011)
55. Xu, C.Y., Inai, R., Kotaki, M., Ramakrishna, S.: Electrospun nanofiber fabrication as synthetic extracellular matrix and its potential for vascular tissue engineering. Tissue Eng. **10**, 1160–1168 (2004)
56. Clupper, D.C., Gough, J.E., Hall, M.M., Clare, A.G., LaCourse, W.C., Hench, L.L.: In vitro bioactivity of S520 glass fibers and initial assessment of osteoblast attachment. J. Biomed. Mater. Res., Part A **67A**, 285–294 (2003)
57. Hsu, F.-Y., Weng, R.-C., Lin, H.-M., Lin, Y.-H., Lu, M.-R., Yu, J.-L., Hsu, H.-W.: A biomimetic extracellular matrix composed of mesoporous bioactive glass as a bone graft material. Microporous Mesoporous Mater. **212**, 56–65 (2015)
58. Quintero, F., Pou, J., Comesana, R., Lusquinos, F., Riveiro, A., Mann, A.B., Hill, R.G., Wu, Z.Y., Jones, J.R.: Laser spinning of bioactive glass nanofibers. Adv. Funct. Mater. **19**, 3084–3090 (2009)
59. Walmsley, G.G., McArdle, A., Tevlin, R., Momeni, A., Atashroo, D., Hu, M.S., Feroze, A. H., Wong, V.W., Lorenz, P.H., Longaker, M.T., Wan, D.C.: Nanotechnology in bone tissue engineering. Nanomed. Nanotechnol. Biol. Med. **11**, 1253–1263 (2015)
60. Tran, N., Webster, T.J.: Nanotechnology for bone materials. Wiley Interdiscip. Rev. Nanomed. Nanobiotechnol. **1**, 336–351 (2009)
61. Yousefi, A.-M., Oudadesse, H., Akbarzadeh, R., Wers, E., Lucas-Girot, A.: Physical and biological characteristics of nanohydroxyapatite and bioactive glasses used for bone tissue engineering. Nanotechnol. Rev. **3**, 527–552 (2014)
62. Yang, Q., Sui, G., Shi, Y.Z., Duan, S., Bao, J.Q., Cai, Q., Yang, X.P.: Osteocompatibility characterization of polyacrylonitrile carbon nanofibers containing bioactive glass nanoparticles. Carbon **56**, 288–295 (2013)
63. Wang, H., Leeuwenburgh, S.C.G., Li, Y., Jansen, J.A.: The use of micro- and nanospheres as functional components for bone tissue regeneration. Tissue Eng. Part B Rev. **18**, 24–39 (2012)
64. Yang, L., Webster, T.J.: Nanotechnology controlled drug delivery for treating bone diseases. Expert Opin. Drug Deliv. **6**, 851–864 (2009)
65. Wu, C., Fan, W., Chang, J.: Functional mesoporous bioactive glass nanospheres: synthesis, high loading efficiency, controllable delivery of doxorubicin and inhibitory effect on bone cancer cells. J. Mater. Chem. B **1**, 2710 (2013)
66. Liang, Q., Hu, Q., Miao, G., Yuan, B., Chen, X.: A facile synthesis of novel mesoporous bioactive glass nanoparticles with various morphologies and tunable mesostructure by sacrificial liquid template method. Mater. Lett. **148**, 45–49 (2015)
67. Wu, C., Chang, J.: A review of bioactive silicate ceramics. Biomed. Mater. **8**, 032001 (2013)
68. Clark, A.E., Pantano, C.G., Hench, L.L.: Auger spectroscopic analysis of bioglass corrosion films. J. Am. Ceram. Soc. **59**, 37–39 (1976)

69. Kasemo, B., Gold, J.: Implant surfaces and interface processes. Adv. Dent. Res. **13**, 8–20 (1999)
70. Jiang, P., Lin, H., Xing, R., Jiang, J., Qu, F.: Synthesis of multifunctional macroporous-mesoporous TiO_2-bioglasses for bone tissue engineering. J. Sol-Gel. Sci. Technol. **61**, 421–428 (2012)
71. Lin, K., Liu, P., Wei, L., Zou, Z., Zhang, W., Qian, Y., Shen, Y., Chang, J.: Strontium substituted hydroxyapatite porous microspheres: surfactant-free hydrothermal synthesis, enhanced biological response and sustained drug release. Chem. Eng. J. **222**, 49–59 (2013)
72. Wu, C., Zhou, Y., Xu, M., Han, P., Chen, L., Chang, J., Xiao, Y.: Copper-containing mesoporous bioactive glass scaffolds with multifunctional properties of angiogenesis capacity, osteostimulation and antibacterial activity. Biomaterials **34**, 422–433 (2013)
73. Wu, C., Zhou, Y., Fan, W., Han, P., Chang, J., Yuen, J., Zhang, M., Xiao, Y.: Hypoxia-mimicking mesoporous bioactive glass scaffolds with controllable cobalt ion release for bone tissue engineering. Biomaterials **33**, 2076–2085 (2012)
74. Zhao, S., Zhang, J., Zhu, M., Zhang, Y., Liu, Z., Tao, C., Zhu, Y., Zhang, C.: Three-dimensional printed strontium-containing mesoporous bioactive glass scaffolds for repairing rat critical-sized calvarial defects. Acta Biomater. **12**, 270–280 (2015)
75. Nielsen, S.P.: The biological role of strontium. Bone **35**, 583–588 (2004)
76. Isaac, J., Nohra, J., Lao, J., Jallot, E., Nedelec, J.-M., Berdal, A., Sautier, J.-M.: Effects of strontium-doped bioactive glass on the differentiation of cultured osteogenic cells. Eur. Cells Mater. **21**, 130–143 (2011)
77. Wu, C., Chang, J.: Multifunctional mesoporous bioactive glasses for effective delivery of therapeutic ions and drug/growth factors. J. Control. Release **193**, 282–295 (2014)
78. Choe, H., Narayanan, A.S., Gandhi, D.A., Weinberg, A., Marcus, R.E., Lee, Z., Bonomo, R. A., Greenfield, E.M.: Immunomodulatory peptide IDR-1018 decreases implant infection and preserves osseointegration. Clin. Orthop. Relat. Res. **473**, 2898–2907 (2015)
79. Balamurugan, A., Balossier, G., Laurent-Maquin, D., Pina, S., Rebelo, A.H.S., Faure, J., Ferreira, J.M.F.: An in vitro biological and anti-bacterial study on a sol–gel derived silver-incorporated bioglass system. Dent. Mater. **24**, 1343–1351 (2008)
80. Rabiee, S.M., Nazparvar, N., Azizian, M., Vashaee, D., Tayebi, L.: Effect of ion substitution on properties of bioactive glasses: a review. Ceram. Int. **41**, 7241–7251 (2015)
81. Yao, Q., Nooeaid, P., Detsch, R., Roether, J.A., Dong, Y., Goudouri, O.-M., Schubert, D. W., Boccaccini, A.R.: Bioglass®/chitosan-polycaprolactone bilayered composite scaffolds intended for osteochondral tissue engineering. J. Biomed. Mater. Res. Part A (2014). doi:10. 1002/jbm.a.35125
82. Helen, W., Gough, J.E.: Cell viability, proliferation and extracellular matrix production of human annulus fibrosus cells cultured within PDLLA/Bioglass® composite foam scaffolds in vitro. Acta Biomater. **4**, 230–243 (2008)
83. Zeimaran, E., Pourshahrestani, S., Djordjevic, I., Pingguan-Murphy, B., Kadri, N.A., Towler, M.R.: Bioactive glass reinforced elastomer composites for skeletal regeneration: a review. Mater. Sci. Eng. C **53**, 175–188 (2015)
84. Moritz, M., Geszke-Moritz, M.: Mesoporous materials as multifunctional tools in biosciences: principles and applications. Mat. Sci. Eng. C Mater. Biol. Appl. **49**, 114–151 (2015)
85. Bretcanu, O., Boccaccini, A.R., Salih, V.: Poly-dl-lactic acid coated Bioglass® scaffolds: toughening effects and osteosarcoma cell proliferation. J. Mater. Sci. **47**, 5661–5672 (2012)
86. Wu, J., Xue, K., Li, H., Sun, J., Liu, K.: Improvement of PHBV scaffolds with bioglass for cartilage tissue engineering. PLoS ONE **8**, e71563 (2013)
87. Yao, Q., Nooeaid, P., Roether, J.A., Dong, Y., Zhang, Q., Boccaccini, A.R.: Bioglass®—based scaffolds incorporating polycaprolactone and chitosan coatings for controlled vancomycin delivery. Ceram. Int. **39**, 7517–7522 (2013)
88. Bellucci, D., Sola, A., Anesi, A., Salvatori, R., Chiarini, L., Cannillo, V.: Bioactive glass/hydroxyapatite composites: mechanical properties and biological evaluation. Mater. Sci. Eng. C **51**, 196–205 (2015)

89. Chen, Y., Chen, H., Shi, J.: In vivo bio-safety evaluations and diagnostic/therapeutic applications of chemically designed mesoporous silica nanoparticles. Adv. Mater. **25**, 3144–3176 (2013)
90. Zhao, Y.N., Trewyn, B.G., Slowing, I.I., Lin, V.S.Y.: Mesoporous silica nanoparticle-based double drug delivery system for glucose-responsive controlled release of insulin and cyclic AMP. J. Am. Chem. Soc. **131**, 8398–8400 (2009)
91. Slowing, I.I., Vivero-Escoto, J.L., Wu, C.W., Lin, V.S.Y.: Mesoporous silica nanoparticles as controlled release drug delivery and gene transfection carriers. Adv. Drug Deliv. Rev. **60**, 1278–1288 (2008)
92. Neumann, A., Christel, A., Kasper, C., Behrens, P.: BMP2-loaded nanoporous silica nanoparticles promote osteogenic differentiation of human mesenchymal stem cells. RSC Adv. **3**, 24222 (2013)
93. Zhu, Y., Kaskel, S.: Comparison of the in vitro bioactivity and drug release property of mesoporous bioactive glasses (MBGs) and bioactive glasses (BGs) scaffolds. Microporous Mesoporous Mater. **118**, 176–182 (2009)
94. Ding, H., Gao, Y.-S., Wang, Y., Hu, C., Sun, Y., Zhang, C.: Dimethyloxaloylglycine increases the bone healing capacity of adipose-derived stem cells by promoting osteogenic differentiation and angiogenic potential. Stem Cells Dev. **23**, 990–1000 (2014)
95. Weidemann, A., Johnson, R.S.: Biology of HIF-1 alpha. Cell Death Differ. **15**, 621–627 (2008)
96. Kang, M.S., Kim, J.-H., Singh, R.K., Jang, J.-H., Kim, H.-W.: Therapeutic-designed electrospun bone scaffolds: mesoporous bioactive nanocarriers in hollow fiber composites to sequentially deliver dual growth factors. Acta Biomater. **16**, 103–116 (2015)
97. Izquierdo-Barba, I., Colilla, M., Vallet-Regí, M.: Nanostructured mesoporous silicas for bone tissue regeneration. J. Nanomater. **2008**, 1–14 (2008)
98. Matsuura, N., Gorelikov, I., Williams, R., Wan, K., Zhu, S., Booth, J., Burns, P., Hynynen, K., Rowlands, J.A.: Nanoparticle-tagged perfluorocarbon droplets for medical imaging. In: Shastri, V.P., Lendlein, A., Liu, L., Mikos, A., Mitragotri, S. (eds.) Advances in Material Design for Regenerative Medicine, Drug Delivery and Targeting/Imaging, pp 87–92 (2009)
99. Kim, Y.-T., Caldwell, J.-M., Bellamkonda, R.V.: Nanoparticle-mediated local delivery of methylprednisolone after spinal cord injury. Biomaterials **30**, 2582–2590 (2009)
100. Cejudo-Guillen, M., Ramiro-Gutierrez, M.L., Labrador-Garrido, A., Diaz-Cuenca, A., Pozo, D.: Nanoporous silica microparticle interaction with toll-like receptor agonists in macrophages. Acta Biomater. **8**, 4295–4303 (2012)
101. Tautzenberger, A., Kovtun, A.: Ignatius Nanoparticles and their potential for application in bone. Int. J. Nanomed. **7**, 4545 (2012). doi:10.2147/ijn.s34127
102. Ma, Z., Ji, H., Hu, X., Teng, Y., Zhao, G., Mo, L., Zhao, X., Chen, W., Qiu, J., Zhang, M.: Investigation of bioactivity and cell effects of nano-porous sol–gel derived bioactive glass film. Appl. Surf. Sci. **284**, 738–744 (2013)
103. Li, Y., Li, B., Xu, G., Ahmad, Z., Ren, Z., Dong, Y., Li, X., Weng, W., Han, G.: A feasible approach toward bioactive glass nanofibers with tunable protein release kinetics for bone scaffolds. Colloids Surf., B **122**, 785–791 (2014)
104. Bi, L., Jung, S., Day, D., Neidig, K., Dusevich, V., Eick, D., Bonewald, L.: Evaluation of bone regeneration, angiogenesis, and hydroxyapatite conversion in critical-sized rat calvarial defects implanted with bioactive glass scaffolds. J. Biomed. Mater. Res. Part A **100**, 3267–3275 (2012)
105. Zhang, Y., Wei, L., Chang, J., Miron, R.J., Shi, B., Yi, S., Wu, C.: Strontium-incorporated mesoporous bioactive glass scaffolds stimulating in vitro proliferation and differentiation of bone marrow stromal cells and in vivo regeneration of osteoporotic bone defects. J. Mater. Chem. B **1**, 5711 (2013)
106. Miguez-Pacheco, V., Hench, L.L., Boccaccini, A.R.: Bioactive glasses beyond bone and teeth: emerging applications in contact with soft tissues. Acta Biomater. **13**, 1–15 (2015)
107. Suzuki, O., Bishop, A.T., Sunagawa, T., Katsube, K., Friedrich, P.F.: VEGF-promoted surgical angiogenesis in necrotic bone. Microsurgery **24**, 85–91 (2004)

108. Day, R.M.: Bioactive glass stimulates the secretion of angiogenic growth factors and angiogenesis in vitro. Tissue Eng. **11**, 768–777 (2005)
109. Peltola, T., Jokinen, M., Rahiala, H., Levanen, E., Rosenholm, J.B., Kangasniemi, I., Yli-Urpo, A.: Calcium phosphate formation on porous sol–gel-derived SiO_2 and CaO–P_2O_5–SiO_2 substrates in vitro. J. Biomed. Mater. Res. **44**, 12–21 (1999)
110. Dai, C., Yuan, Y., Liu, C., Wei, J., Hong, H., Li, X., Pan, X.: Degradable, antibacterial silver exchanged mesoporous silica spheres for hemorrhage control. Biomaterials **30**, 5364–5375 (2009)
111. Lin, C., Mao, C., Zhang, J., Li, Y., Chen, X.: Healing effect of bioactive glass ointment on full-thickness skin wounds. Biomed. Mater. **7**, 045017 (2012)

45S5 Bioglass Based Scaffolds for Skeletal Repair

Anthony W. Wren

Abstract Glass as a material presents significant potential for restoration of bone tissue. Glass can be designed to contain ions that positively influence bone metabolism in addition to stimulating additional pro-healing processes such as angiogenesis. Specifically, Bioglass® (please consult the Editor's note in order to clarify the usage of the terms bioglass, bioactive glass and biocompatible glasses), a SiO_2–CaO–Na_2O–P_2O_5 glass composition has been extensively studied since it was discovered that this particular composition can bond to bone and soft tissue in vivo. This property in particular led to the development of porous scaffolds that can be utilized to permit the ingrowth of bone and soft tissue, in addition to allowing free movement of host cells and physiological fluids that can further improve the healing rate. Many studies and processing methods have been conducted to optimize Bioglass® scaffolds porosity and interconnectivity in addition to improving some of the limitation such as the mechanical integrity. The diversity of studies that have been conducted on this particular composition greatly supports the potential that glassy materials encompass for scaffold materials applied to skeletal repair.

1 Bone Tissue and Skeletal Repair

Bone tissue is a high complex and dynamic connective tissue that is continually being replaced and repaired by our own cells. It protects our vital organs, provides a supporting framework for our body in addition to sites of attachment for soft tissues and contains our marrow which houses many cells in our body including red blood cells, fat cells and cells of our immune system. Bone tissue is also the primary mineral reservoir for calcium homeostasis in addition to other organic chemical messengers such as growth factors and cytokines [1]. Bone can be generally classified into two morphologies, *cortical bone* and *trabecular bone*. Cortical bone is a dense and solid matrix and surrounds the bone marrow space. Trabecular bone

A.W. Wren (✉)
Inamori School of Engineering, Alfred University, Alfred, NY, USA
e-mail: wren@alfred.edu

J. Marchi (ed.), *Biocompatible Glasses*, Advanced Structured Materials 53,
DOI 10.1007/978-3-319-44249-5_7

is composed of a honeycomb like network of trabecular struts which are contained within the bone marrow cavity. Bone has important membranes that form a covering on the outer surface, the *periosteum*, and inner space, the *endosteum*. The periosteum is a fibrous connective tissue that surrounds the outer cortical surfaces, except within the joints. Bone tissue contains blood vessels, nerve fibers and numerous cell type specific to bone metabolism and turnover [1].

Bone is a composite material that contains an organic component (25 %), which is primarily *Type I collagen* (90–95 %) in addition to non-collagenous proteins (bone sialoprotein, osteonectin, osteocalcin), and a mineral phase (70 %) rich in calcium and phosphate, *Hydroxyapatite* (HAp) [2]. During bone formation the initial framework for mineral deposition is a collagen base, *osteoid*. Based on the pattern of collagen formation, two organizations can be identified, *woven bone* and *lamellar bone*. Woven bone is characterized by the haphazard organization of the collagen fibers and lamellar bone is characterized by regular parallel alignment of collagen into sheets (lamellae). The woven bone is produced when osteoblasts, the active bone forming cells, produce osteoid rapidly. This predominantly occurs in fetal bone and during the process of fracture healing. This is subsequently replaced by a process called *bone remodeling* where it is replaced by the more mechanically durable lamellar bone [2].

There are a number of cells that participate in the process of bone remodeling. These are *osteoblasts, osteocytes* and *osteoclasts*. Osteoblasts synthesize new bone matrix and deposit mineral salts on the non-mineral matrix (osteoid) [3]. As time proceeds, bones undergo both longitudinal and radial growth and continual remodeling. Longitudinal growth occurs at the growth plates, where cartilage proliferates in the *epiphyseal* and *metaphyseal* areas of the long bone. The expansion and growth of bone is a process termed *osteogenesis*, which proceeds in three distinct phases, (1) synthesis of extracellular organic matrix (osteoid), (2) matrix mineralization leading to the formation of bone and (3) remodeling of bone by the process of resorption and reformation [2]. Bone remodeling involves osteoclast cells which remove bone matrix and osteoblasts cells which replace bone, osteocytes which reside within the bone matrix, and bone lining cells that cover the bone surface in addition to containing a vascular network. The activities of the cells involved in bone remodeling are regulated by the presence of factors such as RANK and RANKL which promote osteoclastogenesis, in addition to also involving cells such as T-cells and endothelial cells. Figure 1 presents a schematic of the multicellular unit involved in the bone remodeling cycle.

Damage to bone tissue can often require corrective surgery and may require the use of implants or synthetic materials. Bone tissue loss can be incurred through traumatic injury and fracture resulting in bone tissue destruction/removal. In addition diseases such as osteomyelitis (bone infection) and osteosarcoma (bone

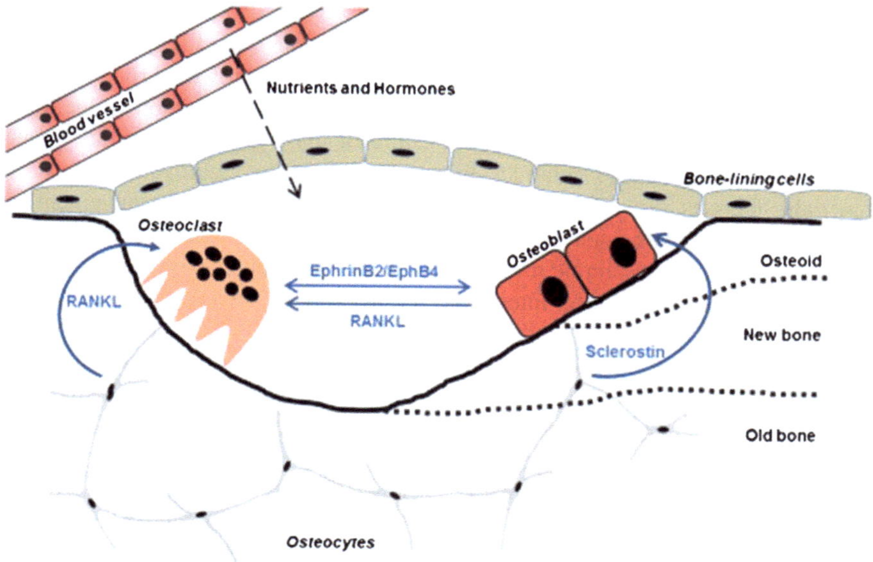

Fig. 1 The bone remodeling cycle involves the combined action of osteoblasts, osteoclasts, bone lining cells and endothelial cells in addition to regulatory factors that mediate a balanced bone remodeling cycle. (Reproduced from Kular et al. [3])

cancer) can require bone tissue to be removed and the resulting void will require filling. The following section highlights the suitability and some of the current glass based materials employed for orthopedic repair.

2 Bioceramic Materials for Skeletal Repair

Today it is estimated that more than 500,000 bone grafting procedures are conducted annually in the United States to repair bone defects in orthopedic surgery, neurosurgery and dentistry [4]. Autologous bone is currently considered the gold standard, however, harvesting the bone is associated with donor site morbidity and availability and with major complications accounting for 8–20 %. Allografts harbor the chances of immune responses and infection while synthetic materials such as bioceramics (*glasses and ceramics*) encompass excellent potential for hard tissue repair [4]. Bioceramics have been applied to many areas of orthopedic and dental medicine primarily due to the ability to (1) incorporate ions into the materials which can stimulate novel properties and responses in physiological systems, and (2) tailor the materials chemistry to control its solubility to facilitate better biocompatibility with the surrounding tissues [5–8]. With respect to applications, bioactive glasses, such as Bioglass®, have been applied to bony defects in vivo, created due to trauma, disease or surgery. Additional applications of bioceramic materials include glass-ceramic scaffolds for cell seeding into bony defects to promote healing [9–11], glass polyalkenoate cements for dental restorations [12–14], hydroxyapatite fillers [15] and glass microspheres for eradicating tumors growths [16, 17].

A benefit of using glass over ceramic materials for this application is due to the materials solubility [7]. The amorphous nature of glass generally permits greater solubility than crystalline ceramics which are primarily employed for scaffold materials. Glasses do not present long range periodic atomic arrangement, in contrast to their ceramic counterparts [18]. The difference in mechanical durability and solubility of glass/ceramic materials is related to the chemistry of the material. Glassy materials consist of an interconnected network of SiO_2 tetrahedron (Si–O–Si) that forms a random network, described as an inorganic polymeric network, where Si^{4+} forms the chain backbone [19]. Silicate glasses are therefore composed of a *network former*, (Si^{4+}) which is accompanied by ions such as Ca^{2+} and Na^{+}, which are termed *network modifiers*. The inclusion of these ions disrupts the continuity of the Si–O–Si network resulting in de-polymerization to Si–O–NBO^{-}, where NBO^{-} are non-bridging oxygen species [20, 21]. The formation of these NBO^{-} species promotes solubility and ion exchange in an aqueous environment, thereby promoting the bioactive response [21]. Weak bonding between the building units and the presence of NBO^{-} facilitate the distortion of the glass structure and the atomic displacement which promotes glass solubility [19, 22].

3 Therapeutic Potential of Bioactive Glasses

One of the attractive properties of employing glasses for hard tissue repair, in addition to being able to control their solubility, is the diversity of ions that can be incorporated and subsequently released in an aqueous media to help alleviate specific medical conditions. The first bioactive glass was developed by Prof. Larry Hench in the late 1960s. This glass, known as 45S5 Bioglass®, contained the composition 45 % SiO_2, 24.5 % Na_2O, 24.5 % CaO, 6 % P_2O_5 (wt%). When this specific composition is immersed in an aqueous environment, dissolution of the glass surface occurs which leads to the release of the ionic constituents contained within the glass. When incorporated in animal models Bioglass® forms a strong interfacial bond with both hard and soft tissues and does not initiate fibrous tissue growth [5, 8]. The specific characteristics that causes this response is attributed to reducing the SiO_2 content to <60 wt%, and by including high amounts of Na_2O and CaO as well as including a relatively high CaO/P_2O_5 ratio. These characteristics make these glass surfaces highly reactive in physiological environments. The bioactivity attributed to this glass is attributed to the formation of a hydroxyl carbonated apatite layer (HCA) on its surface similar to bone mineral [8]. This HCA layer forms as a result of a rapid sequence of chemical reactions on the surface of the implant when in contact with body fluid. There are five proposed reaction stages that lead to the rapid release of soluble ionic species and the formation of a high surface area, hydrated silica and polycrystalline HCA layer on the glass surface [23];

Stage 1: rapid exchange of Na^+ and Ca^{2+} with H^+ or H_3O^+ from solution, causing hydrolysis of the silica groups, which creates silanols (Si–OH), e.g.,

$$Si{-}O{-}Na^+ + H^+ + OH^- \rightarrow Si{-}OH^+ + Na^+(aq) + OH^-$$

The pH of the solution increases as a result of H^+ ions in the solution being replaced by cations.
Stage 2: stage 1 increases the hydroxyl concentration of the solution, which leads to attack of the silica glass network. Soluble silica is lost in the form of $Si(OH)_4$ to the solution, resulting from the breaking of Si–O–Si bonds and the continued formation of silanols at the glass solution interface:

$$Si{-}O{-}Si + H_2O \rightarrow Si{-}OH + OH{-}Si$$

Stages 3–5: condensation and re-polymerization of the silanols groups are then thought to occur, leaving a silica-rich layer on the surface, depleted in alkalis and alkali-earth cations (stage 3). Ca^{2+} and PO_4^{3-} groups then migrate to the surface through the silica-rich layer and from the surrounding fluid, forming a $CaO–P_2O_5$ rich film on top of the silica-rich layer (stage 4). The $CaO–P_2O_5$ film crystallizes as it incorporates OH^- and CO_3^{2-} anions from solution to make a mixed carbonated hydroxyl apatite HCA layer [23].

The bioactive potential of this glass has also stimulated interest in how these ionic dissolution products influence genetic expression [6]. Ion release from Bioglass® is known to influence the cell division cycle where the genes that regulate the cell division cycle are upregulated which enhances osteogenesis. This stimulates osteoblasts to mature more rapidly through a process called osteostimulation [6]. These discoveries have led to the investigation of numerous bioactive glass compositions and ion release studies for skeletal and dental repair. In addition to skeletal applications, ions from bioactive glasses are known to stimulate complimentary metabolic processes such as angiogenesis while also exhibiting antibacterial and anti-inflammatory properties. The discovery of these effects have led to the development for scaffolds for tissue engineering applications that contain trace elements that when released in an aqueous environment, enhance the bioactivity of the scaffold construct and present a positive therapeutic effect to the host cells and tissue.

3.1 *Ionic Dissolution from Vitreous Materials*

A significant amount of literature has been dedicated towards investigating the effect of ionic dissolution products from bioactive glasses on cells and tissues, however, exceptional publications by Hoppe et al. [7] and Rabiee et al. [23] have collated these works into two comprehensive review papers. Inorganic ions such as calcium (Ca), phosphorus (P) and silicon (Si) are well documented and are included in many glass compositions due to their metabolic effects on bone tissue. Ca is known to influence the behavior of osteoblastic cells by stimulating proliferation, differentiation and extracellular matrix production at levels below 10 mmol. Ca also influences bone remodeling by activating intracellular mechanisms that stimulate Ca-Sensing receptors in osteoblasts and is known to be a key regulating agent in bone metabolism [7]. P is also known to be a key regulator of bone formation as it stimulates the expression of matrix Gla (MGP) protein [7]. Si is also known to have positive bone metabolic effects as it has been suggested to influence bone growth processes such as collagen turnover and sialic acid containing extracellular matrix (ECM) proteins such as osteopontin [7]. Additional ions that have been incorporated into bioactive glasses and scaffolds include strontium (Sr), zinc (Zn), copper (Cu), magnesium (Mg) and boron (B). The effect of Sr on bone metabolism has been investigated by Marie et al. These studies showed that Sr exhibits a positive effect on bone growth and metabolism and has been proven to have a positive therapeutic effect in postmenopausal women with osteoporosis when administered the drug strontium ranelate (SR) [24, 25]. Zn is also cited to have beneficial effects as an anti-inflammatory agent in addition to bone metabolism. It has been shown to inhibit bone resorption by suppressing the formation of osteoclasts cells in mouse cultures. It has also been cited to regulate the transcription of osteoblasts differentiation genes such as type I collagen, ALP, osteopontin and osteocalcin [7]. In addition to providing positive biological effects, Zn can also play a diverse role in a glass structure as it can act as a network intermediate where is can assume a network forming or network modifying role [23]. By altering the concentration of Zn within the glass, properties such as the glass transition temperature, solubility and the distribution of non-bridging oxygens can be modified [23] (Fig. 2).

Mg is also known to be essential to bone metabolism where it has been shown to have stimulatory effects on new bone formation. It is contained within mineralized tissue in the human body, 0.44, 1.23 and 0.72 wt% for enamel, dentin and bone respectively [23]. Mg has been cited to interact with integrins of osteoblasts cells which are responsible for cell adhesion and stability [7], however, its incorporation in bioactive glasses has also been cited to severely retard apatite formation on the materials surface as the degradation rate of the glass is decreased [23]. Additionally,

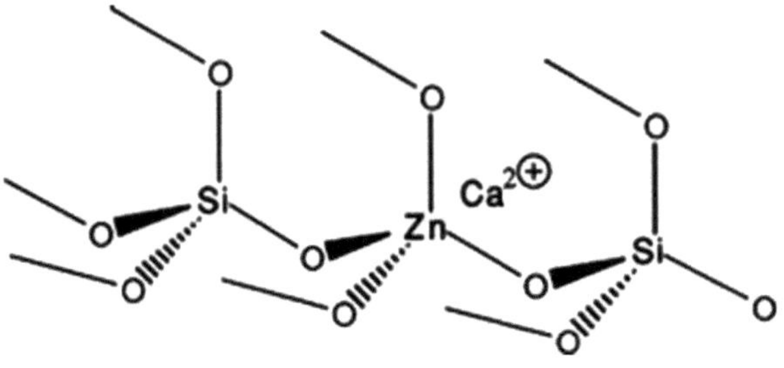

Fig. 2 The incorporation of Zn within a silicate network can form ZnO_4 tetrahedral units charge balanced by calcium ions. (Reproduced from Rabiee et al. [23])

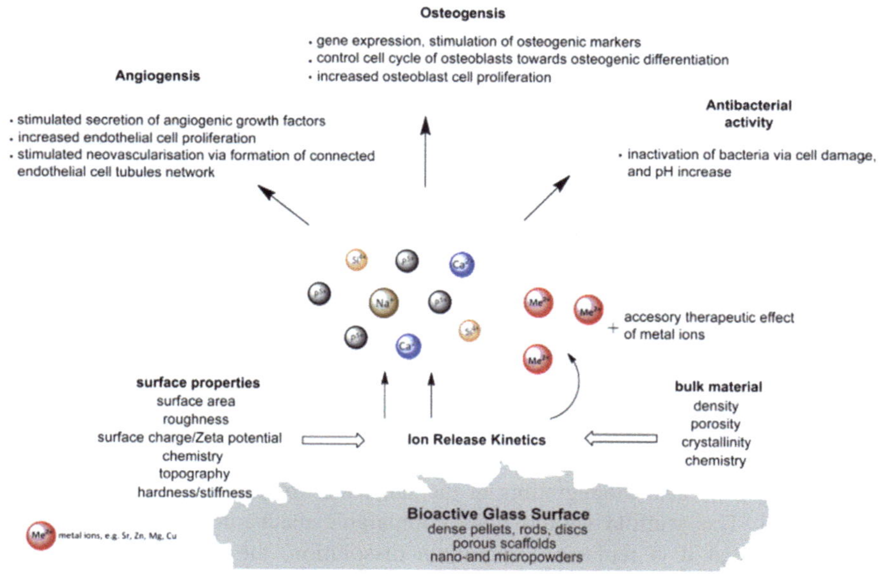

Fig. 3 Ionic dissolution products released from bioactive glasses and a summary of the therapeutic benefits they can impart. (Reproduced from Hoppe et al. [7])

non bone forming or stimulating compounds such as silver (Ag) have stimulated interest as it is cited as having excellent antimicrobial properties when incorporated into a bioactive glass or applied as a coating. However, in certain concentrations, Ag has been proved toxic to cells, i.e. glasses containing 2 wt% Ag, whereas below 1 wt% no toxic influence was observed [23]. Figure 3 presents a schematic of the diversity of ionic dissolution products from glassy materials and a summary of some of the metabolic processes that these ions are known to influence.

4 Ideal Scaffold for Skeletal Restoration

Large bone defects or voids can be treated using a number of strategies. Ideally, an autograft would be used where bone tissue is harvested from other sites in the patient's body. However, this procedure is accompanied by increased morbidity and a second surgery, and only a limited supply of bone tissue is available. Allograft tissue can also be used, however, this comes with the risk of disease transmission and infection and the possibility of tissue rejection. Artificial materials, in particular glasses and ceramics, provide a promising area of research as their composition can be designed to impart specific responses in vivo, and their solubility and mechanical stability can be controlled through the materials chemistry. Some of the current polymer and metallic materials used for orthopaedic surgery lack a number of essential characteristics; the ability to promote self repair, the ability to incorporate a blood supply and the ability to modify their structure in response to environmental factors such as mechanical forces [26]. Tissue engineered scaffold engineering is an approach that utilizes either inorganic or organic materials or a composite of both systems to fabricate a three-dimensional porous structure that can be fabricated from synthetic or natural materials. These scaffolds normally exhibit high porosity and pore interconnectivity [7]. A number of criteria have been suggested for the ideal bone scaffold. The scaffold should be biocompatible or non toxic to the host and act as a three-dimensional template for in vitro and in vivo bone growth. This three dimensional construct should consist of an interconnected macroporous network of pore diameter of at least 100 μm to permit cell movement and migration, tissue ingrowth and vascularisation [26]. The scaffold materials should encourage cell adhesion and should positively influence osteogenesis. This would facilitate the in vitro preparation of the scaffold before implantation. The material should bond to bone tissue without the formation of fibrous tissue creating a stable interfacial bond to the host while also biodegrading at the same rate that the bone tissue is being regenerated. The scaffold should have comparable mechanical properties to the bone tissue that it is replacing, and upon dissolution, the degradation products should be easily metabolized and excreted from the body. The method used to fabricate the scaffold should permit the fabrication of irregular shapes to suit the individuals bone defect, and the materials should be easily sterilized to meet clinical standards [26].

5 Scaffold Synthesis and Processing

Bioactive glass containing scaffolds can fabricated by using micron or nano sized particles to form the scaffold through sintering and controlled heat treatment, or by using the particles as a secondary phase if they are impregnated within a polymer network to impart bioactivity. Synthesis of the particles can be achieved through the traditional melt-quench method or by sol-gel processing. Solgel processing has the advantage of producing high surface area and mesoporous particles (2–50 nm) particles which results in greater adhesion and integration with living tissues [23, 26]. To form scaffolds with these materials a number of methods have been employed which include electrospinning, laser-spinning, flame spray synthesis, microemulaion, gel foaming, gel casting, 3D printing and the polymer foam replication method [23]. The foam replication method uses an organic matrix in addition to the ceramic powders and it subsequently removed using heat treatment. Numerous organic agents have been investigated including polyethylene, sucrose, corn and rice starches [27].

Numerous characterization techniques can be employed for designing and optimizing scaffolds structure and properties in addition to investigating the thermal transitions which occur during heat treatment of the composite materials. Techniques such as hot stage microscopy (HSM) can be used to determine the sintering temperature and the softening and melt temperature of glass and ceramic materials [28]. Differential thermal analysis/thermal gravimetric analysis (DTA/TGA) can be used to determine dehydration and organic removal from the scaffolds post processing. Important transition within the material can be determined such as the glass transition temperature, and the onest and arrest of crystallization. Figure 4 presents some of the thermal transitions identified by Jones et al. when fabricating solgel based 70S30C gel derived foams.

Additional techniques that can provide useful information include high temperature X-ray diffraction (HT-XRD). By employing this technique and using a constant heating rate, the evolution of specific crystal phases can be identified in addition to determining the region where the materials evolve form an amorphous material to a crystalline arrangement [28]. X-ray microtomography can be used to generate 3D images of the scaffold construct in addition to providing critical information on the scaffolds porosity [28]. This is an important characteristic as the porosity of human trabecular bone is cited to be between 80 and 90 % [29]. Nitrogen sorption analysis also yields critical information about pore diameter and pore size distribution, as a minimum of 100 μm is suggested to permit cell migration, tissue ingrowth and vascularization [26]. A study by Jones et al. combines a number of these techniques in addition to bioactivity and mechanical testing, in particular compressive testing. This study employed solgel processing to develop 70S (70 mol% SiO_2) 30C (30 mol% CaO) glasses which were subsequently heat treated a number of temperatures ranging from 600 to 1000 °C. In this study the glasses were foamed with Teepol to produce 3D scaffolds that contained pore diameters within the suggested region ranging from 100 to 500 μm. Compressive testing also revealed mechanical properties comparable to

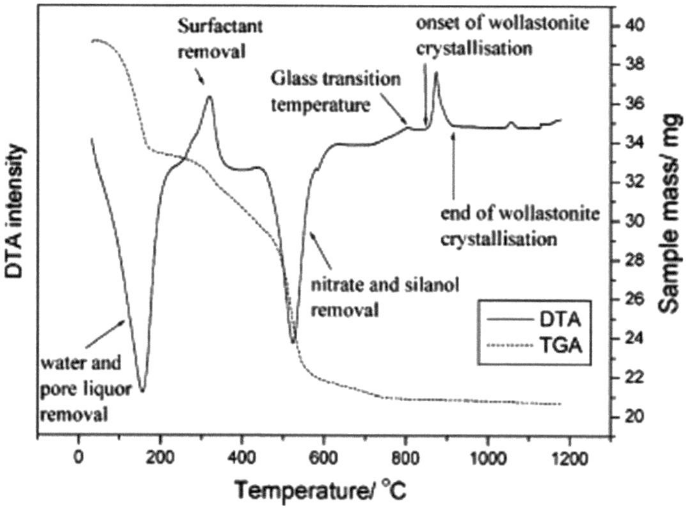

Fig. 4 Thermal transitions and weight loss of 70S30C foams using DTA/TGA. (Reproduced from Jones et al. [26])

human trabecular bone. The compressive strength of the foamed scaffolds was reported to be 2.26 MPa, which lies within the cited strength of porous bone tissue, 2–12 MPa [26].

6 45S5 Bioglass® Based Bone Tissue Scaffolds

Since its introduction in the 1960s, Bioglass® has been applied for hard tissue reconstruction and restoration in orthopedics, maxilla-facial surgery and dentistry. The first Bioglass® based product was the Ossicular Reconstruction Prosthesis tradenamed MEP® and was used to treat conductive hearing loss in the middle ear. Subsequently a monolith, the Endosseous Ridge Maintenance Implant (ERMI®) was marketed to repair tooth roots and to provide a stable ridge for dentures following tooth extraction. Bioglass® products were then synthesized and marketed in particulate form, Perioglas®, Novamin® and Novabone® to fill defects in bone tissue for both orthopedic and dental reconstruction [5, 8]. So due to the bone bonding ability of this particular glass composition, it has been investigated as a potential bone tissue scaffold. The ability of this glass to form a precipitated hydroxyapatite layer on its surface after incubation in physiological fluids makes it a highly desirable scaffold material [8]. Additionally, Bioglass® can easily be resorbed by the body which presents the possibility that the materials will resorb as bone tissue is regenerated. Moreover, Bioglass® has been proven to be non-toxic to human cells and its ionic dissolution products have even been shown to positively influence osteoblasts genes that govern the cell division cycle [6].

However, there are some negative attributed to developing scaffolds from Bioglass®. The ideal porosity of Bioglass® fabricated scaffolds significantly reduces the mechanical behavior of the 45S5 Bioglass® as they are extremely brittle. A compressive strength of 0.27–0.42 MPa is reported for a porous 45S5 Bioglass® body with a porosity of approximately 90 % and a pore size ranging from 510 to 720 μm, a value significantly lower than the reported compressive strength of trabecular bone, 2–12 MPa [27]. Another issue regarding the use of Bioglass® for tissue engineered bone scaffolds is related the processing technique. The traditional foam replication technique requires heat treatment of the scaffold to form stable constructs. This material is reported to fully crystallize prior to densification which can limit its ability to bond to bone tissue as it turns a bioactive glass into an inert material [30]. It has been suggested that crystallization of Bioglass® decreases the kinetics of HA formation rather than inhibiting it [27]. Studies by Bellucci et al. investigated the effect of porosity on Bioglass® based scaffolds which were formed by the foam replication method using polyethylene powders. During processing the sintered Bioglass® was found to crystallize to $Na_2CaSi_2O_6$ and $Na_2Ca_2Si_3O_9$, however, despite crystallization occurring, the scaffold materials were found to form a calcium phosphate (CaP) surface layer when incubated in Simulated Body Fluid (SBF) for extended time periods [27]. SBF is a synthetic fluid that contains a similar ionic composition to that of human blood plasma. It is routinely used to test for bioceramics bioactivity, as the precipitation of a CaP layer on the surface of materials when incubated in SBF for extended time periods is a positive indicator of bone bonding [31].

Studies by Boccaccini et al. have been conducted to form 45S5 Bioglass® scaffolds at different sintering temperatures. This was conducted in order to produce a higher degree of densification within the scaffolds to increase the mechanical integrity, as the kinetics of a highly porous network (increased surface area) can differ significantly from a dense ceramic [30]. For this work they use 5 μm Bioglass® particles to form scaffolds with a polyurethane foam and a polyvinyl alcohol binder (PVA). This study employed a strict heat treatment process where the scaffolds were heated to 400 °C/1 h. Sintering conditions were then specifically designed to be 900 °C/5 h; 950 °C/0–5 h; and 1000 °C/0–2 h. The heating and cooling rates were 2 and 5 °C/min, respectively [30]. This heat treatment schedule resulted in a porous scaffolds, however the cell struts were found to be significantly thicker when sintered at 1000 °C for 1 h than at 900–950 °C for 2–5 h. Figure 5 present SEM images of the 45S5 Bioglass® scaffolds which shows changes in pore structure and strut microstructure [30].

Similarly to the previous study discussed, the crystal phases that were formed post processing were found to be $Na_2Ca_2Si_3O_9$, and similarly to previous studies these scaffolds also formed initial precipitates after 3 days incubation in SBF, which progressed to spherical apatite spheres after 3 weeks. Subsequently the entire surface area of the foams were covered in a distribution of amorphous and crystalline calcium phosphate [30]. The scaffolds tested at 1000 °C for 1 h were found be structurally stable and were found to have mechanical properties ranging from 0.3 to 0.4 MPa in compression, and 0.4–0.5 MPa in bending strength [30]. Further studies to improve the mechanical properties of Bioglass® based scaffolds employed polymer coating of microfibrillated cellulose (MFC) on the exposed surface of the scaffolds. Scaffolds were synthesized by the foam burnout method [32]. Post scaffold fabrication, MFC was added in 5 and 10 wt% additions to PVA solutions and stirred and dried to form a continuous coating along the struts of the scaffold. The PVA/MFC coatings were applied to the scaffolds and subject to compressive testing. The PVA coated scaffolds were 5 times stronger than the uncoated scaffold and the addition of 5 wt% MFC increased the compressive strength tenfold. Additionally, the tensile strength was increased 20-fold also with the addition of 10 wt% MFC. Figure 6 present SEM images of the fractured struts of the MFC coated Bioglass® scaffolds [32].

The strengthening mechanism is due PVA infiltrating the scaffold strut surface defects and hindering the stress concentration in addition to providing stress transfer from the scaffold to the MFC fibers. Furthermore, fracture of MFC fibers contributed to the energy dissipation process which led to the increase of the toughness of the scaffolds [32]. The surfaces of Bioglass® based scaffolds have also been coated or treated to improve their ability to interact with organic compounds such as proteins, a process referred to as surface functionalization [11]. It is understood that cells do not directly adhere to the surfaces of materials, but the preferentially adhere to extracellular matrix component, i.e. proteins such as fibronectin and collagen.

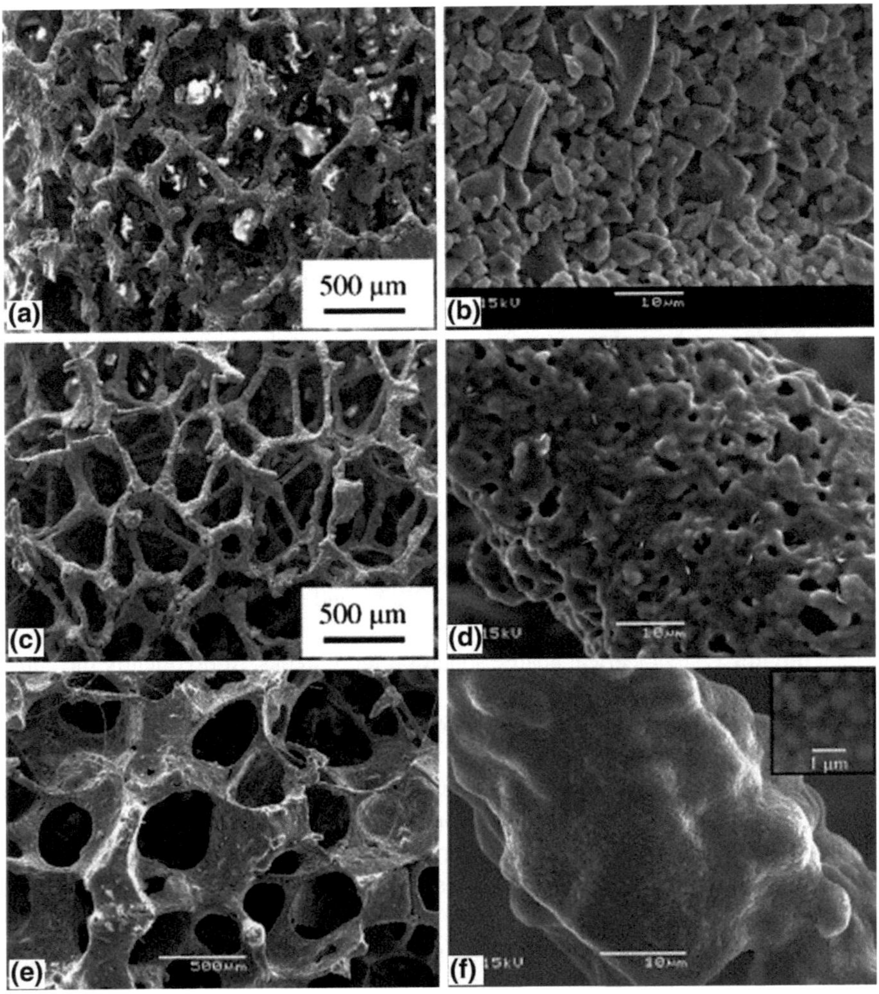

Fig. 5 Bioglass pore size and strut microstructure when processed under, **a**, **b** 900 °C for 5 h, **c**, **d** 950 °C for 2 h and **e**, **f** 1000 °C for 1 h. (Reproduced from Chen et al. [30])

For this work a Bioglass® based scaffold was produced by the foam replication method and was subsequently silanized in 3-aminopropyl-triethoxysilane (APTS) in an effort to surface functionalize the scaffold to maintain its protein binding ability, as partial crystallization can inhibit the bioactivity [11]. This study investigated the efficiency and stability of the surface modification on the scaffolds and determined that the process of surface functionalization, aqueous heat treatment, expedites the reaction of the scaffolds when tested in SBF [11]. Additional, methods of modification of Bioglass® based scaffold surfaces include coating with grapheme in an attempt to improve the scaffolds electrical properties. The grapheme coated scaffolds where synthesized using solgel processing and although these preliminary

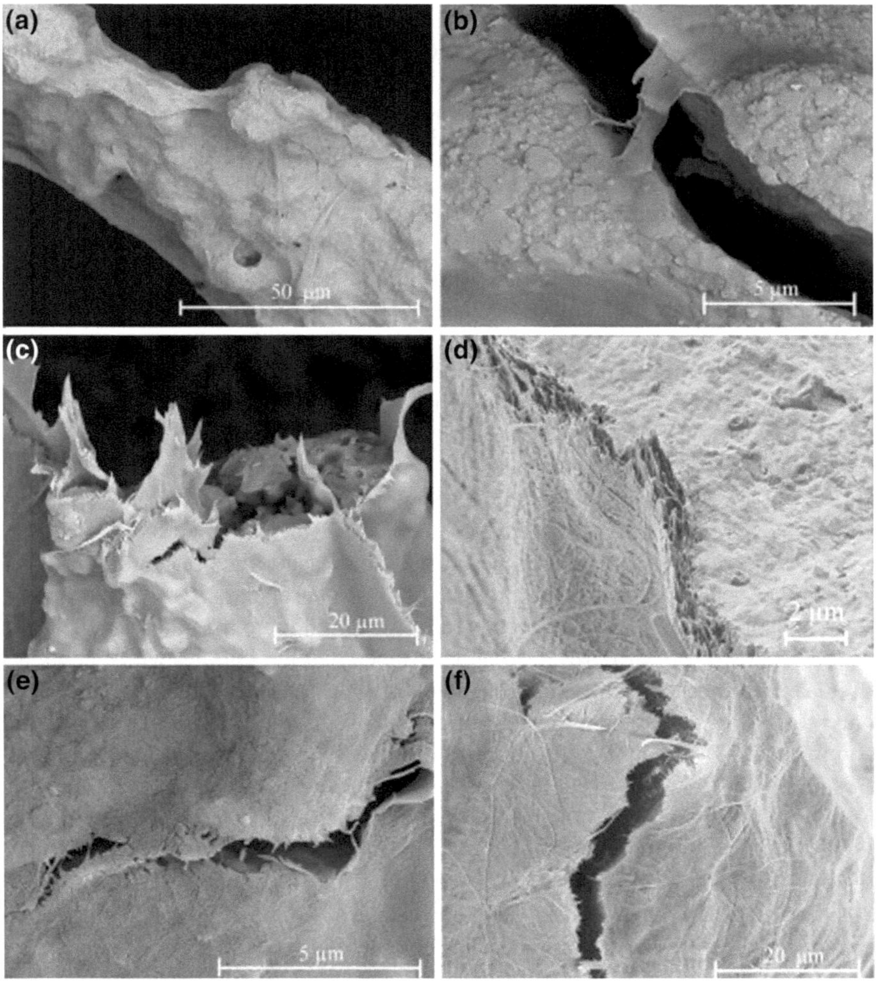

Fig. 6 SEM imaging of fractured coated scaffold struts (**a**), PVA/MFC bridging in a PVA/5 % MFC-coated specimen (**b**), struts fracture of PVA/10 %MFC-coated specimen (**c**), detail of the coating at higher magnification (**d**), bridging by the PVA/MFC pack in PVA/5 %MFC-coated specimen (**e**) and bridging by MFC fibrils only, PVA/10 %MFC-coated specimen (**f**). (Reproduced from Bertolla et al. [32])

studies did not present any significant advantage over the uncoated control, it present a very relevant and interesting hypothesis [33].

A processing method that has been investigated and applied to form higher strength, amorphous Bioglass® based scaffolds is robocasting. This technique is an extrusion based direct writing process that employs high solid paste-like suspensions (inks) to build 3D structures through layer-wise deposition of extruded cylinders. A study by Ferreira et al. used robocasting to produce Bioglass® scaffolds using carboxymethyl-cellulose (CMC) as the single processing additive. Thermal treatment was conducted to burn out CMC which was performed in air and occurred at 400 °C for 1 h. Following the binder removal, the constructs were sintered in air for 1 h at different temperatures up to 1200 °C [34]. The scaffolds contained interconnected porosities ranging from 60 to 80 % and they also achieved compressive strengths comparable to that of trabecular bone tissue (2–13 MPa). In addition scaffolds were sintered at temperatures below the crystallization temperature of 45S5 Bioglass®. This resulted in the ability to produce mechanically suitable Bioglass® based bone tissue scaffolds that retained a vitreous phase, thereby retaining its full bioactivity and therapeutic potential. Figure 7 presents SEM images of the robocast Bioglass®-CMC scaffolds [34].

Additional efforts to preserve the amorphous content of Bioglass® based scaffolds have been made by Russel et al. where they used glass mixtures of Bioglass® and a glass with low crystallization affinity (NC—58.2SiO_2–6.59CaO–18.53Na_2O–6.77MgO–10.1CaF_2 wt%). They used a number of different ratios, NC:Bioglass® 100:0, 70:30, 50:50, 30:70 and 0:100. Samples were sintered at 850 °C, a temperature lower than standard sintering temperatures which are reported up to 1050 ° C. From this study it was determined that by increasing the concentration of NC glass, more dense scaffolds were produced [35]. In particular, 70 wt% additions of NC showed much more dense constructs in addition to forming smaller pore diameters (250–400 μm). SBF testing determined that the samples which contained Bioglass® formed crystalline hydroxyapatite on the surface, while as the concentration of Bioglass® decreased, the formation of an amorphous CaP surface predominated [35]. Even though the addition of NC did reduce the degree of crystallinity, it did not prevent it. The growth of new crystal phases (rich in Mg and F) were evident when examined using X-ray diffraction and resulted in altering the solubility of the scaffolds [35].

Additional studies have been conducted to investigate the potential of Bioglass® based scaffolds to serve as drug delivery vehicles. Studies by Francis et al. have employed poly(3-hydroxybutyrate), P(3HB), to deliver gentamycin, which was encapsulated within P(3HB) microspheres. The drug loaded microspheres were coated on the surface of the Bioglass® scaffolds using a number of methods including agitation, sonication and using binders such as PVA solution. The resulting scaffolds were found to have increased compressive strength and comparable bioactivity to the coating free Bioglass® scaffolds when tested in SBF, in addition to proving a highly effective drug carrier. Figure 8 present the release profiles of gentamycin from the 45S5 Bioglass scaffolds.

Drug release profiles were tested over the period of 30 days and the cumulative rate of gentamycin release (84 %) from the microsphere coated scaffolds was found to occur in a controlled manner which is much more beneficial than the release profile from the microspheres alone, which released 95 % over a time period of 24 h [36].

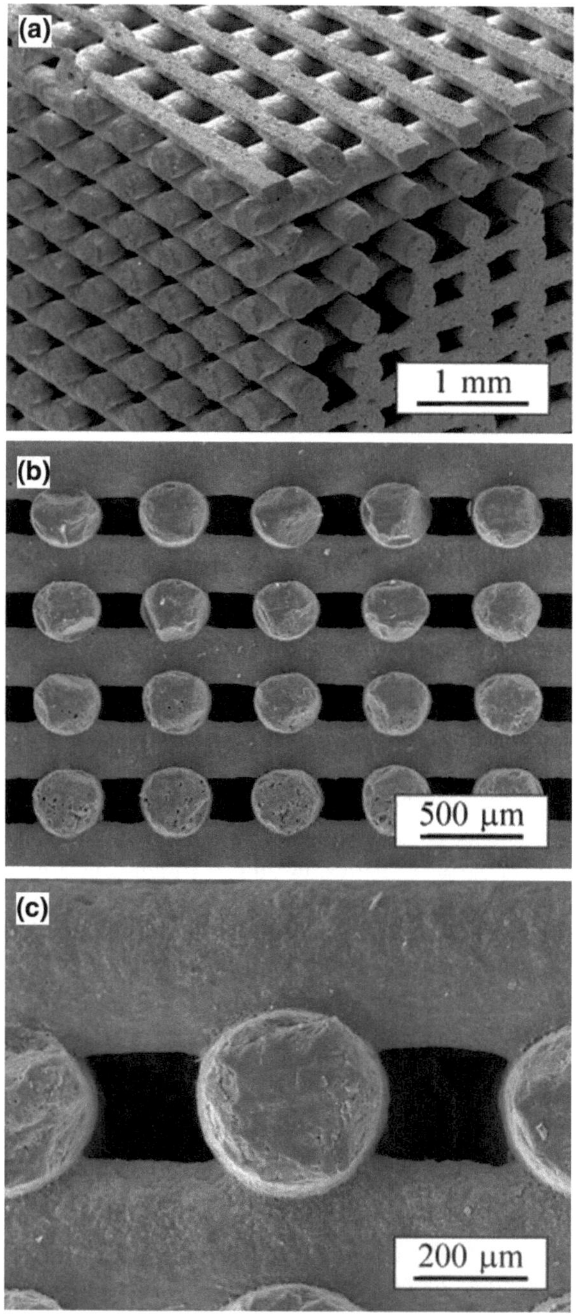

Fig. 7 SEM images of a 45S5 Bioglass® tetragonal mesh scaffold fabricated by robocasting and sintered at 1000 °C for 1 h: **a** corner view of an as-cut sample for use in uniaxial compressive tests and **b**, **c** side views of the same sample. (Reproduced from Eqtesadi et al. [34])

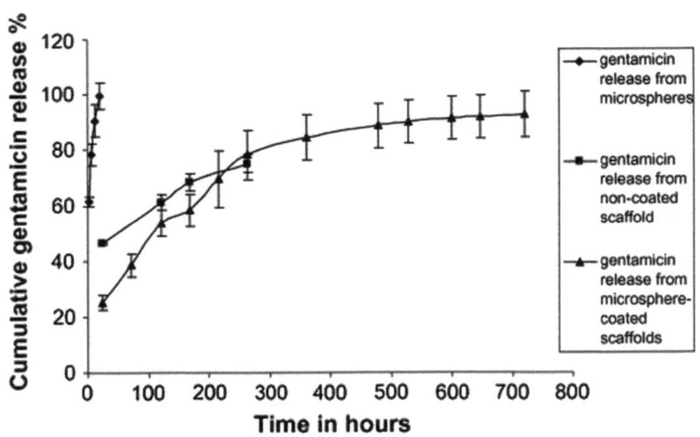

Fig. 8 Release of gentamycin from free microspheres, uncoated 45S5 Bioglass® scaffolds and microsphere-coated composites scaffolds. (Reproduced from Francis et al. [36])

6.1 Bioglass® Scaffolds Influence on Angiogenesis

Another promising area of study is the effect that the ionic dissolution products from bioactive glasses have on angiogenesis. One of the major challenges associated with bone tissue engineering includes vascularisation of the three-dimensional scaffold as the viability of the construct depends on its rapid vascularisation once implanted. To promote blood vessel formation pre-cellularised and pre-vascularised scaffolds can be developed in vitro by seeding scaffolds with co-cultures of endothelial cells, osteoblasts or osteoprogenitor cells. Additionally the incorporation of growth factors into the scaffolds can also influence the growth of blood vessels. A study conducted by Gerhardt et al. investigated the angiogenic potential of Bioglass® particles incorporated into poly(D,L lactide) (PDLLA) [37]. Figure 9 shows the secretion of VEGF by human CCD-18Co fibroblasts. The addition of Bioglass® significantly improved angiogenic signaling compared to the control PDLLA materials.

Composites were formed with micron sized (m-BG) and nano-sized (n-BG) Bioglass® particles. The study investigated the secretion of vascular endothelial growth factors (VEGF) by human fibroblasts in contact with the composite materials. It was shown the highest additions of m-BG or n-BG (20 wt%), human fibroblasts produced 5 times higher VEGF than on pure control PDLLA materials. Additionally, after 8 weeks implanted in rat models the m-BG and n-BG were infiltrated with newly formed tissue and demonstrated higher vascularisation and percentage blood vessel to tissue than PDLLA scaffolds [37]. Further studies by Kent Leach et al. [38] on the angiogenic potential of Bioglass® coated VEGF scaffolds determined that enhanced mitogenic stimulation of endothelial cells was observed particularly in the presence of the bioactive glass coating.

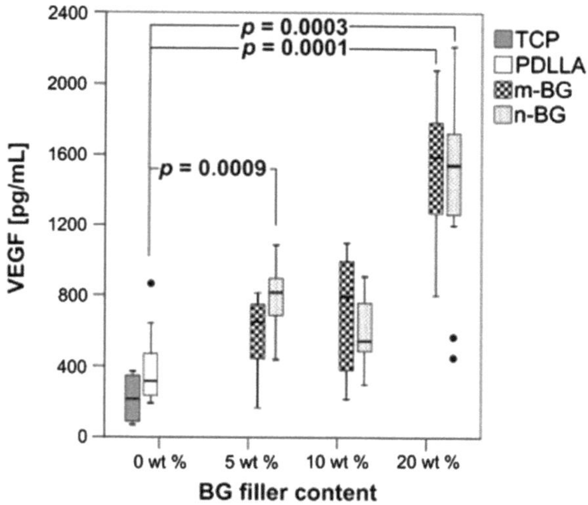

Fig. 9 Influence of BG filler content and particle size on the secretion of VEGF by human CCD-18Co fibroblasts. (Reproduced from Gerhardt et al. [37])

7 Chapter Summary

45S5 Bioglass® is widely regarded as the foundation of bioactive glass based materials. Since its invention and success in early dental applications, it has been heavily investigated and applied, in particular, to skeletal repair for porous, biodegradable bioactive scaffolds. Bioglass® particles can be employed with polymers to form the composite scaffold itself or they can be applied as coatings to the scaffold struts. Numerous synthesis methods and processing conditions can be used to fabricate scaffolds with different critical properties such as porosity and exposed surface area, solubility and mechanical integrity. Additionally, Bioglass® based scaffolds can be modified to deliver therapeutics such as antibiotics and organic compounds to stimulate bones regenerative properties or to positively influence critical wound healing processes such as minimizing the inflammatory response and increasing the rate of blood vessel growth within the scaffolds. These properties, attributed to 45S5 Bioglass®, has greatly supported its incorporation into bioceramic based scaffold materials and has, to a great extent, stimulated interest in developing non-Bioglass® based scaffolds for skeletal repair.

References

1. Martini, F.R.: Fundamentals of Anatomy and Physiology. Pearson Eductaion International, San Francisco (2006)
2. Fogelman, I., Gnanasegaran, G., van der Wall, H. (eds.): Radionuclide and Hybrid Bone Imaging. Springer, Berlin (2013)
3. Kular, J., Tickner, J., Chim, S.M., Xu, J.: An overview of the regulation of bone remodelling at the cellular level. Clin. Biochem. **45**, 863–873 (2012)

4. Faour, O., Dimitriou, R., Cousins, C.A., Giannoudis, P.V.: The use of bone graft substitutes in large cancellous voids: any specific needs? Injury **42**, S87–S90 (2011)
5. Hench, L.L.: The story of bioglass. J. Mater. Sci. Mater. Med. **17**, 967–978 (2006)
6. Hench, L.L.: Genetic design of bioactive glass. J. Eur. Ceram. Soc. **29**, 1257–1265 (2009)
7. Hoppe, A., Guldal, N.S., Boccaccini, A.R.: A review of the biological response to ionic dissolution products from bioactive glasses and glass-ceramics. Biomaterials **32**, 2757–2774 (2011)
8. Jones, J.R.: Review of bioactive glass: from Hench to hybrids. Acta Biomater. **9**, 4457–4486 (2013)
9. Haimi, S., Gorianc, G., Moimas, L., Lindroos, B., Huhtala, H., Raty, S., Kuokkanen, H., Sandor, G.K., Schmid, C., Miettinen, S., Suuronen, R.: Characterization of zinc-releasing three-dimensional bioactive glass scaffolds and their effect on human adipose stem cell proliferation and osteogenic differentiation. Acta Biomater. **5**, 3122–3131 (2009)
10. Vargas, G.E., Mesones, R.V., Bretcanu, O., López, J.M.P., Boccaccini, A.R., Gorustovich, A.: Biocompatibility and bone mineralization potential of 45S5 Bioglass®-derived glass-ceramic scaffolds in chick embryos. Acta Biomater. **5**, 374–380 (2009)
11. Chen, Q.-Z., Rezwan, K., Françon, V., Armitage, D., Nazhat, S.N., Jones, F.H., Boccaccini, A.R.: Surface functionalization of Bioglass®-derived porous scaffolds. Acta Biomater. **3**, 551–562 (2007)
12. Moshaverinia, A., Ansari, S., Moshaverinia, M., Roohpour, N., Darr, J.A., Rehman, I.: Effects of incorporation of hydroxyapatite and fluoroapatite nanobioceramics into conventional glass ionomer cements (GIC). Acta Biomater. **4**, 432–440 (2008)
13. Hatton, P.V., Hurrell-Gillingham, K., Reaney, I.M., Miller, C.A., Crawford, A.: Devitrification of ionomer glass and its effect on the in vitro biocompatability of glass ionomer cements. Biomaterials **24**, 3153–3160 (2003)
14. Hatton, P.V., Hurrell-Gillingham, K., Brook, I.M.: Biocompatability of glass ionomer bone cements. J. Dent. **34**, 598–601 (2006)
15. Ravarian, R., Moztarzadeh, F., Hashjin, M.S., Rabiee, S.M., Khoshakhlagh, P., Tahriri, M.: Synthesis, characterization and bioactivity investigation of bioglass/hydroxyapatite composite. Ceram. Int. **36**, 291–297 (2010)
16. Bortot, M.B., Prastalo, S., Prado, M.: Production and characterization of glass microspheres for hepatic cancer treatment. Proced. Mater. Sci. **1**, 351–358 (2012)
17. Anderson, J.H., Goldberg, J.A., Bessent, R.G., Kerr, D.J., McKillop, J.H., Stewart, I., Cooke, T.G., McArdle, C.S.: Glass yttrium-90 microspheres for patients with colorectal liver metastases. Radiother. Oncol. **25**, 137–139 (1992)
18. Rahaman, M.N., Day, D.E., Sonny Bal, B., Fu, Q., Jung, S.B., Bonewald, L.F., Tomsia, A.P.: Bioactive glass in tissue engineering. Acta Biomater. **7**, 2355–2373 (2011)
19. Shelby, J.E.: Introduction to Glass Science and Technology, 2nd edn. The Royal Socitey of Chemistry, Cambridge (2005)
20. Clark, D.E., Dilmore, M.F., Ethridge, E.C., Hench, L.L.: Aqueous corrosion of soda-silicate and soda-lime-silicate glass. J. Am. Ceram. Soc. **59**, 62–65 (1976)
21. Serra, J., Gonzalez, P., Liste, S., Chiussi, S., Leon, B., Perez-amor, M., Ylanen, H.O., Hupa, M.: Influence of the non-bridging oxygen groups on the bioactivity of silicate glasses. J. Mater. Sci. Mater. Med. **13**, 1221–1225 (2002)
22. Paul A.: Chemistry of Glasses. 2nd edn. Chapman and Hall, London (1990)
23. Rabiee, S.M., Nazparvar, N., Azizian, M., Vashaee, D., Tayebi, L.: Effect of ion substitution on properties of bioactive glasses: a review. Ceram. Int. **41**, 7241–7251 (2015)
24. Marie, P.J.: Strontium ranelate; a novel mode of action optimizing bone formation and resorption. Osteoporos. Int. **16**, S7–S10 (2005)
25. Marie, P.J.: Strontium ranelate: new insights into its dual mode of action. Bone **40**(1), S5–S8 (2007)
26. Jones, J.R., Ehrenfried, L.M., Hench, L.L.: Optimising bioactive glass scaffolds for bone tissue engineering. Biomaterials **27**, 964–973 (2006)

27. Bellucci, D., Cannillo, V., Sola, A., Chiellini, F., Gazzarri, M., Migone, C.: Macroporous Bioglass®-derived scaffolds for bone tissue regeneration. Ceram. Int. **37**, 1575–1585 (2011)
28. Wren, A.W., Coughlan, A., Smale, K.E., Misture, S.T., Mahon, B.P., Clarkin, O.M., Towler, M.R.: Fabrication of CaO–NaO–SiO_2/TiO_2 scaffolds for surgical applications. J. Mater. Sci. Mater. Med. **23**, 2881–2891 (2012)
29. Ochoa, I., Sanz-Herrera, J.A., García-Aznar, J.M., Doblaré, M., Yunos, D.M., Boccaccini, A. R.: Permeability evaluation of 45S5 Bioglass®-based scaffolds for bone tissue engineering. J. Biomech. **42**, 257–260 (2009)
30. Chen, Q.Z., Thompson, I.D., Boccaccini, A.R.: 45S5 Bioglass®-derived glass–ceramic scaffolds for bone tissue engineering. Biomaterials **27**, 2414–2425 (2006)
31. Kokubo, T., Takadama, H.: How useful is SBF in predicting in vivo bone bioactivity. Biomaterials **27**, 2907–2915 (2006)
32. Bertolla, L., Dlouhý, I., Boccaccini, A.R.: Preparation and characterization of Bioglass®-based scaffolds reinforced by poly-vinyl alcohol/microfibrillated cellulose composite coating. J. Eur. Ceram. Soc. **34**, 3379–3387 (2014)
33. Fabbri, P., Valentini, L., Hum, J., Detsch, R., Boccaccini, A.R.: 45S5 Bioglass®-derived scaffolds coated with organic–inorganic hybrids containing graphene. Mater. Sci. Eng., C **33**, 3592–3600 (2013)
34. Eqtesadi, S., Motealleh, A., Miranda, P., Pajares, A., Lemos, A., Ferreira, J.M.F.: Robocasting of 45S5 bioactive glass scaffolds for bone tissue engineering. J. Eur. Ceram. Soc. **34**, 107–118 (2014)
35. Farag, M.M., Rüssel, C.: Glass-ceramic scaffolds derived from Bioglass® and glass with low crystallization affinity for bone regeneration. Mater. Lett. **73**, 161–165 (2012)
36. Francis, L., Meng, D., Knowles, J.C., Roy, I., Boccaccini, A.R.: Multi-functional P(3HB) microsphere/45S5 Bioglass®-based composite scaffolds for bone tissue engineering. Acta Biomater. **6**, 2773–2786 (2010)
37. Gerhardt, L.-C., Widdows, K.L., Erol, M.M., Burch, C.W., Sanz-Herrera, J.A., Ochoa, I., Stampfli, R., Roqan, I.S., Gabe, S., Ansari, T., Boccaccini, A.R.: The pro-angiogenic properties of multi-functional bioactive glass composite scaffolds. Biomaterials **32**, 4096–4108 (2011)
38. Kent Leach, J., Kaigler, D., Wang, Z., Krebsbach, P.H., Mooney, D.J.: Coating of VEGF-releasing scaffolds with bioactive glass for angiogenesis and bone regeneration. Biomaterials **27**, 3249–3255 (2006)

Vitreous Materials for Dental Restoration and Reconstruction

Anthony W. Wren

Abstract Glasses are a highly versatile class of materials that have been utilized for numerous applications in restorative dentistry. Their use in dentistry ranges from reconstruction of the underlying bone tissue used to house or support metallic implants, to glass based adhesive materials for tooth restoration. The destruction of alveolar bone tissue, due to periodontitis or periapical infection, leads to resorption of the underlying bone tissue that needs to support constructs required for implant surgery. The Bioglass based system (SiO_2–CaO–Na_2O–P_2O_5) can provide the required ionic dissolution characteristics to promote mineral deposition in bone tissue which subsequently results in the formation of hydroxyapatite (HAp) and a permanent interfacial bond. The success of this particular composition has resulted in a range of commercial materials that can be applied to procedures such as guided bone regeneration (GBR) and to improve resistance to dentin associated hypersensitivity. Glasses can also be applied in a composite form to aid in the restoration of de-mineralized tooth after carie formation, or to fix metal based constructs to the tooth enamel. The predominant types of glass based dental adhesive materials are glass polyalkenoate cements (GPCs). These materials generally consist of a SiO_2–Al_2O_3–CaO/CaF based glass, and when mixed with a polyalkenoic acid (PAA) and water, set to form a solid matrix. GPCs are commonly used as cavity fillers, liners and as luting agents as they form a strong bond to the mineral phase of tooth, have the ability to release fluoride in the oral environment and have appropriate handling and mechanical properties for their intended application.

1 Dental Anatomy and Tooth Restoration

Each tooth can be divided in two regions, the *crown* and the *root* [1]. The crown is covered with *enamel*, which is the hardest mineral in the human body where is consists of up to 96 wt% hydroxyapatite (HAp) mineral, with the remaining being

A.W. Wren (✉)
Inamori School of Engineering, Alfred University, Alfred, NY, USA
e-mail: wren@alfred.edu

J. Marchi (ed.), *Biocompatible Glasses*, Advanced Structured Materials 53,
DOI 10.1007/978-3-319-44249-5_8

protein and water [2]. The root portion of the tooth is covered with *cementum* [3]. The crown and the root portion join at the at the *cemento-enamel junction* (CEJ) [1]. The bulk of dental tissue is composed of *dentin* which is also a mineralized tissue which contains a higher organic content than its enamel covering. Dentin represents the load bearing component of the tooth and is more similar to bone tissue as it consists of primarily type I collagen fibrils, water and nanocrystallites of HAp [4]. Dentin also contains *tubules* which run perpendicular to the tooth surface that contains *fluids* and *odontoblastic processes* which houses projections of the primary cell type of dental tissues, *odontoblasts*. Odontoblasts are dentin forming cells and are tall columnar cells located between the pulp and the primary dentin [5]. Their functions include secretion of dentin matrix proteins, regulating the mineralization process and they are involved in the transmission of stimuli from the external environment to the pulp [5]. In the center of the tooth is a mineral free cavity that contains dental cells, connective tissue, blood vessels, nerve endings and lymphatics [1]. This region is called the *dental pulp* and its primary function is to form the dentin of the tooth. Dental pulp initially begins as a large chamber which progressively becomes smaller as the tooth matures. The opening of the pulp cavity is located at the *apex;* which is constricted through the *root canal,* and is called the *apical foramen* [1]. The tooth itself is held in place by the *periodontal ligament* which is composed of connective tissue fibers that securely anchors the tooth to the surrounding bone tissue. The two bone structures that house the tooth are the maxilla (*upper jaw*) and the mandible (*lower jaw*) and are the primary bones of the facial skeleton [1]. The maxilla is divided into a left and right section and is fused to the skeleton. The mandible has no osseous union with the skull and is a movable joint. The *alveolar process* makes up the inferior portion of the bone cavities that surrounds the roots of the tooth and provides osseous support [1]. The alveolar process is maintained by the presence of the teeth. Should any tooth be lost, that portion of the alveolar process that supports the missing tooth will be subject to atrophic reduction. Should all of the teeth be lost, the alveolar process will eventually be lost [1].

Dental implants can be separated into two categories called endosteal (endosseous) implants which are incorporated into the bone tissue, or subperiosteal systems, which contact the exterior bone surfaces [6]. Endosteal forms, such as root devices include cylinders, screws, plateaus, blades are placed into the bone tissue [6]. However, in order for these materials to be placed within the bone tissue, it must be in good health. Glass based materials can be applied for dental repair to either promote alveolar bone re-growth to support dental implant devices, encourage re-mineralization of exposed dental tissue surface or restoration of the tooth structure itself after carie formation and destruction of the tooth anatomy. The following section will focus on the application of glass based materials for dental applications that include re-mineralization of the supporting bone tissue and the tooth surfaces.

2 Skeletal Repair to Support Dental Surgery

Forty years or so ago, the transition from bioinert materials to bioactive materials became evident when glasses, that were applied for skeletal repair, stimulated a highly desirable and positive response in the human body. This was the formation of a strong chemical interfacial bond between the glassy material and the hosts bone and soft tissue [7, 8]. This was a significant discovery as this glass composition was initially designed using the SiO–Na_2O–CaO_2 ternary phase diagram for ceramics after the realization that if materials could be designed to form a hydrated calcium phosphate or Hydroxyapatite (HAp) surface layer, they may not be rejected by the body through fibrous scar tissue formation [7]. Dr. Larry Hench was the first to report that these glasses, which he developed as part of a US Army Medical R and D Command funded project, with a specific composition 45 % SiO_2, 24.5 % Na_2O, 24.5 % CaO, 6 %P_2O_5 (termed Bioglass®) formed a direct bond to bone tissue in rat femoral implant models. The small rectangular glass cast implants were inserted into rat femurs and over the course of 6 weeks, formed a strong interfacial bond to the bone as opposed to the control samples which were easily removed [7]. This lead to the development of osteoinductive, osseoconductive and regenerative products for replacement or regeneration of bone structure required for placement of dental devices. Alveolar bone is the primary support construct for teeth and dental implant materials. The loss of teeth and/or alveolar bone tissue through lack of osseous stimulation results in gradual bone loss, which is manifested in both bone density and volume [9] (Fig. 1).

If the tooth and periodontal ligament are removed, the body initiates resorption of the alveolar bone [9, 11]. Osteoclastic activity increases and the alveolar ridge is continually eroded. If this process is not intercepted quickly, there will be a number of negative consequences dealt to the patient. Extensive resorption of the bony processes restricts the quality of the dental restoration available, which will subsequently affect the recipient's quality of life [11]. In order to restore the underlying bone tissue, a number of criteria have been suggested for the ideal implant material to possess to support alveolar ridge restoration [12]. These include no evidence of early resorption of the implanted material; acceptable strength to fill the space without fracture under masticatory forces; strong attachment to the soft and hard tissues at the implant interface; and no adverse reactions to the host [12]. Without intervention and the use of suitable supportive implant materials, severe alveolar bone resorption will occur and this will subsequently require extensive grafting to support dental implants [11]. The ability of glasses to initiate bone reconstruction is related to its biodegradation properties in an aqueous environment. The following section details the methods we can employ to evaluate glasses aqueous potential for skeletal and dental restoration.

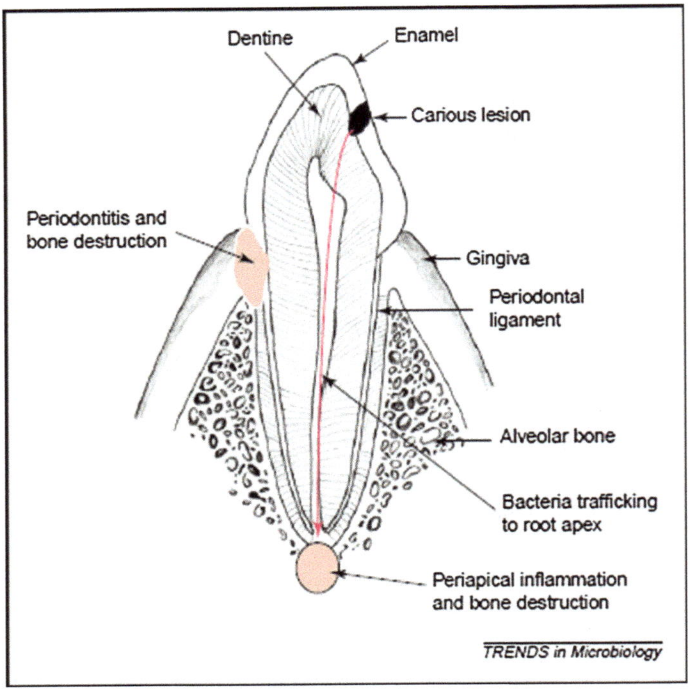

Fig. 1 Anatomy of the alveolar region supporting the tooth. Periodontitis and periapical infection can result in tooth loss which subsequently influences alveolar bone density. (Reproduced from Henderson et al. [10])

3 Aqueous Evaluation of Glasses for Dental Restoration

The initial tests conducted by Hench and associates described critical information about the compositional characteristics required to design glass based biomaterials for positive interactions with hard tissues. The early studies were initially conducted using silicate based glass compositions that contained less than 60 wt% SiO_2. Formulations that contain higher levels of SiO_2 were found to inhibit bone bonding behavior [13]. Similarly, if multivalent cations such as Al^{3+}, Ti^{4+} or Ta^{5+} are added, it reduced the bone bonding potential. Studies by Dr. June Wilson on the interfacial interactions of soft tissues with Bioglass® showed that glasses exceeding 52 wt% SiO_2 will still bone to bone, but not to soft tissues [7]. This discovery, in addition to the high amounts of Na_2O and CaO as well as the relatively high CaO/P_2O_5 ratio, makes these glass surfaces highly reactive in physiological environments [8]. These key compositional characteristics lead to dissolution of the glass surfaces in physiological fluids that leads to the formation of a HA surface layer, which is largely attributed to their ability to bond to mineralized tissues. The mechanism of mineral formation has been widely investigated in vivo and in vitro and has led to the generation of artificial physiological fluids that aim to represent the natural host's aqueous environment. Fluids such as Simulated Body Fluid (*SBF*) [14, 15] and Artificial Saliva (*AS*) mimic the aqueous host environment and are commonly used as a preliminary test for bioceramic's (glass and ceramic based biomaterials) bioactivity. The compositions of SAGF *Artificial Saliva* and *Simulated Body Fluid* are presented in Table 1.

These solutions do not precisely represent the host aqueous environment as the organic components, i.e. soluble proteins, hormones, vitamins, glucose and cellular components are largely absent [13]. *SBF* is a solution that contains an ionic composition that is representative of human blood plasma and is widely used to test dental bioceramics potential to induce mineral deposition for maxillofacial restoration and alveolar bone re-growth. *AS* is difficult to reproduce accurately as saliva is a mixture of a number of natural fluids with varying composition which are secreted by the parotid, submaxillary and sub lingual glands [17]. Its composition also varies among the same individual and is largely subject to parameters such as changes in health condition, diet and time of day [17, 18]. Numerous formulations for simulating AS have been presented, with the earliest formulation being designed by Gal et al. [18]. A review of approximately 60 *AS* compositions are conducted by Gal et al. highlights the compositions that are most commonly used experimentally. *AS* is generally an inorganic fluid that principally contains Ca^{2+}, CO_3, P, Mg^{2+}, K^+, Na^+, Cl^-, SCN^-, NH_4^+ with a pH that ranges between 5.1 and 7.7 [18]. Studies have been conducted to incorporate the glycoprotein organic component of saliva as this imparts the viscosity attributed to natural saliva. This viscosity most likely influences the diffusion rates of solutes and hence the surface reactivity and solubility of bioceramic materials are likely affected by its absence [18]. Both of these synthetic media are extensively used to determine the effect that the ionic dissolution products from bioceramic materials have with respect to the precipitation of an amorphous calcium phosphate (CaP) and/or crystalline Hydroxyapatite

Table 1 Composition of SAGF artificial Saliva [16] and simulated body fluid [15]

SAGF artificial saliva (AS) pH 6.7		Simulated body fluid (SBF) pH 7.4	
Compound	Concentration (mg/l$^-$)	Compound	Concentration (g/l)
NaCl	125.64	NaCl	8.035
KCl	963.90	$NaHCO_3$	0.355
KSCN	189.20	KCl	0.225
KH_2PO_4	654.50	$K_2HPO_4 \cdot 3H_2O$	0.231
$CO(NH_2)_2$	200.00	$MgCl_2 \cdot 6H_2O$	0.311
$CaCl_2 \cdot 2H_20$	227.80	1.0 M-HCl	39 ml
$Na_2SO_4 \cdot 10H_20$	763.20	$CaCl_2$	0.292
NH_4Cl	178.00	Na_2SO_4	0.072
$NaHCO_3$	630.80	Tris	6.118
–	–	1.0 M-HCl	0–5 ml

(Reproduced from Levallois et al. [16] and Kokubo et al. [15])

(HAp) surface layer after incubation and solution exchange over time. Additionally, researchers can employ these media, which is compositionally more similar to our own physiological fluids than either sterile de-ionized water or buffered solutions (TRIS), to investigate properties such as ion release kinetics. The mechanism of HAp layer formation on the surface of bioactive glasses is attributed to a number of stages which involve calcium dissolving from the material into the surrounding solution while a Si-rich intermediate layer forms on the glass surface. Nucleation is possible as the surrounding solution becomes supersaturated due to the dissolution of Ca ions. In addition, the Si-rich intermediate layer presents soluble Si which provides favorable sites for the nucleation sequence. The process of nucleation and growth of the HAp layer is facilitated by the interaction of calcium, phosphate and hydroxide ions [8, 13, 15].

Bioceramics solubility profiles can differ and can be modified by a number of different characteristics which includes; altering the local pH, modifying the chemical composition of the material, increasing or decreasing the degree of crystallinity and by changing the particle size, exposed surface area and porosity of the material [11]. Additional factors such as the Ca/P ratio can also lead to changes in the dissolution characteristics, i.e. the greater the Ca/P molar ratio is, the lower the materials solubility [11]. Modifying the solubility of the materials reflects in the in vivo rate of degradation and the subsequent bioactive response. The ability to modify this process leads to bioceramics being a highly versatile class of materials.

4 Bioglass® Based Dental Restorative Materials

The first Bioglass® based implants were cleared for marketing in the US to treat conductive hearing loss by replacing the bones of the middle ear. This device was called Bioglass® Ossicular Reconstruction Prosthesis and tradenamed MEP®. This device was able to bond to both bone and soft tissue i.e. the tympanic membrane. The success of MEP® led to the development of numerous Bioglass® based hard tissue replacement devices. The devices that are relevant to the field of dentistry and that are applied for restoration of bone tissue required for effective dental surgery is presented in the following section.

4.1 Endosseous Ridge Maintenance Implant (ERMI®)—Monolithic Materials

Due to the success of these early studies the second Bioglass® based device that was given market approval was the Endosseous Ridge Maintenance Implant (ERMI®) device [7]. This device was designed to repair the tooth roots and to provide a stable ridge for dentures following tooth extraction. This was a 45S5 Bioglass®

composition that was fabricated into a cone shaped monolith such that it could be implanted into cavities in the jaw bone following the removal of teeth. Removal of a tooth produces changes in the jaw bone which are followed by gradual bone loss such that the normal shape of the bone tissue, which supported the healthy tooth, change in shape to a narrow knife-edge ridge with reduced height [19]. This morphological change in the bone geometry cannot comfortably support dentures. To prevent this bone loss the Bioglass ERMI® device can be implanted into the cavities and it has been reported that after 1 h of implantation, the formation of a chemical bond to the bone tissue appeared. The prevention of the bone loss provided a much more comfortable and suitable base for dentures [19]. These implants were highly stable and proved more successful than HA tooth root implants. One of the limitations of this device was that they came in pre-fabricated shapes which limited the surgeons to using fixed sized cones for each surgery [8, 13].

4.2 *Perioglas®: 90–710 μm Glass Particles*

The success of the Bioglass® continued with the development of implantable particles which ranged from 90–710 μm in diameter. Particles were preferred as the surgeons could press and compact particles into irregular defects as opposed to using prefabricated monoliths. Perioglas® was initially released by NovaBone Products LLC in 1993 to restore bone loss in the jaw which resulted from periodontal disease and in surgical procedures such as Guided Tissue Regeneration (GTR) [13, 20]. GTR is a surgical technique used to direct and stimulate regeneration of periapical bone tissue. The main problem being that the soft tissues, such as gingival connective tissue or the migration of the oral epithelium into the bone defect, can quickly occur after the insult which can prevent the formation of new trabecular bone [20]. The use of synthetic bone substitutes (such as Perioglas®, Biogran®) in addition to non-absorbable and bioabsorbable membranes (e-PTFE, lactic acid, collagen type I, polyglycolic acid) can be used to facilitate cellular re-growth within the periodontal defect [21]. GTR is a technique for enhancing and directing cell growth to repopulate specific parts of the periodontium that have been damaged by periodontal diseases, tooth diseases, or trauma [22, 23]. Two case studies on the use of Periolgas® have been reported by Lokade et al. where periapical bone tissue was severely reduced after both patients experienced trauma resulting in tooth loss. Initially, severe periapical bone loss was evident in both patients and each was selected for treatment with Perioglas® and a GTR membrane and was observed over 6 months to 1 year [20]. In each case the patients were found to experience a significant decrease in the periapical translucency over time when observed under X-ray which was attributed to new bone deposition [20].

In addition to having bone forming properties, Perioglass® has also been cited to have the additional beneficial effects of being anti-inflammatory and antibacterial [17, 24]. Studies by Wilson et al. were conducted to determine if the cascade of surface reactions in aqueous media that are responsible for the osseointegration process also impart antibacterial properties in a range of oral bacteria. This study evaluated the antimicrobial dissolution effects of Bioglass® when immersed in nutrient broth (*NB*), artifcial saliva (*AS*) or Dulbecco's modifed eagle medium plus 10 % fetal calf serum. Each of the bacteria tested i.e. *Streptococcus sanguis, Streptococcus mutans* and *Actinomyces viscosus,* showed reduced viability following 1 h exposure to Bioglass®, and this effect was found to increase after 3 h [25]. Similar effects were found in a number of other bacteria which include *Porphyromonas gingivalis, Fusobacterium nucleatum, Prevotella intermedia* and *Actinobacillus actinomycetemcomitans.* A considerable reduction in viability was observed with all bacteria tested, in both media, compared to inert glass controls [25]. Additional studies have been conducted to improve the antibacterial response of the Bioglass® by including elements such as silver (Ag). The appeal of the Ag ion is a result of its broad-spectrum antimicrobial efficacy. Ag is particularly effective for treating poly-microbial colonization associated with biomaterial related infections. Bacteria do not generally tend to develop resistance to silver-based materials [26]. Therefore, both metallic and ionic silver have been incorporated into numerous polymer and ceramic biomaterials such as polyurethane, hydroxyapatite (HA) and bioactive glasses. Studies using Ag-modified Bioglass® systems have been conducted by Ferreira et al. where *E. coli* cultures were greatly reduced by incorporating Ag into the Bioglass® system [26]. These modified particles can also be incorporated as a coating on metals such as titanium which is used extensively in both orthopedic and dental surgery [27], to reduce the chances of infection [28]. Septic complications can often result in poor functional outcomes and can ultimately involve revision surgery. Figure 2 shows the comparison of Bioglass® and Ag doped Bioglass® on *E. coli* cultures after 72 h of exposure.

Additionally, the anit-inflammatory response of Bioglass® has been studied by Moldawer et al. where they implanted 50 mg (5 μm Bioglass® particles) intraperitoneally in C57BL/6 mice. Leukocyte and cytokine levels in the peritoneal fluid were subsequently analyzed. This study concluded that exposure to Bioglass®

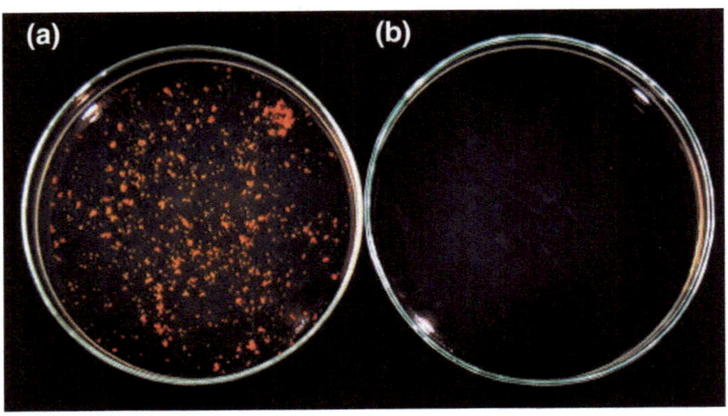

Fig. 2 Image of the effect of **a** Bioglass® and **b** AgBioglass on *E. coli* in culture medium containing 20 mg/ml of Bioglass after 72 h exposure. (Reproduced from Balamurugan et al. [26])

produced an IL-6 response without the associated expression of TNF-α or IL-1α which suppressed the inflammatory response to endotoxin, likely through the early induction of IL-6. Additionally, the Bioglass® did not induce white cell recruitment into the periodontal extract fluids [29]. Studies by Chang et al. investigated the effect of Bioglass® on wound healing using human umbilical vein endothelial cells (HUVEC). They found that in vivo wound healing of full thickness excisional wounds in rats is accelerated by the inclusion of Bioglass® and was associated with reduced inflammation during the initial stages of healing [30]. These properties greatly support the use of the Bioglass® composition for restoration of alveolar bone loss.

Perioglas® has also be used to produce a slurry to assist in root canal surgery prior to insertion of implants. This slurry assists by raising the local pH to levels that become bactericidal [13]. Another application includes re-mineralization of dentin by using an ultrafine particle size. Dentin and enamel are dental tissues that can both suffer the consequences of bacterial biofilm formation as these microbes produce organic acids that can dissolve both of these hard tissue layers. The loss of mineral is normally counterbalanced by deposition of minerals from saliva or oral fluids, a term referred to a re-mineralization. The solubility and osteoconductive properties of the Bioglass® composition makes it a suitable candidate to aid in the dentin re-mineralization process [31]. Vollenweider et al. synthesized nanosized Perioglas® particles using flame spray synthesis and compared the efficacy to the analogous micron-sized controls [31]. This study employed 20–50 nm particles and compared them to the micron-sized analogues. Figure 3 shows the nano and micron sized Perioglas® particles used for this particular study [31].

Dentin bars were prepared from human third molars following extraction and were used to evaluate the re-mineralization efficacy of the glass particles. This study concluded that re-mineralization of the dentin is encouraged by nanometric particles when compared to the commercial sized Perioglas® in terms of mineral weight [31]. However, the mechanical properties of the re-mineralized samples were below the stability of natural dentin, which is suggested to be a consequence of imperfect arrangement of the newly deposited mineral. The increase in mineral content was

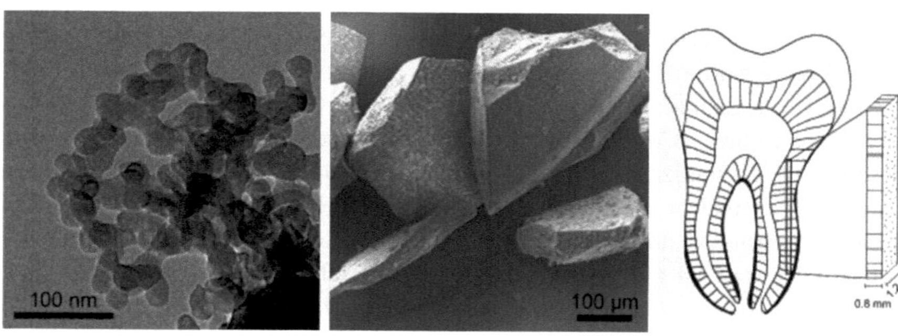

Fig. 3 TEM image of nano and *micon sized* particles in addition to dentin bar from third molar used for testing. (Reproduced from Vollenweider et al. [31])

attributed to the nanosized particles which highlights the importance of particle size in relation to the clinical applications of Bioglass® materials [31].

4.3 *Novamin®: 18 μm Glass Particles*

Another Bioglass® based dental product is NovaMin®, developed by NovaMin Technology, GlaxoSmithKline (Florida, UK). This commercial product employs a much finer particle size that the above mentioned products and has a particle size of approximately 18 μm [13]. The primary aim for this material was to re-mineralize dentin in the tooth to reduce the effects of hypersensitivity which occurs due to gingival exposure [32]. Dentin hypersensitivity is an oral condition where the root of the tooth becomes exposed due to periodontal disease, toothbrush abrasion or cyclic loading fatigue of the thin enamel near the cemento-enamel junction [13]. Dentin accounts for the greatest part of the dental hard tissue and is composed of an organic matrix of collagen and other proteins imbedded with crystalline apatite. The dental tubules (30,000–40,000/mm^2) contain projections of odontoblast cells that reside in the pulpo-dentinal junction in addition to dental fluid [31, 33]. When external stimuli such as rapid changes in temperature or osmotic pressure; fluid is displaced within the dental tubules. The opening of the dentin tubules facilitates hydrodynamic fluid flow which causes changes in pressure that excites nerve endings in the dental pulp which results in hypersensitivity [13, 31, 33]. When micron sized particles of NovaMin® are incorporated into toothpaste, the small particles are known to adhere to the dentine and induce a HAp layer which has the effect of arresting fluid movement within the tubules which subsequently alleviates the pain [13, 32].

Regarding it mechanism of action, the physical efficacy of the Novamin® (and the Bioglass® composition in general) particles begin when the material is subject to an aqueous media [34]. Sodium ions (Na^+) in the glass particles exchange with hydrogen cations (H^+ or H_3O^+) which subsequently facilitates both calcium (Ca^{2+}) and phosphate (PO_4^{3-}) ions to be released from the glass. This series of reactions occurs within very rapidly, and continues when the glass particles are exposed to an aqueous environment. A localized, transient increase in pH occurs which encourages the precipitation of the Ca^{2+} and PO_4^{3-} ions from both the Novamin® glass particles, in addition to the host saliva. This results in the formation of a precipitated calcium phosphate (Ca-P) layer. As the particle reactions proceeds, this layer subsequently crystallizes into hydroxycarbonate apatite, which is chemically and structurally equivalent to biological apatite [32]. The combination of the residual Novamin® particles and the hydroxycarbonate apatite layer results in the physical occlusion of dentinal tubules, which relieves the effects of hypersensitivity [34]. Studies conducted by Curtis et al. on the particle size of Bioglass® based compositions for dentin restoration and hypersensitivity treatment were also conducted and confirmed this effect. This study determined that treatment of the dentin specimens, irrespective of particle size, resulted in the formation of continuous adherent apatite which occluded the previously exposed dentin tubules. This study employed Bioglass® based compositions that were fabricated using melt-derived and sol-gel glass synthesis routes. The mean particles sizes were 3.3 (0.42) and 0.65 (0.19) μm for the melt derived and sol-gel compositions respectively [32]. The dentin samples used were extracted from human wisdom teeth which were cut to produce 1.5 mm thick acellular dentine samples (4.0 $\times$ 3.0 mm). These samples were treated with a slurry of the micron and nano Biolgass® based powders, where the dentin samples were brushed within the slurry for 2 min and a constant load of 3.5 N. This study found that after brushing with a Bioglass® slurry of human saliva, particle agglomeration was identified on the sample surface, while 24 h after the treatment, rod-like projections were found around the previously exposed tubules. These rod-like projections appeared to emanate from within the tubules [32].

Energy Dispersive X-ray (EDX) analysis confirmed the projections to be calcium and phosphate rich which supported the concept of apatite formation. Sections of the samples were cut using Focused Ion Beam (FIB) Spectroscopy and were subsequently analyzed using Scanning Electron Microscopy (SEM). The results of this study is presented in Fig. 4 and presents FIB images which highlight the formation of apatite rods following the application of the nanosized Bioglass® to dentine (Fig. 4a) [32]. Cross sections of the apatite rods that occupy the dentin tubules were sectioned using the ion beam. The apatite rods are indicated using arrows in Fig. 4b, while the fully encased tubules are highlighted using circles. The size of the individual rods were estimated at 25 μm, however, observations using SEM of the transverse sections measured these rods to a depth of 270 μm [32]. This study determined that the apatite deposited on the dentin surface was altered in response to the difference in particle size which resulted in a distinctive morphology. This study concluded that brushing with nanosized Bioglass® particles caused particulate entrapment within the tubules from which the apatite rod formation occurred. Additionally, the rods did not show any evidence of de-lamination which suggests they will remain stable under hydrodynamic flow [32].

This study further highlighted the effect that particle size has on the dissolution characteristics of Bioglass® based materials. This effect was also supported in studies conducted by Wang et al. where they found that nano-sized bioactive glass induced dentin formation more strongly than micron sized glass particles [35]. However, this study also investigated the cellular influence that both particle sizes have on odontogenic cells as materials that can induce odontogenic differentiation and dentin formation is extremely desirable in relation to pulp repair and tooth regeneration [35]. Human dental pulp cells (hDPCs) were isolated from third molars and cultured directly with the micro- and nano-sized glass particles. Figure 5 presents the effect of incubating micron and nano-sized bioactive glass particles with hDPCs [35].

This study determined that the proliferation rate of the hDPCs was significantly increased (Fig. 5) when exposed to the nano-sized particles. Additionally, the cells chemotactic activity was also improved as the mineralization capacity and the expression of odontogenic related proteins (dentin sialophosphoprotein, dentin matrix protein 1 and collagen type 1) and genes were upregulated by the addition of

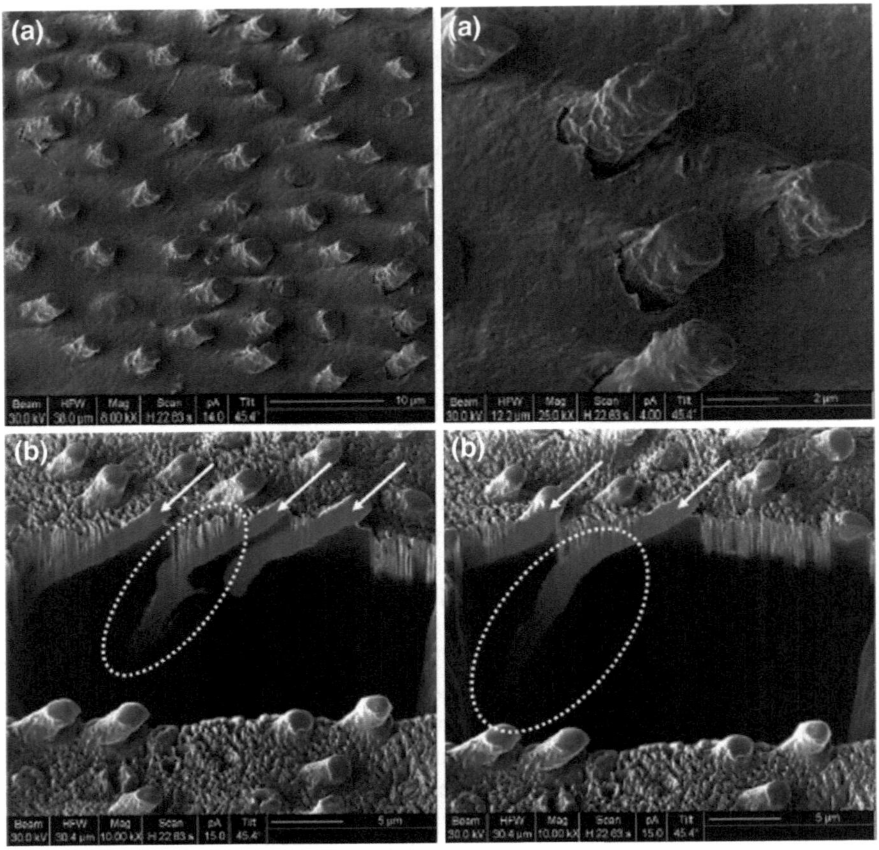

Fig. 4 FIB prepared dentin specimens which present **a** apatite rods projecting from the dentin tubules, and **b** transverse sections of the apatite encased dentin tubules. (Reproduced from Curtis et al. [32])

the bioactive glass and in particular with respect to the nano-sized particulates [35]. The nanoscale glass particles induces dentin formation more strongly than the microscale particles through the combined action of cell migration, surface attachment, polarization, odontogenic differentiation and mineralization of hDPCs, which is due to the nano sized particles having a larger surface area, more binding sites and a faster dissolution rate [35].

Restoration of alveolar bone tissue for dental implant support and re-mineralization of the tooth structure to alleviate hypersensitivity are applications that have seen great success with the use of Bioglass® based glasses. Bioglass materials have been widely investigated due to their ability to bone to bone tissue, however, additional properties such as anti-inflammatory effects and antibacterial efficacy have accelerated interest in these materials where studies have been conducted to explore the effect of the ionic dissolution products on the host cells

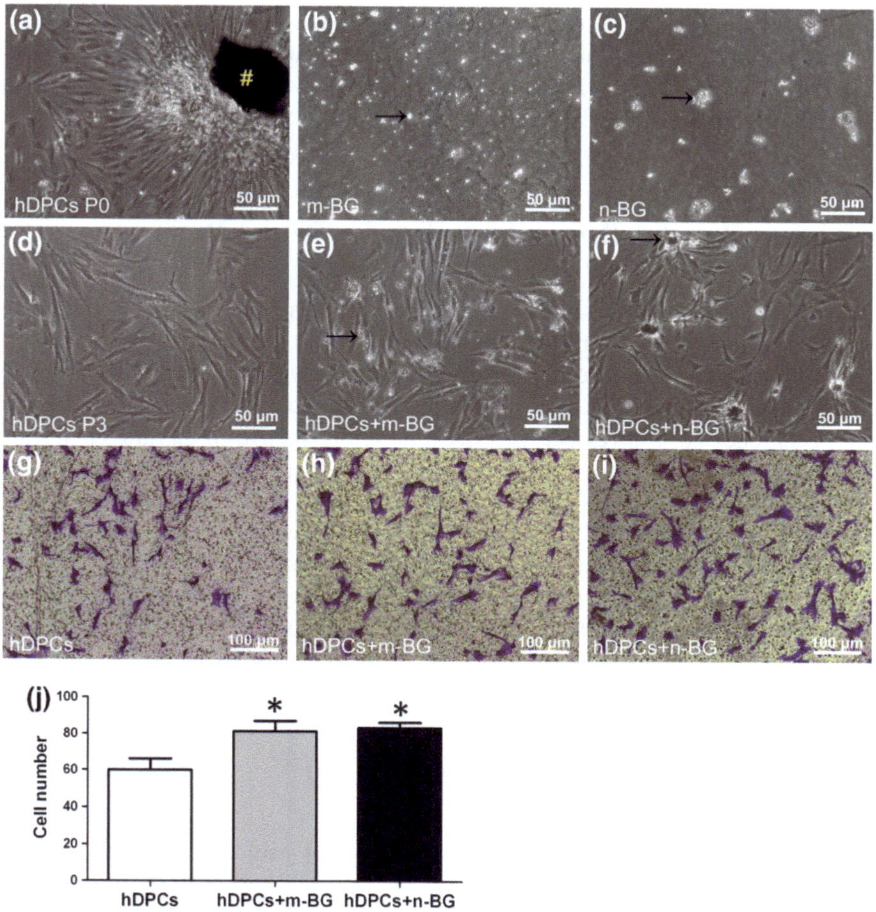

Fig. 5 **a** Primary hDPCs from human third molars. Incubation of micron (**b**, **e**) and nano (**c**, **d**) sized glass coating (0.1 mg/ml^{-1}) of the tissue culture vessel. Where, **e** and **d** indicate third passage and *arrows* indicate glass particle clusters **g** indicates control group while **h** and **i** indicates micron and nano groups by crystal violet staining. (Reproduced from Wang et al. [35])

genetic expression. The bioactive process is now known to stimulate genetic control [36]. Bioactive glasses can enhance osteogenesis through direct control over genes that regulate cell cycle induction and progression towards a mature osteoblast phenotype, a process termed osteostimulation. The effect of this genetic stimulation of the cell cycle of osteoblast progenitor cells is the rapid proliferation and differentiation of osteoblasts [36]. The result is rapid regeneration of bone tissue. The clinical significance is the rapid filling of bone defects with regenerated bone that is structurally and mechanically equivalent to normal healthy bone [36]. In addition to the Bioglass® based materials that are used to reconstruct supportive alveolar bone tissue and the re-mineralization of tooth surfaces, glassy materials are also used for additional purposes in tooth restoration that includes filling caries, lining and sealing applications and luting (bonding) metallic materials to the tooth surfaces. These adhesive properties, with respect to the predominant glass based dental restorative adhesives, will be discussed in the following section.

5 Glass Based Adhesive Materials for Dental Restoration

Adhesive restorative dentistry originated with the work of Buonocore in 1955 in bonding resins to etched enamel. He initially demonstrated that the application of phosphoric acid to enamel resulted in a porous surface which could be infiltrated with a resin, which resulted in a strong micromechanical bond [37]. Adhesive materials and techniques have developed at a rapid rate since then with the first chemically adhesive material, the Zinc Polycarboxylate Cement (ZPC) being produced in the 1960s by Smith, and Glass Polyalkenoate Cements (GPC) following shortly after [38]. The conventional GPCs were then modified in the early 1990s by the addition of a water-soluble resin, to produce resin-modified GPCs (RMGPCs). The resin was added as it is a photo-polymerizable monomer that, when exposed to light, accelerates the setting reaction [39]. Dental adhesive materials that include a glass phase as one of its primary constituents will be considered in the following section.

5.1 Glass Polyalkenoate Cements (GPCs)

Glass-polyalkenoate cements (GPCs) are a class of acid-base adhesive cements used in restorative dentistry that contains a degradable glass as one of its base constituents. GPCs are water-based composite materials which set by an acid-base reaction between a polyalkenoic acid, which is typically polyacrylic acid (PAA), in addition to an alumino-silicate based glass. When the components are mixed together in specific formulations with water, the materials set to form a solid cement-like material. Upon mixing the powder and liquid components, the acidic liquid attacks the basic glass resulting in surface degradation of the glass particles which encourages the release of metal ions (e.g. strontium, calcium, aluminium), fluoride ions and silicic acid. The metal ions react with the carboxyl (COO–) groups on the PAA chains to form a polyacid salt, which becomes the cement matrix, while the surface of the glass becomes a silica hydrogel. The unreacted cores of the glass particles remain as a filler [37, 39, 40]. Figure 6 is a schematic representing the setting reaction of a conventional GPC.

GPCs are extremely versatile materials as the modification of the glass composition, changes in the respective quantities of the powder to liquid ratios or employing PAAs with different molecular weight and concentrations can result in significant changes in the resulting properties which include ion release and solubility, mechanical properties, setting characteristics and interfacial bond strength.

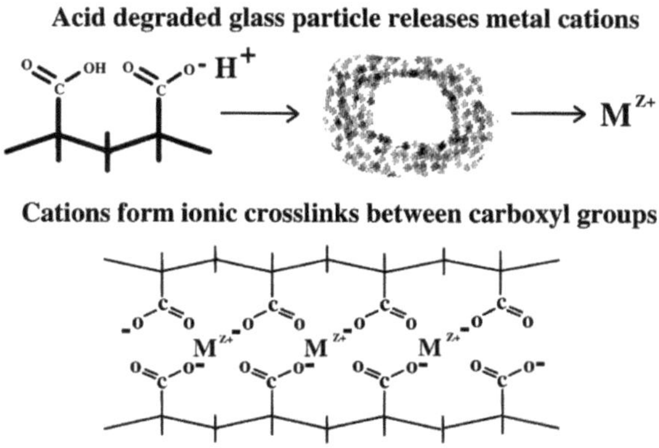

Fig. 6 Setting reaction of GPC where acid degraded glass particles release cations which form ionic crosslinks between carboxyl groups. (Reproduced from De Barra and Hill [41])

5.1.1 Dental Suitability and Applicability

Glass polyalkenoate cements have a unique combination of properties that make them suitable for restoration of dental tissues. GPCs are known to adhere to both tooth mineral and metallic substrates. They can also release beneficial ions, such as fluoride, over extended periods of time which can help prevent secondary carie formation [39]. They are translucent and can be colour matched to tooth surface and they are known to possess high mechanical properties which is preferable for materials in contact with tooth dentin and enamel. GPCs also have the added advantage of not requiring mechanical undercuts for retention which is required for non-adhesive based tooth fillers. The GPC was initially developed as a substitute for dental silicate cements for the aesthetic restoration of front (anterior) teeth [39]. Their applications have now become integrated with many type of dental restoration. They can be classified as Type I GPCs where they are used as luting cements as they are characterized as having a low film thickness and set rapidly. Type II GPCs are restorative cements with sub-types 1 and 2 [37]. Type II-1 GPCs are aesthetic and Type II-2 GPCs are 'reinforced' as they are more wear resistant. Type III GPCs are lining cements and fissure sealants which are characterized as having a low viscosity and rapid set [37].

5.1.2 The Glass Component of GPCs

The glass component plays a significant role in the chemistry and physics of a GPC. It acts as a source of ions for the cement-forming reactions, it controls the setting rate and the resulting strength and also imparts translucent properties [37]. Glasses employed for dental restorative GPCs are based on SiO_2–Al_2O_3–CaO or SiO_2–Al_2O_3–CaF formulations. All contain alumina, silica and an alkaline earth or rare earth oxide or fluoride. The alumina to silica ratio (Al/Si) in the glass is critical to producing an acid degradable glass that can liberate ions which subsequently forms cements [39, 40]. Glasses are generally produced by the traditional melt-quench method and the melt temperature of the glass is dependent on the specific composition. They typically range from 1200 to 1550 °C i.e. SiO_2–Al_2O_3–CaO (1350–1550 °C), SiO_2–Al_2O_3–CaO–P_2O_5 (1370–1450 °C), SiO_2–Al_2O_3–CaO–Na_2O (1200–1350 °C). The glass frit is typically ground to pass through a 45 μm sieve for use as filling materials or a 15 μm sieve for luting applications and annealed between 400 and 600 °C which slows down the reactivity of the glass so GPCs can form [39, 42].

The addition of different alkali or alkali earth metals, lanthanoids, transition metals and non-metals to the glass can significantly influence the properties of the set GPC. The inclusion of sodium into the glass phase is known to improve the translucency of the resulting cement but can affect its hydrolytic stability. The addition of strontium or lanthanum in place of calcium can impart radiopacity to the cements [39]. Also, the addition of fluoride has a number of beneficial properties which includes lowering the processing temperature, improving the handling properties of the cement paste, increase the strength of the cement strength and translucency and also imparts antibacterial properties when used as a filling material [39]. Numerous glass compositions have been investigated and commercialized and in general they consist of the traditional SiO_2–Al_2O_3–CaO or SiO_2–Al_2O_3–CaF based composition with slight modifications to the concentrations or presence/absence of specific elements. Some commercially available GPCs include *Fuji IX* (GC Corporation, Japan), G2 (CDL, UK), G338 (CDL, UK), G2SR (CDL, UK) and Ketac Molar (3M-ESPE, Germany) [43]. Studies by Stamboulis et al. investigated the composition and structure of the glass phase of some of these glasses. The composition of these glasses were investigated using X-ray Fluorescence to determine the Si, Al, P, Na, Sr and La content, whereas the F concentration was investigated using ion-selective electrodes [43] (Table 2).

The setting and formation of a GPC is dependent on the ability of the glass to degrade and release cations in acidic conditions. It is required that ions be liberated from the glass surfaces into an aqueous media to form crosslinks with the polyacid component and this occurs through decomposition of the glass. The introduction of cations that depolymerize the Si–O–Si bonds within the glass structure leads to increased surface dissolution when in aqueous media [39]. These cations, termed *network modifying cations*, disrupt the continuity within the glass network, thereby promoting non-bridging oxygen groups ($–O^-$). The incorporation of network

Table 2 Chemical analysis of glass phase used in commercial GICs (at.%). (Reproduced from Stamboulis et al. [43])

Glass	Al	Si	P	Ca	O	F	Sr	La	Na
Fuji IX	0.129	0.115	0.017	0.000	0.547	0.126	0.056	0	0.010
G2	0.140	0.158	0.011	0.038	0.528	0.192	0.000	0	0.058
G338	0.131	0.098	0.030	0.041	0.536	0.143	0	0	0.055
G2SR	0.168	0.106	0.027	0.031	0.567	0.061	0.061	0	0.007
Molar	0.104	0.104	0.015	0.060	0.515	0.163	0	0.043	0.021

modifiers imparts a net negative charge within the glass network, which is subsequently balanced by positively charged cations such as calcium (Ca^{2+}) and sodium (Na^{+}) [40]. Depending on the concentration of network modifiers introduced, a distribution of connectivity, termed Q-structure (Q1, Q2, Q3, Q4) will be present which represents the breaking of Si–O–Si bonds to form non-bridging oxygens (–O^{-}) in the glass. The Q structure of a glass is determined by the number of bridging oxygens present, a glass with a structure Q4, denotes 4 bridging oxygens species. The use of network modifiers such as the alkaline earth oxides (Ca) induces the formation of two non-bridging oxygens (NBOs) per alkaline earth oxide. Altering or modifying the Q-structure leads to the ability to modify the degradation of the glass surfaces in acidic conditions [39, 40].

With respect to aluminosilicate glasses, the alumina can act as either a network modifier in sixfold coordination or a network former in fourfold coordination. Acting as a network former, the Al^{3+} can replace Si^{4+} as it has a similar ionic radius; however the network acquires a negative charge. If this negative charge accumulates to a high enough degree, the glass becomes susceptible to acid attack. The charge on this glass network also has to be balanced by positively charged network modifying cations. It is therefore hypothesized that the structure of an aluminosilicate glass consists of linked $[SiO_4]$ and $[AlO_4]^{-}$ tetrahedra [40, 44, 45] (Figs. 7 and 8).

Therefore, a negatively charged network of non-bridging oxygens and aluminium sites renders these glasses susceptible to acid degradation [39]. The composition of the glass not only influences the solubility and dissolution characteristics, it also provides the critical inorganic components required for the setting of the resulting GPC [46]. Elements such as Fluorine have been widely investigated and introduced to a number of aluminosilicate based glass compositions which include; SiO_2–Al_2O_3–CaF_2 (1105–1350 °C), SiO_2–Al_2O_3–CaO–CaF_2 (1320–1450 °C), SiO_2–Al_2O_3–CaF_2–$AlPO_4$ (1150–1300 °C), SiO_2–Al_2O_3–CaF_2–$AlPO_4$–Na_3AlF_6–AlF_3 (1100–1300 °C) [39]. Fluorine is thought to disrupt the glass network by replacing bridging oxygens with non-bridging fluorines [47, 48].

Fluorine is also known to impart properties such as reducing the glass transition temperature (Tg), viscosity and refractive index, aids crystallization and increases

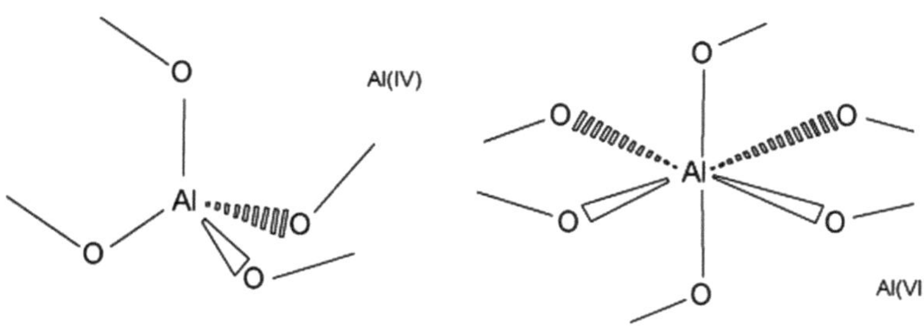

Fig. 7 Representation of aluminium coordination states in glasses and GPCs. (Reproduced from Munhoz et al. [45])

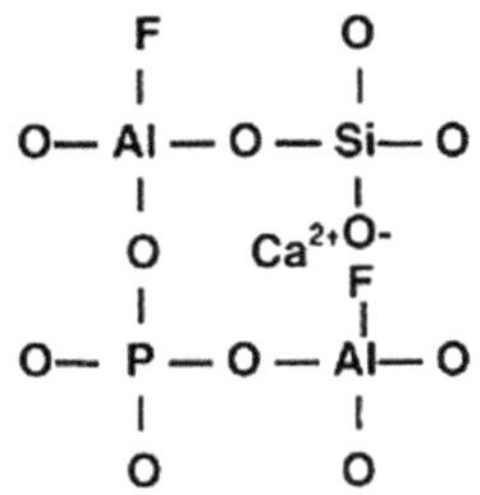

Fig. 8 Schematic showing the structural role of calcium and fluorine in GPCs. The calcium ions disrupt the glass network forming non-bridging oxygens as well as charge balancing charge deficient AlO_4 tetrahedra. Fluorine replaces bridging oxygens and forms non-bridging fluorines. (Reproduced from De Barra and Hill [48])

glass degradability. Its incorporation into a partially soluble acid degradable glass facilitates its release from the cement when a GPC is formed. This is a major advantage for glasses that are applied for dental restoration [47]. Modification of the glass phase of a GPC can be used to influence a number of properties such as the handling and mechanical properties in addition to one of the most important characteristics for dental restorative cements, the adhesive bond strength to the mineralized substrate.

5.1.3 Bonding of GPC to Mineralized Tissues

Bonding of adhesive materials to mineralized tissue under oral conditions presents a number of difficulties. The substrate is a biological tissue and is subject to change. The presence of moisture and water also presents a significant barrier to adhesion. Water competes for the polar surface of the tooth material against any potential polymer adhesive where it tends to hydrolyze any adhesive bond that may form. Bonding of a GPC to dental tissues involves the formation of an ionic bond between the carboxyl (COO^-) groups on the PAA chains and Ca^{2+} ions in the enamel and dentin. As the GPC is mixed and placed on the tooth surface, demineralization of the substrate is minimal as since the tooth hydroxyapatite buffers the acidic effects in addition to PAA being a weak acid [37]. Phosphate anions and calcium cations are displaced from the hydroxyapatite and are absorbed into the unset cement. This interface is referred to as the ion exchange or hybrid layer and is believed to consist of calcium and phosphate ions from the mineralized tissue and aluminium, silicic, fluoride and calcium/strontium ions from the GPC [37]. Measuring the bond strength of the GPC-mineral interface is complicated by the brittle nature of the material. Bond strength tests report on the cohesive failure of the GPC, rather than failure within the ion exchange layer. Bond strength values have been reported in the 3–10 MPa range [37].

5.1.4 Resin Modification of GPCs

The original GPCs are water-based materials that set by an acid-base reaction between a polyalkenoic acid and a fluoro-alumino-silicate glass. The incorporations of resins into the GPC system gave rise to resin modified glass polyalkenoate cements (RMGPCs) and have been investigated to further control the setting reaction, and to overcome some of the shortcomings of conventional GPCs such as moisture sensitivity and low early mechanical strengths [49]. The polymer component in this case can include a modified polyalkenoic acid with a hydrophilic photocurable monomer (e.g. 2-hydroxyethylmethacrylate, 2-HEMA) grafted onto the polymer backbone or a separate photocurable monomer (HEMA) in addition to the polyalkenoic acid and water [49]. The RMGPCs have a dual curing mechanism involving the acid base reaction of the polyalkenoic acid with the glass, which occurs in conventional GPCs, however this reaction can also take place concurrently with light activated polymerisation of the resin monomer. The resin based reaction proceeds by free-radical polymerization of the monomer components after exposure to visible light in the region of 470 nm. The final set RMGPC contains an interpenetrating network of polyalkenoate salts and a poly(HEMA) matrix [49].

Acid Base Reaction

- Calcium-Aluminosilicate Glass + Polyalkenoic Acid − Ca & Al polysalt hydrogel.

Polymerization Reaction

- HEMA + Photochemical Initiator/Activator − PolyHEMA Matrix.

The resulting set RMGPC consists of two matrices: a metal polyacrylate salt and a polymer. Additionally, there is a lack of water in the system as it has been replaced by the HEMA. This lack of water is known to slow down the acid-base reaction, and the final set cement contains an interpenetrating network of polyalkenoate salts and a polyHEMA matrix [39]. RMGPC are known to release clinically relevant levels of fluoride, however, they are also known to swell in aqueous media and the bond strength to dentin and enamel seems less than the traditional GPCs [40]. The bonding mechanism of a RMGPC has been reported to include both ionic interactions between the cements and the dentin surface in addition to a micromechanical interlocking of the polymer with the tooth surfaces. The presence of a hybrid like layer (*H*) has been reported at the RMGPC/dentin interface. In addition, a resin rich non-particulate later (*AL*) is also observed between the hybrid layer and the RMGPC (*RM*) which contains the glass particles [49]. The *AL* was observed to develop over time after the setting phase has completed and is believed to be due to water sorption from the dentin to the maturing cement. This layer was also only observed when applied to deep dentin and was absent from either superficial dentin or enamel [49]. Figure 9 shows the layers that are known to exist between a RMGPC and the dentin substrate.

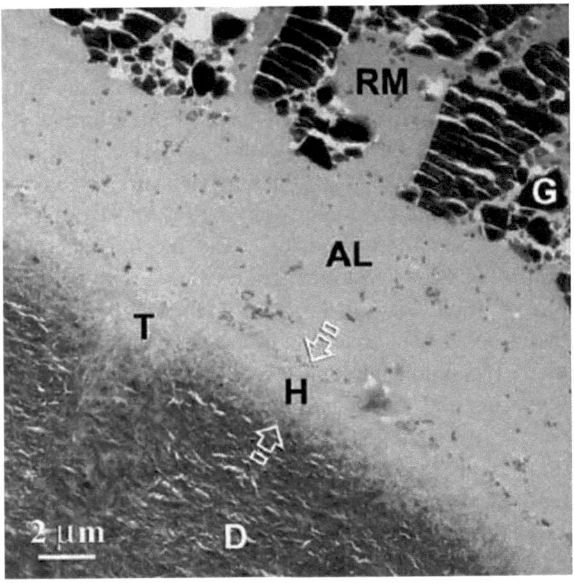

Fig. 9 TEM micrographs of intact unfractured RMGPC (Fuji LC)/dentin interface. This interface shows a distinctive resin-rich, non-particulate absorption layer (*AL*) between the hybrid layer (*H*; between *open arrows*) and the particulate RMGPC. *T* dentinal tubule, *D* intertubular dentine. (Reproduced from Yiu et al. [49])

5.2 Non-vitreous Based Cements for Dental Restoration

In addition to GPCs and RMGPCs, numerous other cements exist for dental applications; however, most differ from GPCs as they do not contain a glass phase. A dental adhesive that does contain a glass phase, similar to GPCs, are glass polyphosphonate cements. These cements also contain an aluminosilicate based glass which is mixed with a concentrated solution of poly(vinyl-phosphonic) acid (PVPA). The main disadvantage of this cement is the susceptibility of the cements to aqueous attack and the inability to achieve sufficient translucency to match that of tooth enamel [39]. Zinc Polycarboxylate Cements (ZPC) are the precursor to GPCs, however, these materials experience an acid-base setting reaction between a Zinc oxide powder and a polyalkenoic acid. ZPCs were the first class of adhesive cements and were employed for luting and lining applications and as a periodontal pack. The main problem attributed to these materials is that their mechanical properties are relatively weak when tested at 37 °C, and they are also subject to plastic behaviour when fully hardened [39]. Zinc oxide can also be mixed with Eugenol, a constituent of the oil found in olive cloves, to form Zinc Eugenol Cements (ZOE). These cements were used in dentistry for temporary cementation of crowns, temporary filling of teeth, as a root canal sealer and as an impression paste. This cement also set via an acid base reaction leading to the formation of a zinc eugenolate chelate. However, similarly to ZPCs, the mechanical properties of ZOE are quite poor [39]. Composite resins are a class of dental materials that contain the organic component Bisphenol-A-glycidylmethacrylate (Bis-GMA), and an inorganic filler which is typically pyrogenic SiO_2 combined with barium silicate or strontium silicate, ground quartz or zirconium dioxide. These materials are the aesthetic material of choice for tooth repair and are widely used for repairing damage caused by caries or trauma [40]. The setting of these materials is light induced or chemically induced, the main disadvantage of composite resin materials being the shrinkage during polymerisation which can be as large as 2–3 wt% volume [40].

6 Chapter Summary

Vitreous materials are currently applied to fulfil a number of applications in restorative dentistry ranging from alveolar bone reconstruction to support dental implants to restoration of the tooth itself through filling cavities and acting as an interfacial bonding agent to adhere metallic constructs to mineralized surfaces. Glasses provide the ability to control the rate of biodegradation and dissolution in an aqueous media, which in turn controls processes such as mineral deposition in bone cavities and the extent of cross-linking within adhesive cements. Additionally, glasses that contain antibacterial properties and positively influence the behavior of the host cells are currently being investigated to further improve the bioactive process and improve healing in vivo. Glass based materials provide a wide range of compositions that leads to countless properties that stems from their versatility as a stand-alone material or as a component within a composite system.

References

1. Nelson, S.J., Ash, M.: Wheelers Dental Anatomy, Physiology, and Occlusion, 9th edn. Elsevier, St. Louis (2010)
2. Scheider, I., Xiao, T., Yilmaz, E., Schneider, G.A., Huber, N., Bargmann, S.: Damage modeling of small-scale experiments on dental enamel with hierarchical microstructure. Acta Biomater. **15**, 244–253 (2015)
3. Jang, A.T., Lin, J.D., Choi, R.M., Choi, E.M., Seto, M.L., Ryder, M.I., Gansky, S.A., Curtis, D.A., Ho, S.P.: Adaptive properties of human cementum and cementum dentin junction with age. J. Mech. Behav. Biomed. Mater. **39**, 184–196 (2014)
4. Bertassoni, L.E., Kury, M., Rathsam, C., Little, C.B., Swain, M.V.: The role of proteoglycans in the nanoindentation creep behavior of human dentin. J. Mech. Behav. Biomed. Mater. **55**, 264–270 (2016)
5. Garces-Ortiz, M., Ledesma-Montes, C., Reyes-Gasga, J.: Scanning electron microscopic study on the fibrillar structures within dentinal tubules of human dentin. J. Endod. **41**(9), 1510–1514 (2015)
6. Ratner, B.D., Hoffman, A.S., Schoen, F.J., Lemons, J.E.: Biomaterials Science: An Introduction to Materials in Medicine, 1st edn. Academic Press, London (1996)
7. Hench, L.L.: The story of Bioglass. J. Mater. Sci. Mater. Med. **17**, 967–978 (2006)
8. Jones, J.R.: Review of bioactive glass: from Hench to hybrids. Acta Biomater. **9**, 4457–4486 (2013)
9. Heinz, S.A., Paliwal, S., Ivanovski, S.: Mechanisms of bone resorption in periodontitis. J. Immunol. Res. (2015). doi:10.1155/2015/615486

10. Henderson, B., Nair, S.P.: Hard labour: bacterial infection of the skeleton. Trends Microbiol. **11**(12), 570–577 (2003)
11. Turkyilmaz, I.: Current Concepts in Dental Implantology. InTechOpen (2015). doi:10.5772/58668
12. Stanley, H.R., Clark, A.E., Hench, L.L.: Alveolar ridge maintenance implants. In: Hench, L. L., Wilson, J. (eds.) Clinical Performance of Skeletal Prostheses, pp. 255–269. Springer, Dordrecht (1996)
13. Abbasi, Z., Bahrololoom, M.E., Shariat, M.H., Bagheri, R.: Bioactive glasses in dentistry: a review. J. Dent. Biomater. **2**(1), 1–9 (2015)
14. Kokubo, T., Kim, H.-M., Kawashita, M.: Novel bioactive materials with different mechanical properties. Biomaterials **24**, 2161–2175 (2003)
15. Kokubo, T., Takadama, H.: How useful is SBF in predicting in vivo bone bioactivity. Biomaterials **27**, 2907–2915 (2006)
16. Levallois, B., Fovet, Y., Lapeyre, L., Gal, J.Y.: In vitro fluoride release from restorative materials in water versus artificial saliva medium (SAGF). Dent. Mater. **14**(6), 441–447 (1998)
17. Aina, V., Bertinetti, L., Cerrato, G., Cerruti, M., Lusvardi, G., Malavasi, G., Morterra, C., Tacconi, L., Menabue, L.: On the dissolution/reaction of small-grain Bioglass® 45S5 and F-modified bioactive glasses in artificial saliva (AS). Appl. Surf. Sci. **257**(9), 4185–4195 (2011)
18. Gal, J.-Y., Fovet, Y., Myriam, A.-Y.: About a synthetic saliva for in vitro studies. Talanta **53**, 1103–1115 (2001)
19. Shi, D.: Biomaterials and Tissue Engineering. Springer, Berlin (2004)
20. Lokade, J., Wankhade, S., Chandak, M., Lanjewar, A.: Guided tissue regeneration principle with inserts of Perioglas in endodontic surgery: two case reports. Int. J. Prosthodont. Restor. Surg. **3**(2), 72–77 (2013)
21. Bashutski, J.D., Wang, H.-L.: Periodontal and endodontic regeneration. J. Endod. **35**(3), 321–328 (2009)
22. Lin, L., Chen, M.Y.H., Ricucci, D., Rosenberg, P.A.: Guided tissue regeneration in periapical surgery. J. Endod. **36**(4), 618–625 (2010)
23. Scantlebury, T., Ambruster, J.: The development of guided regeneration: making the impossible possible and the unpredictable predictable. J. Evid. Based Dent. Pract. **12**(3), 101–117 (2012)
24. Rams, T.E., Roberts, T.W., Tatum Jr., H., Keyes, P.H.: The subgingival microbial flora associated with human dental implants. J. Prosthet. Dent. **51**(4), 529–534 (1984)
25. Allan, I., Newman, H., Wilson, M.: Antibacterial activity of particulate Bioglass® against supra- and subgingival bacteria. Biomaterials **22**(12), 1683–1687 (2001)
26. Balamurugan, A., Balossier, G., Laurent-Maquin, D., Pina, S., Rebelo, A.H.S., Faure, J., Ferreira, J.M.F.: An in vitro biological and anti-bacterial study on a solgel derived silver-incorporated bioglass system. Dent. Mater. **24**(10), 1343–1351 (2008)
27. Lopez, M.M.M., Faure, J., Cabrera, M.I.E., Garcia, M.E.C.: Structural characterization and electrochemical behavior of 45S5 bioglass coating on Ti6Al4 V alloy for dental applications. Mater. Sci. Eng., C **206**, 30–38 (2016)
28. Jurczyk, K., Kubicka, M.M., Ratajczak, M., Jurczyk, M.U., Niespodziana, K., Nowak, D.M., Gajecka, M., Jurczyk, M.: Antibacterial activity of nanostructured Ti-45S5 bioglass-Ag composite against Streptococcus mutans and Staphylococcus aureus. Trans. Non-Ferr. Metals Soc. China **1**, 118–125 (2016)
29. Rectenwald, J., Minter, R.M., Rosenberg, J.J., Gaines, C.G., Lee, S., Moldawer, L.L.: Bioglass attenuates a proinflammatory response in mouse peritoneal endotoxicosis. Shock **17**, 135–138 (2002)
30. Li, H., He, J., Yu, H., Green, C.R., Chang, J.: Bioglass promotes wound healing by affecting gap junction connexin 43 mediated endothelial cell behavior. Biomaterials **84**, 64–75 (2016)

31. Vollenweider, M., Brunner, T.J., Knecht, S., Grass, R.N., Zehnder, M., Imfeld, T., Stark, W. J.: Remineralization of human dentin using ultrafine bioactive glass particles. Acta Biomater. **3**(6), 936–943 (2007)
32. Curtis, A.R., West, N.X., Su, B.: Synthesis of nanobioglass and formation of apatite rods to occlude exposed dentine tubules and eliminate hypersensitivity. Acta Biomater. **6**(9), 3740–3746 (2010)
33. Farooq, I., Moheet, I.A., AlShwaimi, E.: In vitro dentin tubule occlusion and remineralization competence of various toothpastes. Arch. Oral Biol. **60**(9), 1246–1253 (2015)
34. Kumar, A., Singh, S., Thumar, G., Mengji, A.: Bioactive glass nanoparticles (NovaMin®) for applications in dentistry. J. Dent. Med. Sci. **14**(8), 30–35 (2015)
35. Wang, S., Gao, X., Gong, W., Zhang, Z., Chen, X., Dong, Y.: Odontogenic differentiation and dentin formation of dental pulp cells under nanobioactive glass induction. Acta Biomater. **10**(6), 2792–2803 (2014)
36. Hench, L.L.: Genetic design of bioactive glass. J. Eur. Ceram. Soc. **29**(7), 1257–1265 (2009)
37. Tyas, M.J., Burrow, M.F.: Adhesive restorative materials: a review. Aust. Dent. J. **49**(3), 112–121 (2004)
38. Wilson, A.D.: Glass Ionomer Cements, Origins, Developments and Future. Quintessence Publishing Co., Chicago (1998)
39. Nicholson, J.W., Wilson, A.D.: Acid-Base Cements: Their Biomedical and Industrial Applications. Chemistry of Solid State Materials, vol. 3. Cambridge University Press, Cambridge (1993)
40. Nicholson, J.W.: Adhesive dental materials: a review. Int. J. Adhes. Adhes. **18**(4), 229–236 (1998)
41. De Barra, E., Hill, R.G.: Influence of alkali metal ions on the fracture properties of glass polyalkenoate (ionomer) cements. Biomaterials **19**(6), 495–502 (1998)
42. Mount, G.J.: An Atlas of Glass-Ionomer Cements: A Clinician's Guide, 3rd edn. Taylor & Francis, Milton Park (2001)
43. Stamboulis, A., Law, R.V., Hill, R.G.: Characterisation of commercial ionomer glasses using magic angle nuclear magnetic resonance (MAS-NMR). Biomaterials **25**(17), 3907–3913 (2004)
44. Yildirim, E., Dupree, R.: Investigation of Al–O–Al sites in an Na-alumino-silicate glass. Bull. Mater. Sci. **27**(3), 269–272 (2004)
45. Munhoz, T., Karpukhina, N., Hill, R.G., Law, R.V., De Almeida, L.H.: Setting of commercial glass ionomer cement Fuji IX by 27Al and 19F MAS-NMR. J. Dent. **38**(4), 325–330 (2010)
46. Deb, S., Nicholson, J.W.: The effect of Strontium oxide in glass ionomer cements. J. Mater. Sci. Mater. Med. **10**, 471–474 (1999)
47. Stamboulis, A., Hill, R.G., Law, R.V.: Characterization of the structure of calcium alumino-silicate and calcium fluoro-alumino-silicate glasses by magic angle spinning nuclear magnetic resonance (MAS-NMR). J. Non-Cryst. Solids **333**(1), 101–107 (2004)
48. De Barra, E., Hill, R.G.: Influence of glass composition on the properties of glass polyalkenoate cements. Part III: influence of fluorite content. Biomaterials **21**(6), 563–569 (2000)
49. Yiu, C.K.Y., Tay, F.R., King, N.M., Pashley, D.H., Carvalho, R.M., Carrilho, M.R.O.: Interaction of resin-modified glass-ionomer cements with moist dentine. J. Dent. **32**(7), 521–530 (2004)

Special Applications of Bioactive Glasses in Otology and Ophthalmology

Francesco Baino and Isabel Potestio

Abstract The invention of bioactive glasses (please consult the Editor's note in order to clarify the usage of the terms bioglass, bioactive glass and biocompatible glasses) more than 45 years ago posed the basis of modern regenerative medicine introducing the concept that a material implanted in the body can not only form a tight bond with living tissues but also stimulate the growth of new healthy tissue. Bioactive glasses are traditionally used for the repair, reconstruction and augmentation of hard tissues in orthopaedics and dentistry due to their ability to create a tight interface with calcified tissues. Most studies on bioactive glasses and glass-ceramics have been focused on their use in these two clinical fields, however some emerging applications are arising in other medical areas. In fact, available literature indicates that bioactive glasses are able to bond to soft tissues, too, and can exhibit an additional range of highly attractive properties (e.g. angiogenesis, antibacterial effect) which could expand dramatically their potential and impact in science and medicine. This chapter reviews the special applications of bioactive glasses in otology (substitution of middle ear ossicles, cochlear implants, mastoid cavity obliteration) and ocular surgery (orbital implants, artificial cornea, orbital floor repair), in which the ability to bond to soft tissues is a fundamental property. A comprehensive picture of the existing devices for such applications is presented as well as a prospect for the future, with the aim of providing useful stimuli for further research in these two fascinating and crucial areas for patient's life quality.

Keywords Bioglass · Bioactivity · Tissue engineering · Angiogenesis · Antibacterial

F. Baino (✉) · I. Potestio
Applied Science and Technology Department, Institute of Materials Physics and Engineering, Politecnico di Torino, Corso Duca degli Abruzzi 24, 10129 Turin, Italy
e-mail: francesco.baino@polito.it

J. Marchi (ed.), *Biocompatible Glasses*, Advanced Structured Materials 53,
DOI 10.1007/978-3-319-44249-5_9

1 Introduction

The first bioactive glass was developed by Prof. Larry Hench at the University of Florida in the late 1960s. This revolutionary biomaterial, which since then has been known worldwide as "45S5 Bioglass®", consists of a SiO_2 network incorporating Na_2O and CaO as network modifiers and a small amount of P_2O_5 (Table 1) [30]. Since then, many other silicate-, borate-, and phosphate-based glass formulations have been investigated by other research groups for biomedical applications. Silicate bioactive glasses are the most studied and include a wide range of glass compositions such as the Hench's glass 45S5, 13-93 and S53P4. Borate-based systems, such as 13-93B3, are attracting attention due to their faster bioactive kinetics when compared to 45S5 and 13-93 and the ability to control their degradation rate by designing carefully their composition [39]. Phosphate glasses are known to be highly resorbable in the biological fluids [1, 2] and have been proposed as vehicles for the local release of therapeutic metal ions [47]. A selection of some bioactive glass compositions is reported in Table 1; some of them, such as 45S5 Bioglass® and 13-93, are in clinical use and marketed worldwide from many years after receiving FDA approval for medical use.

Bioactive glass-ceramics can be obtained from a parent glass in order to increase the mechanical properties of the material. In fact, controlled heat treatment applied to bioactive glasses of suitable composition can induce the development of crystalline phases in the amorphous matrix, so that the physico-mechanical properties are improved while an adequate bioactivity is retained.

Being inorganic, stiff materials with physical characteristics similar to those of the hard tissues of the body, bioactive glasses and glass-ceramics have been traditionally applied in orthopedics and dentistry to repair diseased bone and teeth; however, a few recent studies have highlighted the potential of these materials to regenerate various types of damaged soft tissues, too [11, 57].

This chapter focuses on the special applications of bioactive glasses and glass-ceramics in ear and eye surgery where they come in contact with both hard and soft tissues. Briefly, applications in otology concern the development of artificial middle ear ossicles and cochlear implants as well as the obliteration of

Table 1 Examples of some bioactive glass and glass-ceramic compositions

Glass	Composition (wt%)							Relevant references
	SiO_2	K_2O	MgO	CaO	B_2O_3	P_2O_5	Na_2O	
45S5 Bioglass®	45.0	–	–	24.5	–	6.0	24.5	[30, 34, 36]
13-93	53.0	12.0	5.0	20.0	–	4.0	6.0	[17]
13-93B3	–	11.1	4.6	18.5	56.6	3.7	5.5	[39]
S53P4	53.0	–	–	20.0	–	4.0	23.0	[43, 62]
58S	58.2	–	–	32.6	–	9.2	–	[71]
Biosilicate®	48.5	–	–	23.75	–	4.0	23.75	[15, 16]

Table 2 Sequence of interfacial reactions leading to the formation of a HA layer on the surface of (silicate) bioactive glass (adapted from Hench [31] with permission by John Wiley and Sons)

Stage	Description
1	Rapid exchange of cations (e.g. Na^+ and Ca^{2+} belonging to glass modifier oxides) with H^+ or H_3O^+ from the surrounding solution, which leads to hydrolysis of silica groups and creation of silanols (Si–OH). The pH of the solution increases as H^+ in the biological fluids are gradually replaced by alkaline cations
2	Attack of the silica network, loss of soluble silica in the form of $Si(OH)_4$ to the solution (resulting from the breaking of Si–O–Si bonds) and continued formation of silanols at the glass-solution interface
3	Condensation and re-polymerization of the silanols, leading to the formation of a silica-rich layer depleted in alkalis and alkali-earth cations on the glass surface
4	Migration of Ca^{2+} and PO_4^{3-} groups to the surface through the silica-rich layer and from the surrounding fluids, thereby forming an amorphous CaO/P_2O_5-rich film on the top of the silica-rich layer
5	Growth and crystallization of the calcium phosphate film to form a HA layer; actually, by incorporation of OH^-, CO_3^{2-} and F^- ions from the solution, a mixed apatitic layer constituted by HA, hydroxycarbonateapatite and fluoroapatite can develop

mastoid cavity, whereas bioactive glasses are used in ophthalmology for the treatment of orbital floor injuries, damaged cornea and anophthalmic socket (orbital implants). Many of these applications exploit the double ability of bioactive glasses to bond to hard and soft tissues [9, 14, 67] as well as the technological versatility of these materials that can be produced in the form of powders, particles, granules, dense bulk or porous structures (scaffolds) of complex shapes and sizes as well as in the form of coatings and in combination with other materials to produce composites [41].

2 Bonding Mechanism of Bioactive Glasses to Hard and Soft Tissues

Traditionally, bioactive glasses are known to bond to host bone and promote the growth of new bone tissue while dissolving over time. The creation of a tight bond with calcified tissues is attributed to the formation of a hydroxyapatite (HA) or apatite-like layer that interacts actively with the collagen fibrils of the damaged bone [29]. This layer of nano-crystalline HA formed on the surface of bioactive glasses upon contact with biological fluids can be considered biomimetic, as it mimics the composition and crystallography of bone mineral phase. Reactions stages leading to the formation of this surface apatite layer are now quite well understood, whereas the biological interactions that occur at the HA-host bone interface still remain partially unclear. The formation of a bond in vivo between this surface nano-HA layer and the host bone is a complex process involving protein adsorption, incorporation of collagen fibrils, adhesion of osteoprogenitor cells, cell differentiation, production of bone extracellular matrix (ECM) and ECM mineralization [33]. Osteogenesis is also related to the action of ion dissolution products released from bioactive glass on the activity of osteoblasts, which are stimulated to produce new bone. Moreover, it has been demonstrated that the intrinsic nanoroughness of the apatite layer provides in itself a surface suitable for osteogenic cell attachment and proliferation [41].

The HA layer forms following solution-mediated dissolution of the bioactive glass according to a process that resembles the corrosion of conventional glasses [68]. Accumulation of dissolution products causes both the chemical composition of the glass surface and the pH of the solution to change, thus providing surface sites and a pH favourable to HA nucleation. Hench and co-workers proposed five stages for HA formation on the surface of (silicate) bioactive glasses in body fluid in vivo or in simulated body fluid (SBF) in vitro [22, 30, 31, 34], as summarized in Table 2. Once the HA layer has formed, proteins adsorb to it, and cells attach, differentiate and produce bone matrix.

It is now well accepted that there are two kinds of interactions—extracellular and intracellular—which occur in the body upon implantation of bioactive glasses. Extracellular interactions are determined by the material surface features; in general, different surfaces have different protein adsorption properties [5]. For instance, surface nanoroughness and negatively charged silanols exposed by (silicate) bioactive glasses play an important role in promoting the adsorption of proteins and collagen on the material surface. Intracellular interaction occurs between the protein ligands formed on the implant surface and cell receptors that determine the degree of cellular adhesion, differentiation and proliferation [5]. A key role is played by the (bio)availability of different ions; for instance, release of Si and Ca ions from glass surface has been demonstrated to promote osteogenesis exerting specific effects at the genetic level in osteoblasts (increased DNA synthesis, enhanced alkaline phosphatase activity and osteocalcin release) [35].

Another important property of bioactive glasses is the "osteoproductive ability", i.e. new bone can form on the glass surface away from the implant-bone interface [81]. The term "osteoproduction" was coined to distinguish this process from "osteoinduction", which refers to bone growth in ectopic (non-bony) sites (e.g. muscle). It is worth pointing out that other biomaterials used for bone repair (e.g. calcium phosphate ceramics) are defined "osteoconductive", i.e. they simply provide a biocompatible interface along which bone migrates; these implant elicit only an extracellular response at their interface [18].

The surface reaction kinetics of bioactive glasses are mainly controlled by the material composition.

In the early studies on bioactive glasses, Hench and co-workers investigated a series of glasses (including the well-known 45S5 Bioglass®) in the quaternary SiO_2–CaO–Na_2O–P_2O_5 system with a constant 6 wt% of P_2O_5 [30]. The relationship between glass composition and (possible) type of bond with living tissues for this system is shown in Fig. 1. For glasses with up to about 53 mol% of SiO_2, HA crystallization on the glass surface occurs within 2 h from implantation. These glass compositions develop quickly a bond with bone and, very interestingly, can

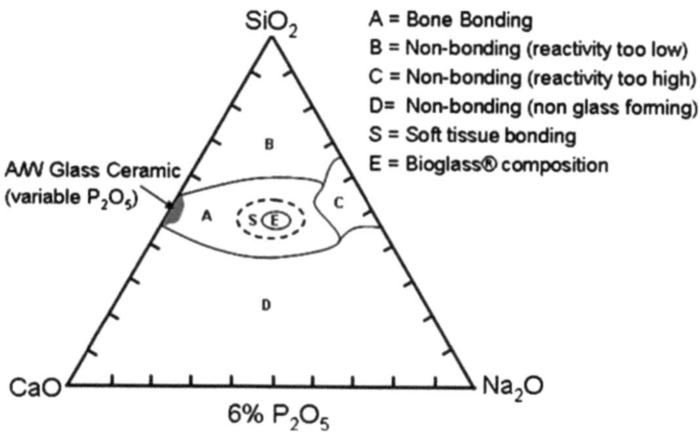

Fig. 1 Compositional diagram for tissue bonding of silicate bioactive glass (reproduced from [34] with permission by Springer)

also form a tight bond with collagenous soft tissues. Glasses with SiO_2 content between 53 and 58 mol% require longer times (2–3 days) to form the nano-crystalline HA layer. Compositions exceeding 60 mol% of SiO_2 do not form a surface apatite layer either in vitro or in vivo even after 4 weeks. Additional network modifiers, e.g. MgO and K_2O, can allow tuning the material bioactivity in order to speed up the bioactive kinetics and increase the thickness of the HA surface layer [65]. Borosilicate glasses with high content of B_2O_3 are highly bioactive but undergo fast degradation in aqueous media due to high reactivity [39]. It was reported that Al_2O_3 and other oxides of multivalent metallic elements such as Ta_2O_5, TiO_2 and ZrO_2 can inhibit the bone-bonding ability of silicate and borosilicate glasses [4, 27]. This negative effect on the glass bioactivity is attributed to a decreased reactivity of the glass network in aqueous media, to the precipitation of multivalent ions in the form of oxides, hydroxides or carbonates, and to the shift of the isoelectric point of the surface from negative to positive at physiological pH [18].

45S5 Bioglass® was invented with the clear scope of developing a material that would not form an interfacial layer of scar tissue but instead would form a living bond with calcified tissues [34]. Since then, most applications of bioactive glasses have been addressed mainly to bone repair in orthopaedics and dentistry, as their physico-mechanical properties (e.g. stiffness) seemed close to those of hard tissues. However, it was demonstrated that a special subset of bioactive glass compositions can bond to soft tissues, too, and recent studies pointed out that some of the characteristics that make bioactive glasses highly attractive materials for bone repair could be wisely exploited for emerging applications in soft tissue engineering [11, 57]. The first comprehensive study on this challenging topic was reported by Wilson et al. [82], who investigated the interactions and biocompatibility of several bioactive glass compositions (including 45S5 Bioglass®) in vitro and in vivo (region S of Fig. 1). In vitro tests were performed by culturing diverse cell types from mice, rats, hamsters, chickens and humans onto solid and powdered bioactive glass samples, whereas in vivo testing was carried out by implanting powdered and solid glass samples subcutaneously, intramuscularly and in the peritoneal cavity of dogs and donkeys. The in vivo tests revealed soft tissue growth and adhesion around 45S5 Bioglass® implants without any signs of inflammatory reaction. This early set of experiments paved the way for the first clinical application of 45S5 Bioglass® in the reconstruction of middle ear ossicles, where the glass was required to bond to both hard and soft tissues [36].

Since then, research on bioactive glasses has been continuously going on, pushing the potential applications well beyond bone substitution [11, 57]. This chapter reviews the special applications of bioactive glasses in ear and eye surgery, with the aim of providing a stimulus for further research in these two fascinating and crucial areas for patient's life quality.

3 Applications in Otology

Otological applications of bioactive glasses and glass-ceramics include the reconstruction of middle ear small bones (ossicles), the development of cochlear implants —both these applications require a material that bonds to both hard and soft collagenous tissues—and mastoid cavity obliteration—for which the "classical" bone-bonding ability is required.

3.1 Reconstruction of Middle Ear Small Bones

The auditory ossicles of middle ear can be irreversibly damaged by chronic infection, which leads to problems in sound conduction from the tympanic membrane to the cochlea with moderate-to-high functional discomfort to the patient. Before the mid 1970s, the preferred material in the middle ear surgery was alumina due to its inertness with living tissues. This paradigm on the use and properties of biomaterials—the more inert the better—changed radically with the advent of bioactive glasses.

The first bioactive material used to reconstruct injured small bones of the ear was Ceravital®, which identifies a set of SiO_2-based glass-ceramic formulations [63]. The intention was to exploit the material bioactivity to form an osseous junction between the implant and the remaining ossicular chain, thereby avoiding a fibrous encapsulation. Animal studies demonstrated the suitability of Ceravital® that neither elicited inflammation of middle ear tissues nor affected negatively cochlear functions [14]. Initially, Ceravital® implants were covered by mucosa in the same way as the reference alumina implants (non-degradable) were. When implant biodegradation occurred and new bone formation continued, defects in the implant surface were refilled with new bone. This eventually led to the formation of a osseous layer surrounding the implant with a thickness up to 40 μm; since this layer was covered by mucosa, it protected the implant from further degradation. Good post-surgical outcomes in guinea pigs were also reported in a subsequent study by Zikk et al. [87] who documented just a temporary hearing loss that solved spontaneously within 20 days from operation and a transient inflammation due to the biochemical reaction between the implanted Ceravital® granules and the middle ear tissues (Fig. 2a). Ceravital® implants have been clinically used in human patients with generally good long-term results (8 years of follow-up), although some concerns about the durability of the implant, which tends to resorb over time, still linger on [64].

45S5 Bioglass® was proposed for the reconstruction of middle ear small bones due to its proved capability to bond to both calcified and soft collagenous tissues [82], hence it was thought able to bond to both bone and eardrum. Cast 45S5 Bioglass® implants (similar to truncated cones, Fig. 2b) received the approval by FDA for clinical use in 1985 and were then marketed under the commercial name of "MEP®" or "Bioglass® Ossicular Reconstruction Prosthesis" [32, 55, 56, 83]. In vivo performance of MEP® was compared to that of alumina implant and it was shown that the former had a longer survivability due to the formation of a tight bond with both the collagen fibres of the tympanic membrane (on one end) and the remaining bone of the stapes footplate (on the other end), whereas the latter gradually erode the eardrum and were finally extruded within 2–3 years from implantation [50].

The strength of the bonds between implant and hard/soft tissues was highlighted in a study by Rust et al. [67], who reported that the implant remained safely

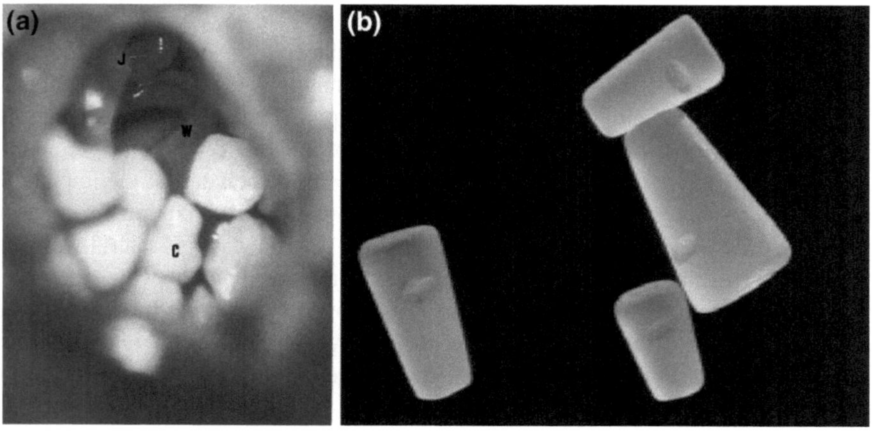

Fig. 2 Bioactive glasses and glass-ceramics used for the reconstruction of middle ear small bones: **a** Ceravital® granules with size 0.3–0.7 mm (*C*) in the middle ear of a guinea pig (*J* incudo-stapedial joint, *W* round window) (reproduced from Zikk et al. [87] with permission by Springer); **b** components of a 45S5 Bioglass® ossicular prosthesis (reproduced from Hench [32] with permission by John Wiley and Sons)

anchored on both ends in the correct position and did not observed micro-movements at the implant-tissue interface over a maximum follow-up of 126 months. Furthermore, from a functional viewpoint, sound conduction was generally excellent without excessive fibrous tissue growth that could impair sound transmission.

More recent studies, however, have reported some concerns about the long-term durability and fate of MEP® implants in vivo. For example, Bahmad and Merchant [7] observed that 45S5 Bioglass® implants tend to be progressively reabsorbed within the middle ear and break down into small fragments after many years from operation (14 years of follow-up). Bioglass® bioinstability in vivo was probably the main reason why these implants were taken off the US market several years after introduction in clinical use; nevertheless, later on these devices are still distributed in some European countries. In summary, caution should be followed in the use of bioactive glass ossicular implants (45S5 Bioglass® and Ceravital®) and further long-term investigations are highly desirable to achieve more definite conclusions.

The use of glass ionomer cement produced by an exothermic reaction between a $CaO–Al_2O_3–SiO_2–CaF_2$ glass and a polyalkenoic acid solution was also proposed for application in middle ear surgery. Both animal and clinical studies in human patients showed that the material was coated with a mucosal layer within a short time, was well-tolerated by middle ear tissues without eliciting an inflammatory response and was not prone to undesirable resorption [26, 52]. However, the use of ionomer cement as an implantable material in ear surgery has been progressively abandoned due to the risk of lethal intoxication of aluminium ions after contact with brain liquor [28].

In recent years, other less popular bioactive glasses have shown potential suitability for the repair of auditory small bones. Biosilicate® was recently assessed to be well-tolerated in the middle ear of guinea pigs (no signs of toxicity to ear structures, including cochlea, were reported after 90 days of follow-up) [76]. Bioverit® granules were also implanted in the middle ear: this material tended to be coated with an epithelial layer and to exhibit a minimal to moderate osteogenic response without eliciting an inflammatory response [13]. The advantage of Bioverit® is the possibility of varying the degree of bioactivity: therefore, implants were developed with different Bioverit® compositions at each end of the implant to induce osseous integration at the malleus and to avoid bony fixation in the oval niche. The antibacterial effect of Bioverit® against gram-negative bacteria was also reported [44]; this is a key added value for an implant material which deserves further investigation in the future. Recently, Bioverit® implants have been also coated with a nanostructured silica layer to improve the bone-bonding ability, and promising results after implantation in the middle ear of mice and rabbits were reported [77, 79].

3.2 Cochlear Implants

In the 1980s, 45S5 Bioglass® was experimented to anchor cochlear implants to the temporal bone of diseased patients who underwent irreversible damage to sensory hair cells in their cochleas, thus becoming completely deaf. Cochlear implants allow patients to understand speech and auditory stimuli from the environment for normal relational activities, although sounds are typically perceived at lower frequencies compared to natural hearing. A cochlear implant is constituted by a microphone, a speech processor to selectively filter sound and prioritize audible speech, a transmitter placed on the external part of the ear, and a receiver anchored in the temporal bone to convert the signals into electric impulses that are sent to an array of electrodes implanted in the cochlear region and connected to the auditory nerve system [23]. A prototype developed at the University College London comprised a 45S5 Bioglass® sleeve that bonded to the temporal bone and protruded through the skin (forming a bond with collagenous soft tissues, too), thus acting as a percutaneous, hermetic and stable seal that protected the interior electronics [80]. This device was sold under the commercial name of Bioglass®-EPI (extracochlear percutaneous implant) till the late 1990s; then, the 45S5 Bioglass® sleeve was replaced by a titanium pedestal exerting a mechanical fixation to the bone. This modification was due to some concerns about the long-term mechanical stability, integrity and durability of the implant since the bioactive glass tended to be progressively reabsorbed over time with [24].

3.3 Mastoid Cavity Obliteration

Bioactive glasses and glass-ceramics in a powder/granule form have been recently proposed for mastoid cavity obliteration, a surgical procedure following the treatment of chronic suppurative otitis and cholesteatoma that continue to affect a large number of patients worldwide, especially in developing countries. This application exploits the well-known ability of bioactive glasses to bond to calcified tissues and promote new bone growth. The mainstay of treatment for cholesteatoma is a surgical procedure of mastoidectomy; however, this approach involves the formation of a mastoid cavity which is unnatural as well as anatomically and physiologically unsatisfactory [53]. In fact, the presence of an open cavity in the mastoid bone causes several problems including chronic discharge, dizziness due to exposure of semicircular canals to direct thermal stimulation by air/water entering the cavity, need for periodic cleaning of the cavity by an expert surgeon, difficulty in placing auditory prostheses, and unsightly appearance due to large meatoplasty [54].

The concept of mastoid obliteration for eliminating the cavity-related problems was first introduced one century ago by Mosher [59] who described the use of a postauricular soft tissue flap for obliteration. Since then, a number of biomaterials have been proposed for mastoid obliteration including bone, cartilage, fat, HA and, in recent years, bioactive glasses with promising results.

Leatherman and Dornhoffer [48] performed tympanic bulla obliteration in Mongolian gerbils (rats) by using commercial 45S5 Bioglass® particulate. Histologic evaluation was performed nine weeks after implantation to evaluate new bone formation around the implanted material. Wound healing occurred without complications and the formation of mature trabecular bone was observed around the implanted 45S5 Bioglass® granules. Extensive neovascularization was also detected within the graft material without any sign of inflammatory response or evidence of short-term resorption.

A group of researchers from Finland reported a series of studies in human patients who received S53P4 glass granules as mastoid obliteration biomaterial [70, 73, 74]. All the treated ears became dry and no cases of biomaterial-associated infection were reported. Significant reduction (or even complete elimination) of the mastoid cavity was successfully achieved in the majority of the patients. These results demonstrate that S53P4 is a valuable material for mastoid obliteration surgery, can be successfully used also in highly problematic cases (chronic infection in the mastoid associated with low pH), do not degrade after surgery and prevents further postoperative infections.

4 Applications in Ophthalmology

Due to its biocompatibility and transparency to visible light, glass has been used since centuries in ophthalmology for fabricating external lenses to correct refractive deficiencies of the eye. In these "traditional" applications, glass has been employed as an optical element of ophthalmic devices; on the contrary, the idea behind the use of bioactive glasses and glass-ceramics for orbital floor repair, enucleation and corneal surgery lies on a completely different approach, i.e. the improvement of biointegration which is crucial for the postoperative success of the implanted device.

4.1 Orbital Implants

In the management of ocular malignancies, removal of the natural eye (through enucleation[1] or evisceration[2]) is necessary when the pathology cannot be treated effectively in other ways. There are several reasons for taking this drastic measure

---

[1]The enucleation operation involves removal of the eyeball in its entirety by cutting the extraocular muscles and severing the optic nerve close to the globe.

[2]In the evisceration method the eye contents are removed whereas the sclera, the Tenon's capsule, the extraocular muscles and the optic nerve are spared.

and the most common include eyes damaged due to trauma, painful blind eyes, severe intraocular infection or malignant intraorbital tumours. Since visual contact plays a key role in human interactions, maintaining a life-like artificial eye (ocular prosthesis) is extremely important for the patient. Therefore, following the removal of the diseased eye, an orbital implant is inserted into the patient's anophthalmic socket in the same position as the eye in order to provide satisfactory volume replacement and, thus, prevent a contracted, sunken appearance. To provide maximum motility of the device, at the time of operation the extraocular muscles are either attached directly onto the implant or indirectly by suturing them to a wrapping material over the implant (wrapping materials usually include human sclera or Vicryl mesh). Then, the anterior tissues—Tenon's capsule and conjunctiva—are closed and antibiotics are applied. An ocular prosthesis is eventually fitted over the orbital implant and, although vision is not restored, the aesthetic appearance of the natural eye can be reproduced.

Since the first study reported by Mules [60], who described in detail the surgical placement of a hollow glass sphere in an eviscerated socket [60], a number of materials and designs have been developed and are still objects of ongoing research to manufacture a successful orbital implant. An ideal orbital implant should exhibit a number of key characteristics, including (i) biocompatibility, (ii) non-degradability (the implant should ensure permanently socket volume replacement and support to surrounding soft tissues), (iii) adequate compressive resistance that can withstand handling during operation, (iv) ease of fabrication and availability at a reasonable cost, (v) ability to be sterilized without undergoing degradation, and (vi) good motility transmitted to the ocular prosthesis [12, 42].

In recent years porous implants, such as polyethylene (PE), HA and alumina, have gained prominence since their interconnecting porous architecture allows them to act as a passive framework for fibrovascular tissue penetration. This involves two important advantages: (i) the porous implant is mechanically anchored to the soft tissues of the orbit, which decreases the risk of postoperative instability, and (ii) vascular supply enables immune surveillance which diminishes postoperative infections. However, there are still drawbacks to the existing orbital implants which include the risk of migration and extrusion, postoperative infections as well as low motility [19]. Hence, the development of new biomaterials and strategies which enable an improved outcome of eye replacement is more than ever desirable.

From a biological point of view, bioactive glasses and glass-ceramics have suitable properties for this specific application. These materials are capable of enhancing angiogenesis and fibrovascularization, and therefore they could show good potential in promoting healing of soft tissue surrounding the implant as well as reducing postoperative complications of anophthalmic surgery such as migration and extrusion.

Various silicate bioactive glass and glass-ceramic compositions have been proposed for manufacturing orbital implants in the form of single-phase materials or added as fillers to a polymer matrix in order to improve its mechanical proprieties (e.g. increase of strength) and bioactivity.

In an experimental study carried out by a group of Chinese researchers [84, 85], bioactive glass-ceramic porous sphere were implanted in enucleated rabbits. After 6 months of implantation, the authors encountered no implant-rejection and, by means of histological analysis, found fibrovascular tissue throughout approximately 90 % of the implant pores. These promising results led the researchers to further investigate the clinical outcomes of the glass-ceramic porous implants in 102 human patients (success rate of 96.1 %).

In 2012, Brandao et al. [15] placed 45S5 Bioglass® and Biosilicate® non-porous cone implants (Fig. 3a) in rabbit anophthalmic sockets to assess their biocompatibility. The anophthalmic socket was examined postoperatively by biochemical evaluations and orbit computed tomography scanning. After that, the orbital content was removed and histological studies were conducted at different experimental stages (7, 90, 180 days postoperatively) in order to evaluate tissue repair reaction and chemical changes in the biomaterial surface due to the contact with living tissue. The study showed that 45S5 Bioglass® and Biosilicate® implants do not lead to orbit infection or fluid accumulation and no signs of systemic toxicity were observed. Additionally, the implants proved capable of bonding to soft tissue. Therefore, the authors concluded that the implants show good potential and might be recommended as a safe implant to restore ocular volume.

It is worth pointing out that attention should be paid on the use of soluble glasses as orbital implants. Orbital implants, in fact, are regarded as being permanent and, thus, should ensure appropriate volume replacement for the patient's lifetime without undergoing volume loss [9].

Moreover, the mechanical properties of bioactive glass orbital implants is an issue that needs to be considered as these materials are considerably stiffer compared to natural ocular globe and soft orbital tissues. The use of mechanically rigid orbital implants is advantageous during the operation as the surgeon can easily maneuver and position the implant into the anophthalmic cavity with high precision and control. Nevertheless, stiffness mismatch between host material and

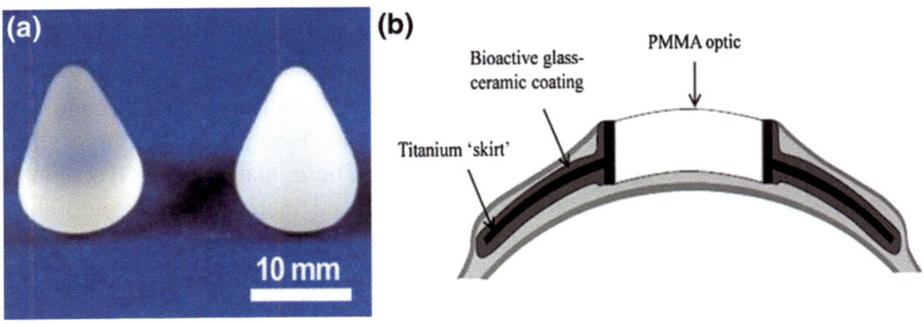

Fig. 3 Examples of application of bioactive glasses/glass-ceramics in ocular surgery: **a** conical orbital implants made of 45S5 Bioglass® (*left*) and glass-ceramic Biosilicate® (*right*) (reproduced from Brandao et al. [15] under a Creative Commons Attribution License); **b** artificial cornea (keratoprosthesis) comprising a PMMA lens and a titanium skirt coated with a bioactive A/W glass-ceramic (reproduced from Linnola et al. [49] with permission by Elsevier)

surrounding soft tissues, in combination with the repetitive movement of the implant by the extraocular muscles, might contribute to the erosion of the conjunctiva—which covers the front of the implant—and the consequent implant exposure. One approach that aims to overcome this problem is the use of bioactive glass as second phases added to a polymer matrix, to produce a composite porous implant which makes the best of both materials. The basic idea is to use the glass particles as stimulators of fibrovascular ingrowth and the polymeric substance, due to its pliable nature, as a compliant support.

A commercial example is Medpor-Plus orbital implant, which is a combination of porous PE and 45S5 glass particles (Novabone®) in a 70:30 ratio. Naik et al. [61] investigated the fibrovascular ingrowth of Medpor-Plus implants in comparison with porous PE implants (Medpor). Ten patients underwent enucleation followed by implantation of 5 Medpor-Plus implants in a first group and of 5 Medpor implants in a second. By means of a MRI study, the authors found a statistically significant increase in the rate of fibrovascularization of PE implants with the Novabone® particulate. Another research group examined the overall postoperative outcomes in 170 patients who underwent placement of a porous PE/bioactive glass composite implant after enucleation or secondary implantation and reported a success rate of 94.7 % [51].

A different approach that is currently under investigation to enhance the performance of orbital implants is the use of a surface coating that has an antibacterial effect. The use of a Cu-doped mesoporous bioactive glass (Cu-MBG) coating over a porous HA implant was recently proposed by a group of Chinese researchers [86]. Briefly, Cu-MBG coatings with 0–5 mol% of CuO were prepared by soaking porous HA scaffolds into a Cu-MBG sol precursor, then air dried to undergo ageing and finally calcined. The objective of this study was to exploit the high specific surface area of the MBG to enhance the drug uptake (and release) capacity of the implant while delivering antibacterial copper ions as the MBG degrades. Preliminary in vitro analyses validated the twofold effect of the proposed system, thus opening new perspectives for the prevention and treatment of implant-related infections.

Silver nanocluster/silica glass composite coatings have been also applied via radio-frequency sputtering on the surface of PMMA ocular prostheses to be coupled with orbital implants [10], and the material elicited a potent antibacterial effect in vitro due to the release of silver ions for 1 month.

4.2 *Orbital Floor Repair*

The orbital floor, which is particularly delicate and extremely thin, is the most common site of maxillofacial bone fracture during facial trauma. In the surgical repair of orbital floor fractures, restoring the original anatomical structure of the orbit is extremely important in order to provide support to the orbital contents and avoid serious complications such as diplopia,[3] extraocular movement limitation, and enophthalmos[4] [72]. Many materials, categorized as autogenous, allogenic and alloplastic (artificial), have been used to manufacture implants for the anatomical reconstruction of the orbital floor in the hope of achieving the best clinical outcome.

Autogenous implants include grafts of bone, cartilage, and fascia lata. Autogenous bone graft has long been considered the "gold standard" option for orbital floor reconstruction due to its proven long-term efficacy and reliability [58]. The successful outcome of a bone graft is the result of its excellent combination of osteogenic, osteoconductive and osteoinductive properties which enable full integration of the material once it is implanted. The graft can be positioned as such, held in position by means of titanium screws or plates, or used in combination with synthetic material. One of the major concerns of using autogenous bone graft is associated to the harvesting of the graft from the donor site, as this increases surgical time and the risk of infection, bony defect at the donor site and neurovascular damage. Furthermore, there are issues about the limited availability of autogenous grafts [21].

Allografts (i.e. the transplant of tissue from one individual to another of the same species, including those from cadaveric donors) are an alternative option to autografts; however, the risk of immunogenic rejection and disease transmission are still partially unresolved issues, and ethical/religious issues can arise, too.

Synthetic materials have been introduced to reduce some limitations of autologous and allogenic grafts. Man-made grafts, in fact, are always readily available without the need for donors and additional operations. Porous HA, PE and composite thereof (Hapex®) are the most commonly used [8]. Their open-pore structure allows vascularization as well as soft tissue and bone ingrowth which stabilize the implant in the defect and eliminate the need for fixation screws and sutures. However, concerns about the fragile nature of HA and the non-osteoinductivity and high infection rate of PE make these implants less attractive compared to autologous bone grafts [78].

A few research groups from Finland have investigated the aptness of plates manufactured from the silicate bioactive glass S53P4 for orbital floor reconstruction, with the aim of improving implant biointegration that is essential for a successful clinical outcome.

The first study was carried out by Suominen and Kinnunen [75] who compared the behaviour of S53P4 implants with that of autologous grafts. Besides demonstrating that S53P4 is associated with minimal risk of postoperative complications, the group reported no sign of implant resorption as well as firmer bonding with the host bone compared to bone grafts. To further examine the effectiveness of S53P4 implants, Kinnunen et al. [43] compared the postoperative outcomes of S53P4 and

[3]It is commonly-known as "double vision". Due to the misalignment of visual axes, the images fall on non-corresponding areas of the two retinas and the patient sees a double image of the same object.

[4]Recession of the eyeball within the orbit. This anomaly may be congenital or due to trauma, such as blow-out fracture of the orbit, and may persist after the repair of orbital floor fracture.

cartilage orbital floor grafts in 28 patients (14 receiving the glass plate and 14 implanted with the autograft); the results showed no sign of implant-related complication in the S53P4 group while a few complications (e.g. diplopia) occurred in the cartilage group.

Aitasalo et al. [3] carried out a review of 36 patients who had undergone placement of S53P4 orbital floor graft. Postoperative examinations were performed at 1 and 3 months after surgery in all cases and at 1 year after surgery in twenty-eight of the patients (82 %). Overall, patients achieved good cosmetic and functional outcomes without any sign of implant resorption. Furthermore, through the use of CT-scan imaging, the authors demonstrated the presence of osseous tissue surrounding the implanted plates. More recently, similar results were reported by Peltola et al. [62] who reviewed the clinical outcomes of 49 patients over a follow-up of 2 years. The selection of the suitable plate size and shape compatible with the dimensions of the bone defect was performed using stainless steel templates. This method allowed the correct definition of the implant design to adequately cover the defect and, thus, no mechanical fixation (i.e. screws) was needed.

The results of these studies highlight the suitability of the bioactive glass S53P4 for orbital floor fracture repair, which could represent a promising alternative to conventional autologous implants. Through stimulation of patient's own tissue, bioactive glass provides a healing-promoting environment, leading to biological fixation of the prosthetic element and reducing the incidence of extrusion. This effectively eliminates the need for invasive screws or threading to fix implants in place. However, the brittleness and rigidity of glass and the fact that S53P4 material cannot be shaped and moulded during operation remain the major limitations compared to autografts [62].

4.3 *Artificial Cornea*

The cornea is the transparent front part of the eye that protects the anterior chamber, the iris and the pupil. It is the major optical element that focuses visible light onto the retina, accounting for about 2/3 of focusing power. The cornea can be affected by several disorders (traumatic or biologic), some of which, despite treatment, may cause irreversible visual consequences. The replacement of a severely damaged or diseased cornea with a keratoprosthesis (artificial cornea) is an alternative approach to corneal transplants from donor eyes (keratoplasty) and is the only feasible route for restoring vision in patients suffering from Stevens-Johnson syndrome, repeated transplanted graft failure, glaucoma or chronic ocular inflammation [6].

An artificial cornea typically consists of a transparent optical core which transmits light from the exterior of the eye onto the retina, and a peripheral rim commonly known as keratoprosthesis "skirt" which anchors the implant to the recipient cornea. An ideal artificial cornea should fulfil a complex set of requirements. Firstly, it should consist of materials that promote integration with the corneal epithelium, stroma and endothelium. A continuous epithelial layer is essential for creating a barrier to infection, whereas stromal anchorage leads to improved retention of the prosthesis. In addition, the materials should exhibit appropriate nutrient and fluid permeability, absence of toxicity, and light transparency as well as low light scattering with respect to the optical part [20, 37].

Most of the keratoprostheses implanted today are totally made of inert polymeric materials, although different alternatives have emerged in order to achieve better biointegration of the device in the host tissue, thus ensuring the long-term success of implant bonding to corneal tissues. Among these, the osteo-odonto-keratoprosthesis (OOKP) constitutes a well-recognized option. The traditional procedure involves the use of a canine tooth and surrounding alveolar bone (harvested from the patient) to act as a carrier for a PMMA optical lens [25]. Despite the fact that bone and tooth show biocompatibility in the ocular environment, the complexity of the multi-stage surgical technique does represent a disadvantage. Furthermore, it has been highlighted by many researchers that the dentine frame undergoes partial resorption, which can be a problem since it may lead to loosening of the optical core and ultimately loss of the prosthesis [66].

In recent years, a great deal of research effort has gone into developing prosthetic skirts manufactured from different bioactive glass and glass-ceramic formulations. These materials are capable of tightly bonding to soft tissues and, therefore, could show good potential in reducing postoperative complications of OOKP implantation such as extrusion. Besides promoting tissue response towards full integration, the use of these biomaterials allows the production of totally synthetic devices, thus overcoming the need of autologous grafting. In an attempt of avoiding the need of tooth extraction, a glass-ceramic belonging to the Ceravital® system was the first bioactive material to be experimented for the fabrication of an alternative anchorage frame around OOKP [38]. Unlike dental lamina, the ceramic disk perfectly conforms to the shape of the corneal surface, thereby overcoming the problem of flattening of the anterior chamber. Nevertheless, these preliminary investigations were interrupted due to the tendency of the material to gradually dissolve over time when exposed to the ocular environment eventually leading to the failure of its supporting function.

Krause [45] tested the intracorneal biocompatibility of Bioverit® glass-ceramics in a rabbit model. The in vivo tests were able to demonstrate the successful incorporation of the materials into corneal tissues without toxic or immune reactions indicating their suitability for porous skirts.

Linnola et al. [49] used a bioactive glass-ceramic coating in an effort of overcoming a recurrent problem encountered with the use of keratoprostheses, i.e. the growth of epithelium between the corneal stroma and the prosthesis material into the anterior chamber which could lead to infections, implant extrusion and secondary glaucoma. The investigated devices consisted of a PMMA optical cylinder surrounded by a peripheral rim of titanium either uncoated or coated with a SiO_2–CaO–MgO–P_2O_5-based A/W glass-ceramic (Fig. 3b). The authors evaluated the outcomes of A/W glass-ceramic coated and uncoated kerathoprostheses in 22 New Zealand albino rabbits (11 for each of the two groups) and compared both materials in terms of epithelial ingrowth. This was more predominant with the uncoated kerathoprostheses, thus supporting the idea that the bioactive glass-ceramic was able to rapidly anchor the prosthesis to the corneal tissue preventing epithelial down-growth from the surface along the prosthesis into the interior of the eye. Despite this positive effect, the coating encountered problems of degradation and detachment and, therefore, the studies were discontinued.

These early experiment have paved the way for an intense research in this field and in more recent years several other researchers have explored the suitability of bioactive glass and glass-ceramic formulations for the fabrication of kerathoprosthesis skirts. Santos et al. [69] investigated a porous phosphate glass ($65P_2O_5$–$15CaO$–$10CaF_2$–$10Na_2O$ mol%)-reinforced hydroxyapatite (GRHA) and assessed its physicochemical and biological behaviors through several in vitro tests. Poly (vinyl alcohol) was used as a pore-forming agent to obtain a material characterized by a mean pore size of 110 μm which is within the desired range for an artificial cornea (50–150 μm). Materials with adequate pore size allow fibrovascularization to occur and produce results, in terms of tight fixation, that are superior compared to materials in the dense form. Furthermore, under physiological pH conditions no mass loss was found and, therefore, the authors concluded that the porous GRHA shows outstanding potential deserving further in vivo studies.

With the aim of replacing the human tooth and bone in OOKP support, which is characterized by the aforementioned degradation problems, Laattala et al. [46] investigated the behavior of four different PMMA/bioactive glass composite materials. Particles of 45S5 Bioglass®, S53P4, 1-98 ($5.9Na_2O$–$7.1K_2O$–$7.6MgO$–$23.9CaO$–$0.9B_2O_3$–$0.9P_2O_5$–53.8–SiO_2 mol%) as well as a slowly dissolving experimental glass FL107 (composition $10Na_2O$–$6MgO$–$16CaO$–$2B_2O_3$–$2P_2O_5$–$64SiO_2$ wt%) were incorporated in a PMMA matrix and the resulting composites were then compared on the basis of glass dissolution. The concept behind this study was to exploit the glass bioactivity as well as the surface porosity left behind after glass degradation for new tissue ingrowth, offering good prosthesis fixation. The PMMA matrix, moreover, is a stable structure that will not undergo volume loss for the patient's lifetime.

With a similar aim in mind, Huhtinen et al. [40] investigated the suitability two silico-boro-phophate bioactive glass compositions, 1-98 and 28-04 ($4.9Na_2O$–$7.2K_2O$–$9.0MgO$–$16.2CaO$–$2.6B_2O_3$–$60.1SiO_2$ mol%). None of the porous bioactive glasses elicited an inflammatory response and, in the course of biological in vitro tests, the keratocytes exhibited a typical elongated morphology that suggested a good adhesive potential. However, material dissolution was reported to be a problem. These authors, thereby, suggested the use of a backbone structure able to maintain the optical part in place following the bioactive glass dissolution.

5 Summary and Outlook

A lot of experimental work carried out mainly over the last two decades has shown how the meaning of the word "bioactivity" has evolved and expanded throughout time. Initially developed to refer to the repair or replacement of skeletal hard connective tissues, today it is also used to indicate the ability of those materials that can bond to soft tissues, promote wound healing and stimulate angiogenesis. Special bioactive glasses and glass-ceramics that lie within a particular compositional range have been found to exhibit these fascinating properties, thus showing promise for application in soft tissue engineering.

As discussed in this chapter, bioactive glasses and glass-ceramics have shown to be suitable materials for applications in ear and eye surgery. This is largely due to their versatile nature: in fact, their physico-chemical, mechanical and bioactive properties can be designed by varying the glass composition (type and amount of inorganic oxides) or applying appropriate processing routes. The use of these fascinating materials as parts of complex otologic and ocular devices has already been exploited to a certain extent, although they have not yet reached their full potential. Bioactive glasses are known to bond both to bone, which is a key property for implants used in the repair of orbital floor fractures and mastoid cavity obliteration, and to soft collagenous tissues, which is crucial for middle ear and cochlear implants. Furthermore, through the release of appropriate ionic dissolution products, porous bioactive glasses could stimulate angiogenesis and fibrovascular in-growth, which are essential to guarantee an adequate motility of orbital implants and reduce the risk of infections. It has been also demonstrated that porous bioactive glasses can stimulate the adhesion and proliferation of keratocytes, which make them promising candidate materials for a new generation of smart keratoprostheses.

Looking at the future, problems of stiffness mismatch with soft tissues still have to be solved; in this regard, tailoring of polymer/glass composites could be a valuable strategy. Moreover, bioactive glasses and glass-ceramics could improve the performance of otologic and ocular implants imparting them key extra-functionalities, such as antibacterial properties via the release of appropriate metal ions (e.g. copper and silver) and controlled drug release (e.g. mesoporous glasses) to elicit, for example, an anti-inflammatory effect at the implant site. We foresee a bright future for bioactive glasses that will indeed lead to exciting advances in human health and life-quality.

References

1. Ahmed, I., Lewis, M., Olsen, I., Knowles, J.C.: Phosphate glasses for tissue engineering: part 1. Processing and characterisation of a ternary-based P_2O_5–CaO–Na_2O glass system. Biomaterials **25**, 491–499 (2004)
2. Ahmed, I., Lewis, M., Olsen, I., Knowles, J.C.: Phosphate glasses for tissue engineering: part 2. Processing and characterisation of a ternary-based P_2O_5–CaO–Na_2O glass fibre system. Biomaterials **25**, 501–507 (2004)

3. Aitasalo, K., Kinnunen, I., Palmgren, J., Varpula, M.: Repair of orbital floor fractures with bioactive glass implants. J. Oral Maxillofac. Surg. **59**, 1390–1395 (2001)
4. Andersson, O.H., Liu, G., Karlsson, K.H., Juhanoja, J.: In vivo behaviour of glasses in the SiO_2–Na_2O–CaO–P_2O_5–Al_2O_3–B_2O_3 system. J. Mater. Sci. Mater. Med. **1**, 219–227 (1990)
5. Anselme, K., Davidson, P., Popa, A.M., Giazzon, M., Liley, M., Ploux, L.: The interactions of cells and bacteria with surfaces structured at the nanometre scale. Acta Biomater. **6**, 3824–3846 (2010)
6. Avadhanam, V.S., Smith, H.E., Liu, C.: Keratoprostheses for corneal blindness: a review of contemporary devices. Clin. Ophthalmol. **9**, 697–720 (2015)
7. Bahmad Jr., F., Merchant, S.N.: Histopathology of ossicular grafts and implants in chronic otitis media. Ann. Otol. Rhinol. Laryngol. **116**, 181–191 (2007)
8. Baino, F.: Biomaterials and implants for orbital floor repair. Acta Biomater. **7**, 3248–3266 (2011)
9. Baino, F.: How can bioactive glasses be useful in ocular surgery? J. Biomed. Mater. Res. A **103**, 1259–1275 (2015)
10. Baino, F., Ferraris, S., Miola, M., Perero, S., Verné, E., Coggiola, A., Dolcino, D., Ferraris, M.: Novel antibacterial ocular prostheses: proof of concept and physico-chemical characterization. Mater. Sci. Eng. C **60**, 467–474 (2016)
11. Baino, F., Novajra, G., Miguez-Pacheco, V., Boccaccini, A.R., Vitale-Brovarone, C.: Bioactive glasses: special applications outside the skeletal system. J. Non-Cryst. Solids **432**, 15–30 (2016)
12. Baino, F., Perero, S., Ferraris, S., Miola, M., Balagna, C., Verné, E., Vitale-Brovarone, C., Coggiola, A., Dolcino, D., Ferraris, M.: Biomaterials for orbital implants and ocular prostheses: Overview and future prospects. Acta Biomater. **10**, 1064–1087 (2014)
13. Beleites, E., Neupert, G., Augsten, G., Vogel, W., Schubert, H.: Rasterelektronenmikroskopische Untersuchungen des Zellwachstums auf maschinell bearbeitbarer Biovitrokeramik und Glaskohlenstoff in vitro und in vivo. Laryngo-Rhino-Otol. **64**, 217–220 (1985)
14. Blayney, A.W., Bebear, J.P., Williams, K.R., Portmann, M.: Ceravital in ossiculoplasty: experimental studies and early clinical results. Am. J. Otol. **100**, 1359–1366 (1986)
15. Brandao, S.M., Schellini, S.A., Moraes, A.D., Padovani, C.R., Pellizzon, C.H., Peitl, O., Zanotto, E.D.: Biocompatibility analysis of Bioglass® 45S5 and Biosilicate® implants in the rabbit eviscerated socket. Orbit **3**, 143–149 (2012)
16. Brandao, S.M., Schellini, S.A., Padovani, C.R., Peitl, O., Hashimoto, E.: Biocompatibility analysis of Bioglass® 45S5 and Biosilicate® cone in rabbit eviscerated cavity. Rev. Bras. Oftalmol. **72**, 21–25 (2013)
17. Brink, M., Turunen, T., Happonen, R., Yli-Urpo, A.: Compositional dependence of bioactivity of glasses in the system Na_2O–K_2O–MgO–CaO–B_2O_3–P_2O_5–SiO_2. J. Biomed. Mater. Res. **37**, 114–121 (1997)
18. Cao, W., Hench, L.L.: Bioactive materials. Ceram. Int. **22**, 493–507 (1996)
19. Chalasani, R., Poole-Warren, L., Conway, R.M., Ben-Nissan, B.: Porous orbital implants in enucleation: a systematic review. Surv. Ophthalmol. **52**, 145–155 (2007)
20. Chirila, T.V., Hicks, C.R., Dalton, P.D., Vijayasekaran, S., Lou, X., Hong, Y., Clayton, A.B., Ziegelaar, B.W., Fitton, J.H., Platten, S., Crawford, G.J., Constable, I.J.: Artificial cornea. Prog. Polym. Sci. **23**, 447–473 (1998)
21. Chowdhury, K., Krause, G.F.: Selection of materials for orbital floor reconstruction. Arch. Otolaryngol. Head Neck Surg. **124**, 1398–1401 (1998)
22. Clark, A.E., Pantano, C.G., Hench, L.L.: Auger spectroscopic analysis of Bioglass corrosion films. J. Am. Ceram. Soc. **59**, 37–39 (1976)
23. Douek, E., Fourcin, A.J., Moore, B.C.J., Clarke, G.P.: A new approach to the cochlear implant. Proc. R. Soc. Med. **70**, 379–383 (1977)
24. Downing, M., Johansson, U., Carlsson, L., Walliker, J.R., Spraggs, P.D., Dodson, H., Hochmair-Desoyer, I.J., Albrektsson, T.: A bone-anchored percutaneous connector system for neural prosthetic applications. Ear Nose Throat J. **76**, 328–332 (1997)

25. Falcinelli, G., Falsini, B., Taloni, M., Colliardo, P., Falcinelli, G.: Modified osteo-odonto-keratoprosthesis for treatment of corneal blindness: long-term anatomical and functional outcomes in 181 cases. Arch. Ophthalmol. **123**, 1319–1329 (2005)
26. Geyer, G.: Implantate in der Mittelohrchirurgie. Eur. Arch. Otorhinolaryngol. **1**, 185–221 (1992)
27. Gross, U., Strunz, V.: Interface of various glasses and glass-ceramics in a bony implantation bed. J. Biomed. Mater. Res. **19**, 251–271 (1985)
28. Hantson, P., Mahieu, P., Gersdorff, M., Sindic, C.J., Lauwerys, R.: Encephalopathy with seizures after use of aluminium-containing bone cement. Lancet **344**, 1647 (1994)
29. Hench, L.L., Paschall, H.A.: Direct chemical bonding of bioactive glass-ceramic materials and bone. J. Biomed. Mater. Res. Symp. **4**, 25–42 (1973)
30. Hench, L.L., Splinter, R.J., Allen, W.C., Greenlee, T.K.: Bonding mechanisms at the interface of ceramic prosthetic materials. J. Biomed. Mater. Res. **2**, 117–141 (1971)
31. Hench, L.L.: Bioceramics—from concept to clinic. J. Am. Ceram. Soc. **74**, 1487–1510 (1991)
32. Hench, L.L.: Bioceramics. J. Am. Ceram. Soc. **81**, 1705–1728 (1998)
33. Hench, L.L., Polak, J.: Third-generation biomedical materials. Sci. **295**, 1014–1017 (2002)
34. Hench, L.L.: The story of Bioglass®. J. Mater. Sci. Mater. Med. **17**, 967–978 (2006)
35. Hench, L.L.: Genetic design of bioactive glass. J. Eur. Ceram. Soc. **29**, 1257–1265 (2009)
36. Hench, L.L., Greenspan, D.: Interactions between bioactive glass and collagen: a review and new perspectives. J. Aust. Ceram. Soc. **49**, 1–40 (2013)
37. Hicks, C.R., Fitton, J.H., Chirila, T.V., Crawford, G.J., Constable, I.J.: Keratoprostheses: advancing toward a true artificial cornea. Surv. Ophthalmol. **42**, 175–189 (1997)
38. Hoffmann, F., Harnisch, J.P., Strunz, V., Bunte, M., Gross, U.M., Manner, K., Bromer, H., Deutscher, K.: Osteo-Keramo-Keratoprothese: eine Modifikation der osteo-odontokeratoprothese nach Strampelli. Klin Monbl Augenheilkd **173**, 747–755 (1978)
39. Huang, W., Day, D.E., Kittiratanapiboon, K., Rahaman, M.N.: Kinetics and mechanisms of the conversion of silicate (45S5), borate, and borosilicate glasses to hydroxyapatite in dilute phosphate solutions. J. Mater. Sci. Mater. Med. **17**, 583–596 (2006)
40. Huhtinen, R., Sandeman, S., Rose, S., Fok, E., Howell, C., Fröberg, L., Moritz, N., Hupa, L., Lloyd, A.: Examining porous bio-active glass as a potential osteo-odonto-keratoprosthetic skirt material. J. Mater. Sci. Mater. Med. **24**, 1217–1227 (2013)
41. Jones, J.R.: Review of bioactive glass: from Hench to hybrids. Acta Biomater. **9**, 4457–4486 (2013)
42. Jordan, D.R.: Anophthalmic orbital implants. Ophthalmol. Clin. N. Am. **13**, 587–608 (2000)
43. Kinnunen, I., Aitasalo, K., Pollonen, M., Varpula, M.: Reconstruction of orbital floor fractures using bioactive glass. J Craniofac.-Maxillofac. Surg. **28**, 229–234 (2000)
44. Koscielny, S., Beleites, E.: Untersuchungen zum Einfluss von Biokeramiken auf biologische Leistungen von Mikroorganismen. HNO **49**, 367–371 (2001)
45. Krause, A.: Intracorneal biocompatibility of glass ceramics. Contactologia **14**, 28–31 (1992)
46. Laattala, K., Huhtinen, R., Puska, M., Arstila, H., Hupa, L., Kellomäki, M., Vallittu, P. K.: Bioactive composite for keratoprosthesis skirt. J. Mech. Behav. Biomed. Mater. **4**, 1700–1708 (2011)
47. Lakhkar, N.J., Lee, I.H., Kim, H.W., Salih, V., Wall, I.B., Knowles, J.C.: Bone formation controlled by biologically relevant inorganic ions: role and controlled delivery from phosphate-based glasses. Adv. Drug Deliv. Rev. **65**, 405–420 (2013)
48. Leatherman, B.D., Dornhoffer, J.L.: Bioactive glass ceramic particles as an alternative for mastoid obliteration: results in an animal model. Otol. Neurotol. **23**, 657–660 (2002)
49. Linnola, R.J., Happonen, R., Andersson, O.H., Vedel, E., Yli-Urpo, A.U., Krause, U., Laatikainen, L.: Titanium and bioactive glass-ceramic coated titanium as materials for keratoprosthesis. Exp. Eye Res. **63**, 471–478 (1996)
50. Lobel, K.: Ossicular replacement prostheses. In: Hench, L.L., Wilson, J. (eds.) Clinical Performance of Skeletal Prostheses, pp. 214–236. Chapman and Hall, London (1996)

51. Ma, X., Schou, K.R., Maloney-Schou, M., Harwin, F.M., Ng, J.D.: The porous polyethylene/bioglass spherical orbital implant: a retrospective study of 170 cases. Ophthal. Plast. Reconstr. Surg. **27**, 21–27 (2011)
52. Maassen, M.M., Zenner, H.P.: Tympanoplasty type II with ionomeric cement and titaniumgold-angle prostheses. Am. J. Otol. **19**, 693–699 (1998)
53. Males, A.G., Gray, R.F.: Mastoid surgery: quantifying the distress in a radical cavity. Clin. Otolaryngol. **19**, 194–198 (1994)
54. Mehta, R.P., Harris, J.P.: Mastoid obliteration. Otolaryngol. Clin. N. Am. **39**, 1129–1142 (2006)
55. Merwin, G.E.: Bioglass middle ear prosthesis: preliminary report. Ann. Otol. Rhinol. Laryngol. **95**, 78–82 (1986)
56. Merwin GE (1990) Review of bioactive materials for otologic and maxillofacial applications. In: Yamamuro T, Hench LL, Wilson J (eds) Handbook on Bioactive Ceramics: Bioactive Glasses and Glass-Ceramics, pp. 323–328. CRC Press, Boca Raton
57. Miguez-Pacheco, V., Hench, L.L., Boccaccini, A.R.: Bioactive glasses beyond bone and teeth: emerging applications in contact with soft tissues. Acta Biomater. **13**, 1–15 (2015)
58. Mok, D., Lessard, L., Cordoba, C., Harris, P.G., Nikolis, A.: A review of materials currently used in orbital floor reconstruction. Can. J. Plast. Surg. **12**, 134–140 (2004)
59. Mosher, H.P.: A method of filling the excavated mastoid with a flap from the back of the auricle. Laryngolscope **21**, 1158–1163 (1911)
60. Mules, P.H.: Evisceration of the globe with artificial vitreous. Trans. Ophthalmol. Soc. UK **5**, 200–206 (1885)
61. Naik, M.N., Murthy, R.K., Honavar, S.G.: Comparison of vascularization of Medpor and Medpor-plus orbital implants: a prospective, randomized study. Ophthalmic Plast. Reconstr. Surg. **6**, 463–467 (2007)
62. Peltola, M., Kinnunen, I., Aitasalo, K.: Reconstruction of orbital wall defects with bioactive glass plates. J. Oral Maxillofac. Surg. **66**, 639–646 (2008)
63. Reck, R.: Preliminary report: tissue reaction to glass ceramics in the middle ear. Clin. Otolaryngol. **6**, 63–65 (1981)
64. Reck, R., Storkel, S., Meyer, A.: Bioactive glass-ceramics in middle ear surgery: an 8-year review. Ann. N. Y. Acad. Sci. **523**, 100–106 (1988)
65. Renghini, C., Giuliani, A., Mazzoni, S., Brun, F., Larsson, E., Baino, F., Vitale-Brovarone, C.: Microstructural characterization and in vitro bioactivity of porous glass-ceramic scaffolds for bone regeneration by synchrotron radiation X-ray microtomography. J. Eur. Ceram. Soc. **33**, 1553–1565 (2013)
66. Ricci, R., Pecorella, I., Ciardi, A., Della Rocca, C., Di Tondo, U., Marchi, V.: Strampelli's osteo-odonto-keratoprosthesis. Clinical and histological long-term features of three prostheses. Br. J. Ophthalmol. **76**, 232–234 (1992)
67. Rust, K.R., Singleton, G.T., Wilson, J., Antonelli, P.J.: Bioglass middle ear prosthesis: long-term results. Am. J. Otol. **17**, 371–374 (1996)
68. Sanders, D.M., Hench, L.L.: Mechanisms of glass corrosion. J. Am. Ceram. Soc. **56**, 373–377 (1973)
69. Santos, L., Ferraz, M.P., Shirosaki, Y., Lopes, M.A., Fernandes, M.H., Osaka, A., Santos, J. D.: Degradation studies and biological behavior on an artificial cornea material. Invest. Ophthalmol. Vis. Sci. **52**, 4274–4281 (2011)
70. Sarin, J., Grenman, R., Aitasalo, K., Pulkkinen, J.: Bioactive glass S53P4 in mastoid obliteration surgery for chronic otitis media and cerebrospinal fluid leakage. Ann. Otol. Rhinol. Laryngol. **121**, 563–569 (2012)
71. Sepulveda, P., Jones, J.R., Hench, L.L.: Bioactive sol-gel foams for tissue repair. J. Biomed. Mater. Res. A **49**, 340–348 (2002)
72. Shin, J.W., Lim, J.S., Yoo, G., Byeon, J.H.: An analysis of pure blowout fractures and associated ocular symptoms. J. Craniofac. Surg. **24**, 703–707 (2013)
73. Silvola, J.T.: Mastoidectomy cavity obliteration with bioactive glass: a pilot study. Otolaryngol. Head Neck Surg. **147**, 119–126 (2012)

74. Stoor, P., Pulkkinen, J., Grénman, R.: Bioactive glass S53P4 in the filling of cavities in the mastoid cell area in surgery for chronic otitis media. Ann. Otol. Rhinol. Laryngol. **119**, 377–382 (2010)
75. Suominen, E., Kinnunen, I.: Bioactive glass granules and plates in the reconstruction of defects of the facial bones. Scand. J. Plast. Reconstr. Surg. Hand Surg. **30**, 281–289 (1996)
76. Tanaka Massuda, E., Lisboa Maldonado, E., Teixeira de Lima, J., Jr, Peitl O., Hyppolito, M. A., Apparecido de Oliveira, J.A.: Biosilicate® ototoxicity and vestibulotoxicity evaluation in guinea-pigs. Braz. J. Otorhinolaryngol. **75**, 665–668 (2009)
77. Turck, C., Brandes, G., Krueger, I., Behrens, P., Mojallal, H., Lenarz, T., Stieve, M.: Histological evaluation of novel ossicular chain replacement prostheses: an animal study in rabbits. Acta Otolaryngol. **127**, 801–808 (2007)
78. Villarreal, P.M., Monje, F., Morillo, A.J., Junquera, L.M., Gonzalez, C., Barbon, J.J.: Porous polyethylene implants in orbital floor reconstruction. Plast. Reconstr. Surg. **109**, 877–885 (2002)
79. Vogt, J.C., Brandes, G., Ehlert, N., Behrens, P., Nolte, I., Mueller, P.P., Lenarz, T., Stieve, M.: Free Bioverit II implants coated with a nanoporous silica layer in a mouse ear model—a histological study. J. Biomater. Appl. **24**, 175–191 (2009)
80. Walliker, J., Carson, H., Douek, E.E., Fourcin, A., Rosen, S.: An extracochlear auditory prosthesis. In: Bansai, P. (ed.) Proceedings of Cochlear Implant Symposium 90, p. 265. Durer, Germany (1987)
81. Wilson, J., Low, S.B.: Bioactive ceramics for periodontal treatment—comparative studies in the Patus monkey. J. Appl. Biomater. **3**, 123–129 (1992)
82. Wilson, J., Pigott, G.H., Schoen, F.J., Hench, L.L.: Toxicology and biocompatibility of bioglasses. J. Biomed. Mater. Res. **15**, 805–817 (1981)
83. Wilson, J., Douek, E., Rust, K.: Bioglass middle ear devices: ten year clinical results. In: Wilson, J., Hench, L.L., Greenspan, D. (eds.) Bioceramics, pp. 239–246. Pergamon/Elsevier, Oxford (1995)
84. Xu, X., Huang, Z., Wang, C.: Clinical study of bioactive glass ceramics as orbital implants. Bull. Hunan Med. Univ. **22**, 440–442 (1997)
85. Xu, X., Wang, C., Huang, T., Ding, L., Huang, Z., Zhang, X.: An experimental study of bioactive glass ceramics as orbital implants. Bull. Hunan Med. Univ. **22**, 25–28 (1997)
86. Ye, J., He, J., Wang, C., Yao, K., Gou, Z.: Copper-containing mesoporous bioactive glass coatings on orbital implants for improving drug delivery capacity and antibacterial activity. Biotechnol. Lett. **36**, 961–968 (2014)
87. Zikk, D., Rapoport, Y., Bloom, J., Himelfarb, M.Z.: Auditory brain-stem responses in guinea pigs following middle ear implantation of Ceravital. Eur. Arch. Otorhinolaryngol. **248**, 102–104 (1990)

Biocompatible Glasses for Cancer Treatment

Renata Deliberato Aspasio, Roger Borges and Juliana Marchi

Abstract Treatment of cancer is an old issue in the history of medicine. Millions cases are reported every year, as well as millions of cancer-related deaths are also registered. The development of new technologies is changing this scenario, and new cancer treatment techniques have been included in the clinical routine. Among these techniques, hyperthermia and brachytherapy have an interesting prominence. Hyperthermia has been suggested as an auxiliary therapy for cancer treatment, while brachytherapy offers the opportunity of delivering high dose beta radiation emission into the cancerous tissue. In this chapter, we pointed out the use of biocompatible glasses (please consult the Editor's note in order to clarify the usage of the terms bioglass, bioactive glass and biocompatible glasses) for cancer treatment by either hyperthermia or brachytherapy. A quick review about hyperthermia is provided, and the main compositions of biocompatible glasses used in hyperthermia are discussed regarding their magnetic and biological properties. In addition, few glasses with suitable radiological properties with potential application in prostate cancer and liver cancer are reviewed, as well as new possible glasses composition are considered from the point of view of Monte Carlo and molecular dynamics simulations.

1 Therapies for Cancer Treatment

There are more than 100 different types of cancer. The genetic material of a cell may suffer damages or changes, producing mutations that affects cell growing and division process. This process might affect vital organs, even resulting in death. According to International Agency for Research on Cancer, from World Health Organization, 14.1 million new cancer cases and 8.2 million cancer-related deaths

R.D. Aspasio · R. Borges · J. Marchi (✉)
Center for Natural Science and Humanities (CCNH), Federal University of ABC (UFABC), Santo André, Brazil
e-mail: juliana.marchi@ufabc.edu.br

J. Marchi (ed.), *Biocompatible Glasses*, Advanced Structured Materials 53,
DOI 10.1007/978-3-319-44249-5_10

occurred in 2012, compared with 12.7 million and 7.6 million, respectively, in 2008, showing a significant increase of cases around the world [1].

There are different forms of cancer treatment, being the most common in the clinical practice [1]:

1. Surgery for the tumor removing;
2. Radiotherapy by using radiation to cleavage tumor's DNA and other important biomolecules;
3. Chemotherapy by using drugs to interfere on cell cycle [1].

However, in most cases such procedures are aggressive, leading to a decrease in the response of the immunological system, and causing undesired symptoms or side effects, such as pain, hair loss, nausea, fatigue, and risk of infection [1]. In order to solve these problems, new more effective and less invasive therapies are being studying around the world. Among them, brachytherapy and hyperthermia are promising therapies, and deserve special attention [1].

Hyperthermia is a term used to describe heat application techniques, and is usually associated with other techniques already well established, especially radiotherapy and chemotherapy. Only in 1970, hyperthermia was considered as a clinical therapy [1]. Nowadays, hyperthermia is in Phase II clinical trial in European countries like Germany, Spain and Netherlands [2–4].

The treatment is based on heating targeted tissues at temperature between 41 and 46 °C, causing the destruction of the malignant cells, while healthy cells do not suffer any non-reversible damage. Then, this treatment shows no very undesirable side-effects [3, 5, 6]. This treatment will be successful when three conditions are satisfied:

(a) The temperature of the heated tumor tissues is kept at and above 41 °C after the first heating;
(b) During a specified time, the tumor tissue is heated up to 43 °C and then kept at that temperature for another given time;
(c) The surrounding normal cells are maintained at temperature below 46 °C [7].

The heat used in hyperthermia treatment can be by either localized or regional. When it is localized, microwave antennae applicators, ultrasound beans, small magnetic seeds, and radiofrequency plate applicators worm up the cancer cell. When it is regional, the most common technique is the application of heated perfusates (hot water). However, due to heating up large areas of body, it exposes normal tissues to temperature elevation to which can produces risks and systemic physiologic responses. In this sense, the usage of localized hyperthermia has been more emphasized, mainly by using magnetic seeds [8, 9].

If magnetic particles are used in cancer treatment, according to the particle size used, hyperthermia can be also classified into four different types of magnetic hyperthermia: intracellular hyperthermia; extracellular hyperthermia; magnetic fluid hyperthermia; hyperthermia using magnetic materials in bulk [10].

Intracellular hyperthermia is a technique that uses the insertion of fine particles (1–100 nm), such as magnetite (Fe_3O_4) with morphology of needles or rods, as heat mediators with superparamagnetic properties, using a non-invasive technique, like injection [11]. When a fluid containing magnetic particles with subcritical size is inserted in the human body, the cells can easily incorporate these particles since the diameter is adequate for endocytose. Extracellular hyperthermia using magnetic particles is similar to the previous one, but using larger particles (magnitude of micrometers) with ferromagnetic properties, and heat effect similarly to superparamagnetic particles [12]. Magnetic fluid consists of ultramicroscopic particles (~ 100 Å) of magnetic oxides. These particles can be stabilized by surfactants to prevent agglomeration, thus obtaining stable colloidal suspensions in water. Ferrofluid particles consisting of superparamagnetic Fe_3O_4 and other magnetic particles modified or coated with different types of biocompatible polymers are the most common example [13]. Finally, hyperthermia can be also carried out by using magnetic materials in "bulk", which are surgically inserted in the tumor site implant [14].

Considering all of these previous mentioned classifications of magnetic hyperthermia, the principle that induces the cancer cells death is the same. Under an alternating external magnetic field, the magnetic material releases heat, which is originated due to (1) the magnetic hysteresis loss process during reorientation of spins; it causes an irreversible magnetization, and consequently conversion of magnetic energy into heat [15] or (2) by frictional losses due to the rotation of the particles in an environment with sufficiently low viscosity [16], allowing the conversion of mechanical energy into heat. Moreover, both mechanisms depends on the thermal conductivity and heat capacity of the medium surrounding the material, which will allow the heat absorption, and the consequent weakening and/or destruction of cancer cells while preserving healthy ones [17].

Nowadays, the molecular basis of hyperthermia is still under investigation. There are different mechanisms of antitumor activity induced by local hyperthermia including loss of membrane integrity, protein denaturation, upregulation of heat shock, activation of immune cells, vessel destruction and tissue necrosis [18, 19]. These mechanisms are illustrated in Fig. 1.

Tumor cells are not capable of dealing with high temperatures like healthy tissue. The microenvironment of cancer presents a reduced blood flow by vessel destruction, favoring hypoxia, acidosis and intratumoral energy deprivation. The hyperthermia temperatures above 42 °C leads to loss of membrane integrity, reduction of cancer blood flow and vessel destruction, leading to tissue necrosis. In addition, the high temperature leads to protein denaturation [3, 4, 18]. The upregulation of heat shock proteins mechanisms is consisted of induction of a cytotoxic cell-activation, leading to a cytotoxic effect in tumor cells. The activation of immune cells can be observed by the sensitization of the lymphocyte function due the heat, occasioning an immunological response to combat the tumor [18]. Then, all these mechanisms works together for an efficient treatment.

Many cellular effects are important for thermal inactivation, such as the inhibition of nucleic acid synthesis, the blockage of malignant cells in mitosis, and depression or inhibition of the oxidative metabolism depressing anaerobic

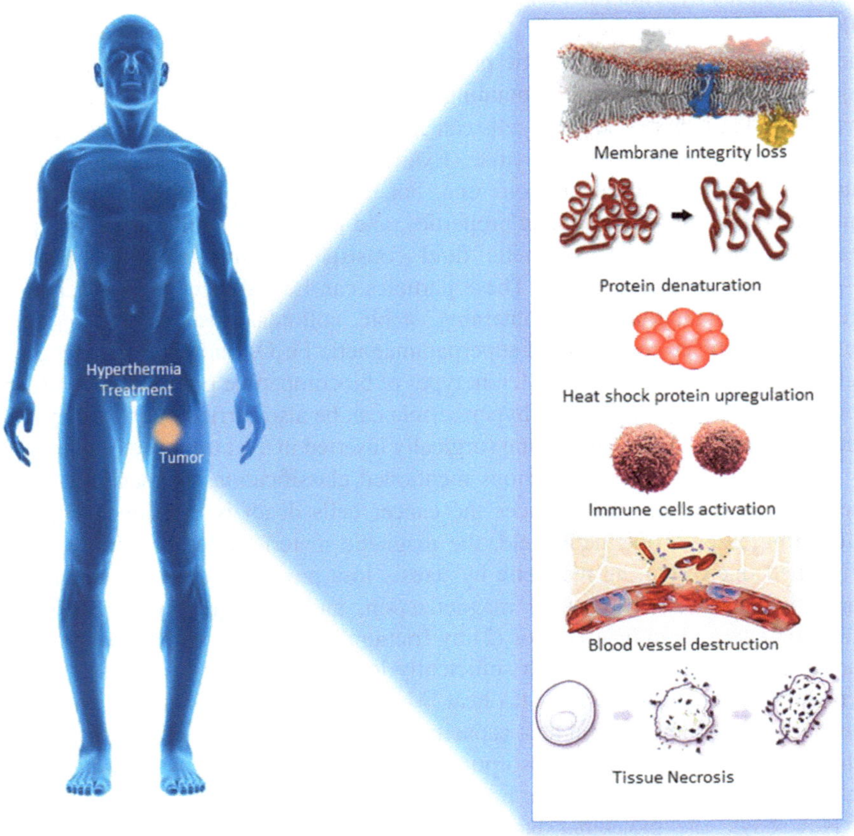

Fig. 1 Different mechanisms of antitumor activity induced by local hyperthermia of tumors

glycolysis. Extracellular effects also contributes to the tumor cells death, such as insufficient nutrition, which inhibits cell proliferation, and changes tumor cell metabolism [20, 21].

Additionally, the increase in tumor temperature can alter the permeability and fluidity of the plasma membrane, allowing greater oxygen and chemotherapeutic drugs uptake by these cells, potentiating the effect of treatments by radiotherapy and chemotherapy, respectively [3, 4]. Thus, the increase of the temperature in the treatment can induce tumor cell death not only by thermal stress, but also by potentiation of ionizing radiation and chemotherapeutic drugs [2, 4].

Another interesting technique is brachytherapy, which is a radioactive-based technique for cancer treatment that has became more popular in clinical practices. Radiotherapy is classified into external and internal radiotherapy, being the last one the brachytherapy. Briefly, in external radiotherapy, the radioactive source is placed out of the patient (Fig. 2). Therefore, high dose of beta and/or gamma rays from the radioactive source goes toward the cancer tissue, passing also through healthy

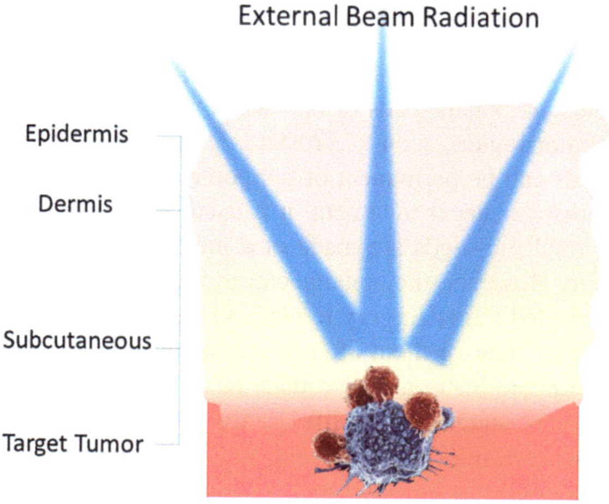

Fig. 2 Scheme demonstrating tissue absorption of external beam radiation. It is observed the radiation emitted damages both tumor and healthy cells through electron excitation and release of energy

tissues. This process may damage either the healthy or the cancer tissue. Treatment using external radiotherapy may take repetitive patient visit to the hospital, because it is carried out on an outpatient basis. In addition, because of the total dose is divided into several smaller doses, the treatment can last from 5 to 8 weeks, being this time based on the size and location of the cancer cells, the type of cancer, the reason for the treatment, the patient's general health, and other treatments that the patient is getting [22].

Usually, healthy tissues can absorb up to 60 % of the total radiation in external radiotherapy, being it an issue to be taken into account, because healthy cell are damaged [22]. On the other hand, in brachytherapy, radioactive seeds are placed in the cancerous tissue, i.e., inside the patient's body (Fig. 3). The advantage of brachytherapy, over other conventional radiotherapy techniques, is its high dose

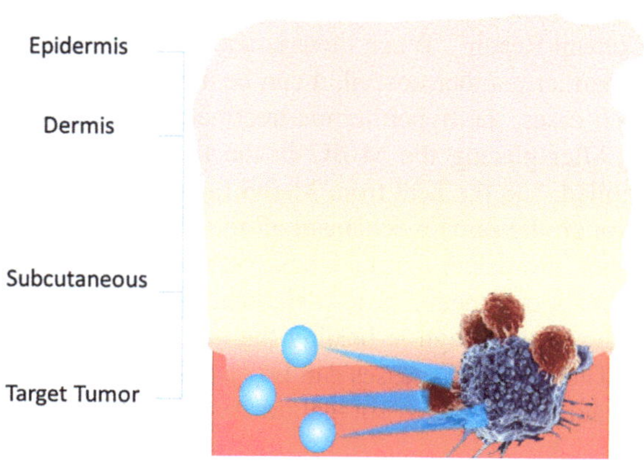

Fig. 3 Schematic figure illustrating the principle of brachytherapy: radioactive seeds (*blue spheres*) emitting beta and/or gamma rays into the target tumor

delivered into the tumor, due to the seed's proximity to the cancer. Brachytherapy is also classified into intracavitary or interstitial. The first is applied in patients cavities, such as uterus, esophagus and rectum, over a pre-calculated time, and then removed. In the second, small seeds or thin wires made of radioactive material are placed into the tumor region, such as prostate, tongue, brain or breast. Interstitial brachytherapy seeds can be permanent or temporary, and it usually depend on the target tissue. In prostate cancer treatment, it is used permanent seeds, for example. The most commercialized seeds are made of a metallic capsule containing ^{125}I as radioactive element. However, the metallic capsule is inert to the tissue, and in most of the cases it is needed a first surgery to place them into the cancerous tissue, and an another surgery to remove them after the treatment. In order to overcome this problem, new resorbable materials have been researched to replace these metallic capsules, consequently increasing the life quality of patients [23].

Glasses and glass-ceramics materials can be considered promising materials to use in these alternatives techniques due to their bioactive and biocompatible behavior. It is possible to incorporate and crystallize magnetic phases into the glass matrix for hyperthermia, as well as the use of radioactive elements as radioactive seeds for brachytherapy. The glass bioactive behavior allows the tissue regeneration, while the magnetic phase or the radioactive seeds allow the cancer treatment for bone cancer, for example. In the next sections biocompatible glasses applied to hyperthermia and brachytherapy will be further covered.

2 Magnetic Biocompatible Glasses for Hyperthermia Treatment

Magnetic biocompatible glasses (M-BG) have been evaluated as potential materials for treatment of bone cancer by hyperthermia. Biocompatible glasses with bioactive behavior are known for their use in bone tissue regeneration, as reviewed on the Chapters "Bioactive Materials: Definitions and Application in Tissue Engineering and Regeneration Therapy" and "An Introduction and History of the Bioactive Glasses", and deeply discussed on the Chapter "45S5 Bioglass Based Scaffolds for Skeletal Repair". When there is a magnetic phase in the glass structure, acting as a hyperthermia thermoseed, it can be used as a material for bone cancer treatment. In such cases, the hyperthermia treatment is allied with bone tissue regeneration [5].

After placing the M-BG in the tumor region, an alternating magnetic field is applied, and the heat from M-BG raises the temperature of the surrounding tissues through the same mechanism aforementioned for ferromagnetic particles. After the tumor shrinkage, the malignant cells can remain around the tumor site, leading to tumor recurrence. These malignant cells can be destroyed to prevent the tumor recurrence through re-heating the implanted material when needed [24].

The bioactive glasses can be synthetized by melting or by sol–gel process. The advantage of using sol–gel method instead of melting is the higher bioactive behavior exhibit by such glasses [25–27]. This improved bioactivity can be explained in terms of their higher textural properties (surface area and porosity), which have a large influence on the reactivity with the surrounding physiological fluids [28]. The magnetic phase of the M-BG can be obtained through heat treatment of the glass system for the crystallization of magnetic phases (Fig. 4 illustrates the melting process and Fig. 5 illustrates the sol–gel process) or by the incorporation of magnetic nanoparticles in the glass matrix (Fig. 6) [29, 30]. The advantage of the magnetic nanoparticles incorporation is due their higher superficial contact area leading to a better magnetization than the magnetic phase crystallized by heat

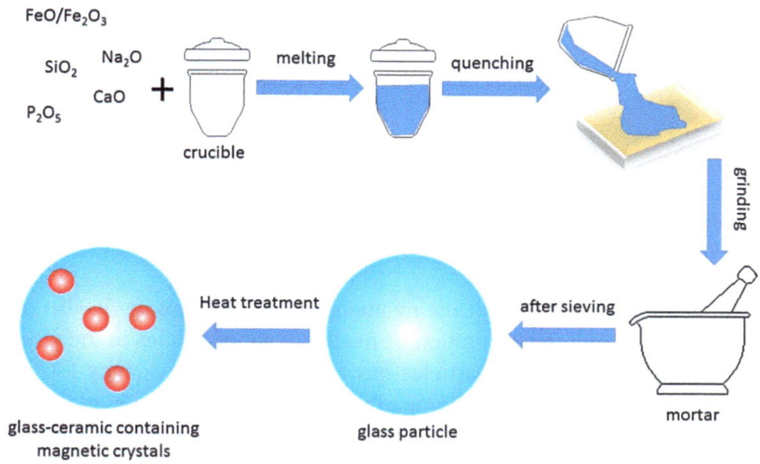

Fig. 4 Schematic representation of M-BG synthesis through melting-quenching method followed by heat treatment in order to nucleate magnetic crystals

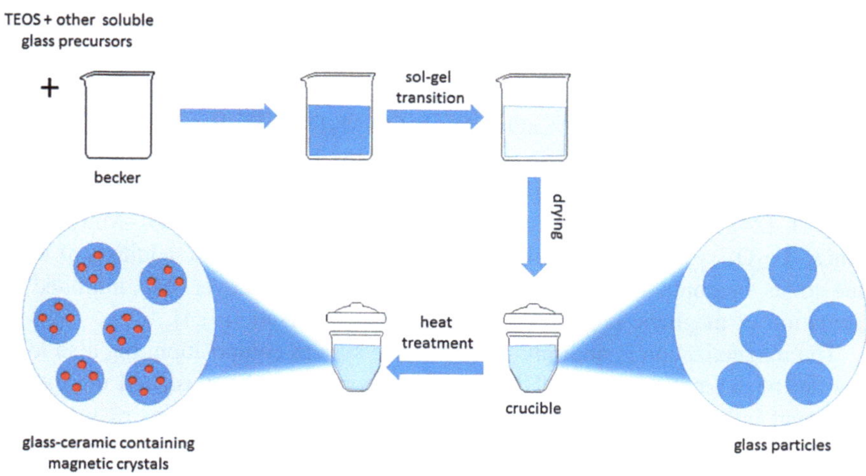

Fig. 5 Obtainment of M-BG through sol–gel method followed by heat treatment in order to nucleate magnetic crystals

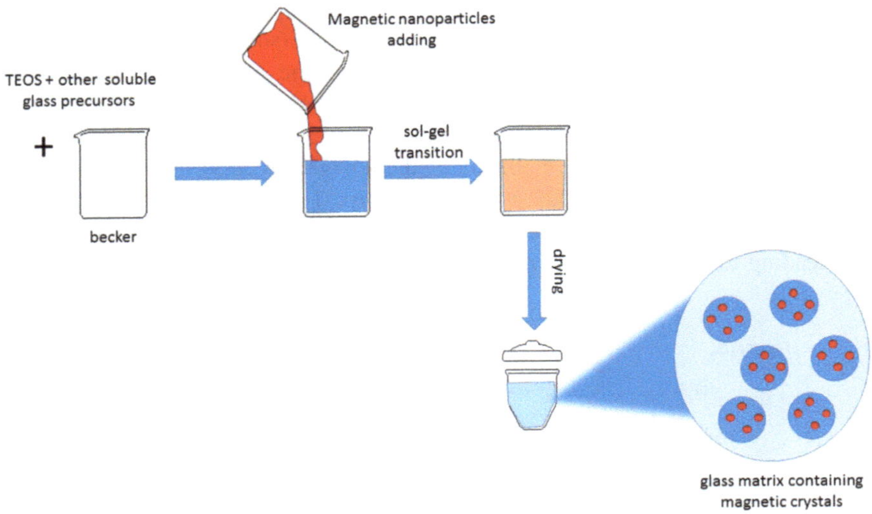

Fig. 6 Obtainment of M-BG through sol–gel method in which the magnetic nanoparticles are added during the synthesis, and the glass is nucleated surround them

treatment, and a better control of the magnetic phase morphology is also provided. However, the uniformly incorporation of magnetic nanoparticles in the glass matrix can be challenging, once nanoparticles has an aggregation tendency [30].

The studied of magnetic biocompatible glasses started with in 1991, when Kokubo et al. [31] developed glasses in the $CaO–SiO_2–B_2O_3–P_2O_5$ system doped with iron oxides II and III through melting-quenching method. The glasses were thermally treated, forming glass ceramics with the formation of β-wollastonite ($CaO{\cdot}SiO_2$) and magnetite (Fe_3O_4), being it the first approached biocompatible glasses with magnetic properties that could be applied to cancer treatment by hyperthermia [31].

Since then, several studies have studied glasses on similar systems, and the glass composition has shown to play an important role on the magnetic properties. Da Li et al. [32] studied the system $CaO–SiO_2–P_2O_5–MgO–CaF_2–Fe_2O_3$ through sol–gel method, where Mg was used to dope ferrite. This Mg ferrite glasses led to larger hysteresis loop, leading to a higher magnetization than Fe ferrite. In another study, Li et al. [24] evaluated the magnetic properties of $CaO–SiO_2–P_2O_5–MnO–CaF_2–MnO_2–Fe_2O_3$ system by sol–gel method. The motivation for the addition of Mn is due to its biocompatibility and high magnetization. However, Mn inhibited the formation of magnetic phases, decreasing the magnetization [24].

The magnetization is not only limited to the system composition, but also to the amount of magnetic element. The iron oxide content in the glass and the thermal treatment influences the microstructure and the magnetic properties of the M-BG [29]. Eniu et al. [33] studied the $CaO–P_2O_5–SiO_2–Fe_2O_3$ system with posterior thermal treatment. They noticed magnetite (Fe_3O_4) crystals was the major magnetic phase, and different iron oxides such as γ-Fe_2O_3 and α-Fe_2O_3 also appears as minorities. These results indicate that the experimental conditions must be controlled to achieve magnetic bioceramics with potential hyperthermia application and bioactive behavior, as long as these additional oxide phases have a lower magnetization than magnetite [33]. In 2007, Singh et al. [34] studied the influence of magnetic phase concentration (2, 4, 6, 8 and 10 % in moles of Fe_2O_3) in the CaO–SiO_2–P_2O_5–Na_2O–Fe_2O_3 system obtained by melting process with posterior heat treatment (to convert Fe_2O_3 into Fe_3O_4 as the magnetic phase). The best result was for the sample containing 10 mol% (corresponding 8.64 wt% of Fe_2O_3), which exhibits the highest magnetization of 7.95 emu/g, illustrated in Fig. 7. This magnetization makes the system a potential biomaterial for hyperthermia treatment. The authors noticed the magnetization in the samples was associated with the iron oxide molar concentration that, in turn, is related to the amount and crystallite size of magnetite phase present in them [34]. Other authors [35] observed the same behavior for the system SiO_2–Na_2O–CaO–P_2O_5–FeO–Fe_2O_3 studied with different concentrations of magnetic phase. The maximum magnetization measured (31.5 emu/g, under a magnetic field of 12 kOe) was for the sample with the highest concentration of magnetic phase in the composition (34 wt%). Thus, it is possible to suggest the magnetization increases with the concentration of magnetic phase. However, higher concentration of magnetic phase decreases the bioactivity behavior of the biomaterial, so to combine the desired bioactivity with enough magnetization is one of the main challenges in M-BG development [24].

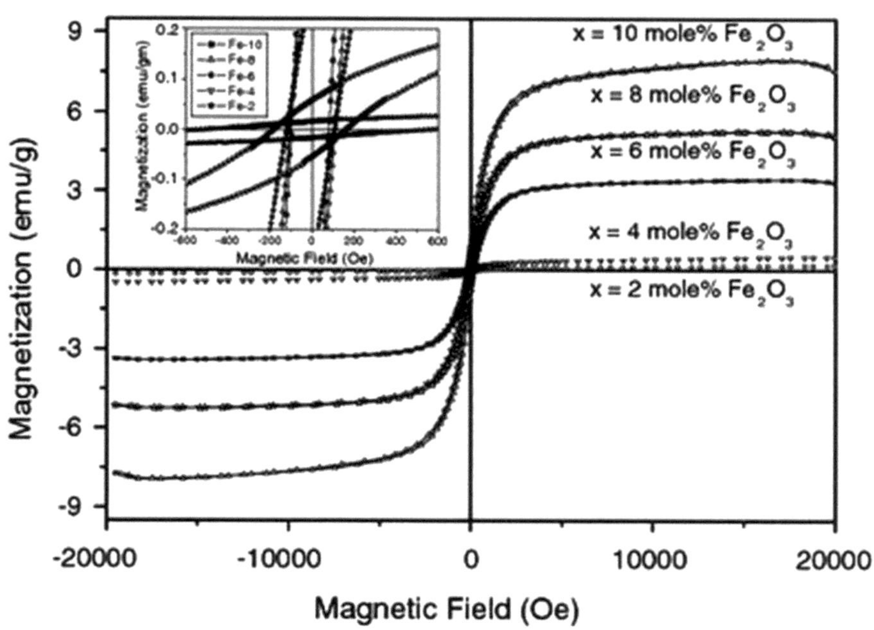

Fig. 7 Magnetic hysteresis loops of glass-ceramics with different iron oxide concentration under magnetic field of ±20 kOe [34]

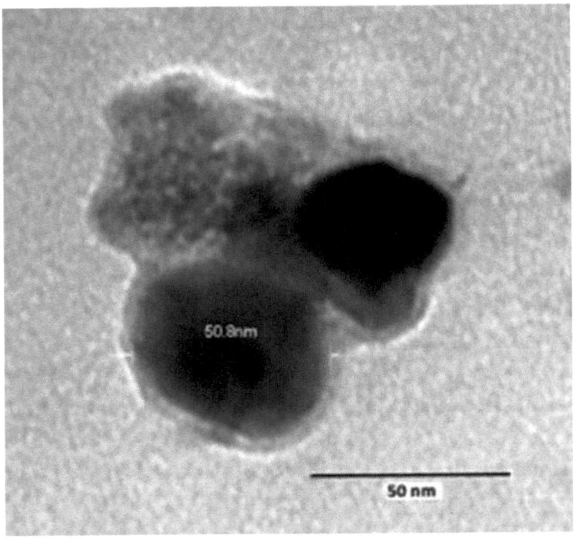

Fig. 8 TEM of polymer/magnetic bioactive glass composite [36]

Once the control of heat treatment is the main step to obtain better magnetic properties, some works have explored the development of glasses matrixes containing magnetic nanoparticles. Wang et al. [30] developed borosilicate bioactive glass scaffolds loaded with different amounts (5–15 wt%) of Fe_3O_4 magnetic nanoparticles (MNPs) in order to obtain a biomaterial with bone tissue ability, and able to destroy residual tumor cells by hyperthermia. They observed the material capability to generate heat was related to the amount of MNPs in the scaffolds [30].

Magnetic bioactive glasses can also be used in polymer/magnetic bioactive glass composites, resulting in a magnetic drug delivery carrier, bringing together hyperthermia and drug delivery system. Jayalekshmi et al. [36] developed a system of chitosan-gelatin with magnetic bioactive glass nanoparticles as a potential material for drug delivery and hyperthermia, prepared through sol–gel method. In that case, the drug could be dispersed in the polymer matrix. The magnetic bioactive glass nanoparticle was in the range of 43–51 nm. The morphology of the magnetic BG nanoparticle can be seen after TEM analysis (Fig. 8). These composite nanoparticles have a structure of iron oxide inside the polymer-bioglass matrix. The advantage of use nanoscale bioactive glasses instead of micron-sized is due their superior osteoconductivity [37]. The magnetization measured was 6.369 emu/g. The results revealed that the composite can be applicable for drug delivery allied with hyperthermia treatment [36].

3 Bioacompatible Glasses as Radioisotope Vectors

In 2003, it was reported the first biocompatible glass used as radioisotope vector, which was developed to replace ^{125}I seeds used in prostate cancer treatment by brachytherapy [38]. The union of biocompatible glasses with radiotherapy is still a new research field within the biocompatible glasses science [38–40]. In fact, there are just few research groups around the world studying the development of biocompatible glasses containing radioisotope. This sort of research sometimes is restricted to places that offers nuclear facilities, mainly because of the experimental procedures involved in the nuclear characterization of these materials, such as neutron activation. This procedure is shown in Fig. 9, which neutrons are generated in a nuclear reactor, and a material containing the desired isotope is exposed to these neutrons. As reaction product, it is obtained radioisotopes and beta and/or gamma rays.

For the development of the first bioactive glass-based seeds, scientists [38] assumed a biodegradable glass would be better for this treatment, because the ^{125}I seeds are temporary, and a second surgery is needed to remove them. Then, they developed a glass based on SiO_2–CaO system incorporated with samarium [38]. The objective was to obtain glasses containing ^{153}Sm radioisotope after neutron activation. ^{153}Sm was chosen because this element has a shorter half-life than ^{125}I (46.27 h and 54.9 days, respectively) being suitable for a resorbable material with chemical durability lower than seven months. Their results showed a samarium concentration between 4.5 and 11.5 wt% in the glass structure would be required to achieve the same activity as ^{125}I implants. In addition, considering this glass would be processed using enriched ^{153}Sm, the amount of Sm diminishes to concentrations between 1.5 and 4.5 wt% [38]. In other works, Roberto et al. [41] showed these implants can emit 130 Gy of β-ray dose, considering a flux activation of 2×10^7n cm^{-2} s^{-1}, and 1 g of biocompatible glass implant, being these values suitable for prostate cancer treatment [39, 40]. The biodegradability of these glasses was also evaluated through rabbit's liver model, using X-ray radiography images to monitor the glass durability in vivo. After seven months, there was found no traces of glass in radiography images, as shown in the Fig. 10 [41].

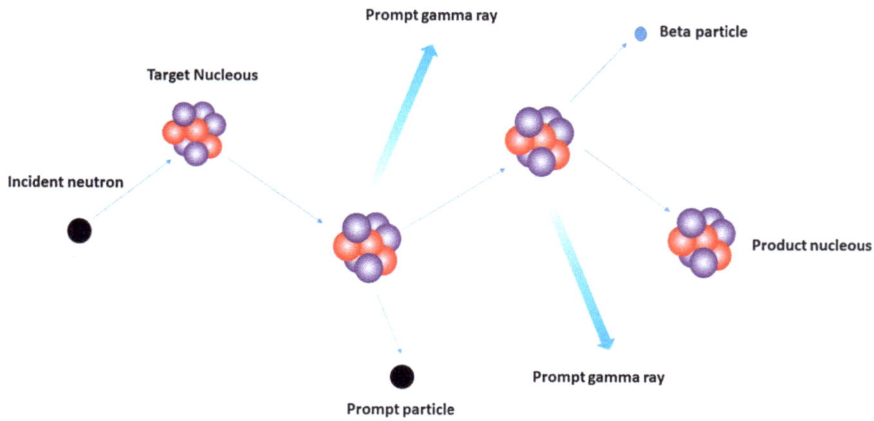

Fig. 9 Schematic representation of nuclear reaction between a target nucleus and an incident neutron, leading to the formation of a radioisotope and the emission of beta particles and/or gamma rays

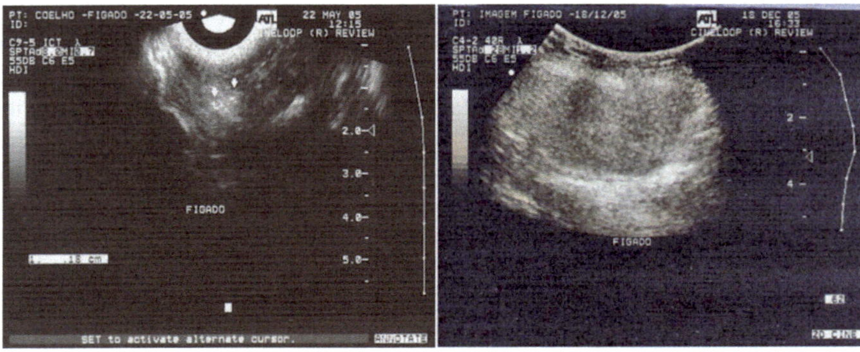

Fig. 10 Radiography showing **a** ^{153}Sm biodegradable glass seed in a liver (as indicated by the *white narrows*) just after implantation, and **b** the same liver after 7 months, when it is not possible to observe any seeds due to their degradation [41]

Another recent work developed by Nogueira and Campos [42] studied a system where Zr, Ba and Ho are incorporated into the bioactive glasses structure. The Zr and Ba were used to improve the visibility of the seeds by radiography, once these elements are suitable contrast agents. The radiography is the most used clinical technique to evaluate the radioactive seeds degradation. Ho was added because it emits higher energy than Sm, being able to diminish the amount of doping elements in the bioactive glass structure, or developing a material that emits higher energy, being able to treat small cancers in shorter time [42, 43].

In another study, Sadeghi et al. [44] emphasized the interesting features of ^{153}Sm in prostate brachytherapy when trapped within a biodegradable glass structure. The authors carried out computational simulations, through Monte Carlo code, in order to evaluate the dose rate in function of distance for a material doped with ^{153}Sm. ^{142}Pr beta emitter source was used as a benchmark to validate the simulation method accuracy and dose calculation. It was also included data about other materials based on ^{32}P and ^{90}Sr/^{90}Y beta emitter for comparison purposes. They concluded beta doses using ^{153}Sm has a shorter distance effectiveness when compared to the other ones (Fig. 11), as well as a higher initial dose rate. Such results

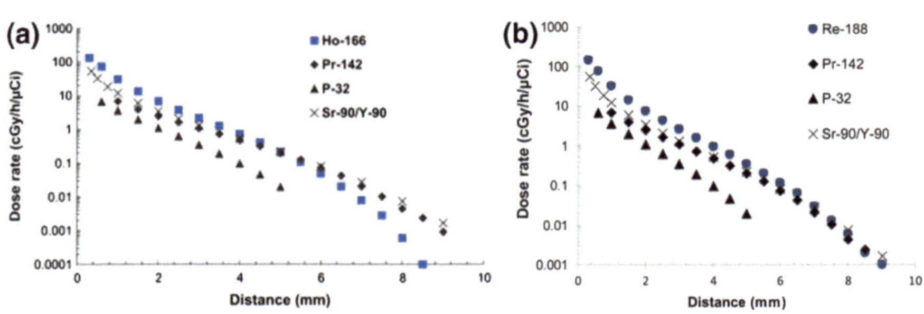

Fig. 11 Comparison the dose rate in function of distance for different beta emitters [45, 46]

suggest ^{153}Sm would enable a less radiation effect on healthy tissues, diminishing the side effects of radiotherapy, and also decreasing the treatment time due to the higher initial dose.

Similar Monte Carlo code simulations were carried out by Hosseini et al. [45], who evaluated the beta dose of ^{166}Ho-based biodegradable glass seed, and by Khorshidi et al., who evaluated ^{188}Re-based biodegradable glasses seed [46]. These authors used the same parameters as Sadegui et al. [44], and they were focused on hepatic cancer treatment. Both of the aforementioned authors led to conclusions similar to Sadegui et al., i.e., both ^{166}Ho and ^{185}Re have a shorter dose distance, and a slight higher initial dose, as showed in the Fig. 11. In all of these cases, the authors approached using the formalism of AAPM TG-60 (American Association of Physicist in Medicine, Task Group—60) report, which recommends a dosimetry protocol for interstitial brachytherapy sources and parameters of beta emitters, enabling to calculate the dose rate, the radial dose function, and the two dimensional anisotropy function of the materials [47].[1]

Since 2011, molecular dynamics studies have suggested ^{90}Y-based bioresorbable glasses (^{90}Y-BG) as potential materials for radiotherapy. The first study carried out by Christie et al. [48] evaluated how yttrium addition into the glass structure would affect the surface reactivity of bioactive glasses. Their challenge was to find out a high surface reactivity typical of BG with a slow release of yttrium, in order to avoid radioactive elements into the bloodstream. Their results showed two distinct behaviors induced by yttrium addiction:

1. the formation of a fragmented silicate network that leads to a lower durability and loss of bioactivity;
2. a yttrium-mediated strong association of dissociated silica fragments that leads to a higher durability and bioactivity.

Therefore, they concluded that an ideal ^{90}Y-BG should be a composition that equilibrate these two aforementioned factors. In a further work [49], it was showed the possibility of overcoming this problem through adding more amount of silica to the glass structure (62 mol%), and also increasing the amount of yttria up to 12 mol %, but keeping the network connectivity surround 2.6. Higher yttrium content in the glass structure would lead to more fragmented silicates, but at the same time the energy of yttrium-mediated cross-linked silicate bonds will increase, and, thus, decrease the glass solubility, enhancing the biocompatibility. The Fig. 12 shows the yttrium-mediated cross-linked silicate bonds, which are very important in ^{90}Y-BG. Although simulations have shown the success of Y-BG, it is still needed experimental dada that supports molecular dynamic simulations.

[1]The AAPM TG-60 should be taken into account in works involving brachytherapy, and more details about this approach can be found in: Amols et al. [47].

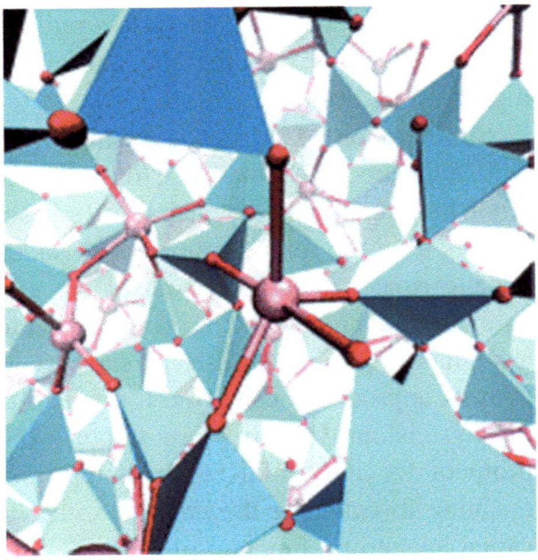

Fig. 12 Yttrium-mediated cross-linked silicate bonds. Silica tetrahedral are shown in *blue*, oxygen atoms in *red*, and yttrium in *pink*. Sodium and calcium atoms were omitted for an easier visualization [49]

4 Challenges and Perspectives

As mentioned before, one of the main challenges of producing magnetic bioactive glasses is combining bioactivity and magnetization properties. The presence of the magnetic phase into the glass matrix decreases the bioactivity and iron can be easily segregated, forming nonmagnetic precipitates while sintering. The possible cytotoxicity of the magnetic phase acts as a limiting factor for their applications [24]. However, the use of low concentrations of iron oxide can be a disadvantage, leading to not enough sufficient amount of magnetic phase to generate heat demanded when under an alternating external magnetic field, affecting the effectiveness of the treatment [34].

Nowadays, the proposal of magnetic biocompatible bioactive glasses focuses on improved biocompatible and magnetic properties, in order to enhance both. The development of new materials with greater degradation rates is also suggested in order to completely degrade the material after their use as therapeutic agents, avoiding immune reactions or the need for a second surgery for removal.

Regarding BG as radioisotope vectors, it is observed new glasses composition have been suggested as suitable compositions for cancer treatment; however, nowadays most of the works are based on simulations and not in experimental data. In this sense, new works involving in vitro and in vivo tests would be appreciated, and would give us a better idea about radiological parameters that lead to effective treatment. At the same time, simulation methods, like the AAPM TG-60, are reliable tools to evaluate compositions beforehand, avoiding experimental failure or even money expends. Clinical test will give us a better feedback about the usage of biocompatible glasses as resorbable seeds for brachytherapy in a near future.

References

1. Nielsen, O.S., Horsman, M., Overgaard, J.: A future for hyperthermia in cancer treatment. Eur. J. Cancer **37**, 1587–1589 (2001)
2. Wust, P., Hildebrandt, B., Sreenivasa, G., Rau, B., Gellermann, J., Riess, H., Felix, R., Schlag, E.P.M.: Hyperthermia in combined treatment of cancer. Lancet Oncol. **3**, 487–497 (2002)
3. Jiang, Y., Ou, J., Zhang, Z., Qin, Q.H.: Preparation of magnetic and bioactive calcium zinc iron silicon oxide composite for hyperthermia treatment of bone cancer and repair of bone defects. J. Mater. Sci. Mater. Med. **22**, 721–729 (2011)
4. Cui, Z., et al.: Molecular mechanisms of hyperthermia-induced apoptosis enhanced by docosahexaenoic acid: Implication for cancer therapy, pp. 1–8. Chemico-Biological Interactions, Japan (2014)
5. Arcos, D., Real, P., Vallet-Regí, M.: Biphasic materials for bone grafting and hyperthermia treatment of cancer. J. Biomed. Mater. Res. A **65**(1), 71–78 (2003)
6. Shah, S.A., Hashmi, M.U., Alam, S., Shamim, A.: Magnetic and bioactivity evaluation of ferrimagnetic $ZnFe_2O_4$ containing glass ceramics for the hyperthermia treatment of cancer. J. Magn. Magn. Mater. **322**, 375–381 (2010)
7. Li, J.: Physics of Tumor Hyperthermia, pp. 1–6. Science Publisher, Beijing (2008)
8. Baronzio, G.F., Hager, E.D.: Hyperthermia in Cancer Treatment: A Primer, pp. 3–4. Medical Intelligent Unit, Springer & Landes Bioscience, New York (2006)
9. Oleson, J.R., Dewhirst, M.W.: Hyperthermia: an overview of current progress and problems. Curr. Probl. Cancer **8**(6), 1–62 (1983)
10. Giri, J., Ray, A., Dasgupta, S., Datta, D., Bahadur, D.: Investigation on Tc tuned nano particles of magnetic oxides for hyperthermia applications. Bio-Med. Mater. Eng. **13**(4), 387–399 (2003)
11. Gilchrist, R.K., Medal, R., Shorey, W.D., Hanselman, R.C., Parott, J.C., Taylor, C.B.: Selective inductive heating of lymph nodes. Ann. Surg. **146**, 596–606 (1997)
12. Yanase, M., Shinkai, M., Honda, H., Wakabayashi, T., Yoshida, J., Kobayashi, T.: Intracellular hyperthermia for cancer using magnetite cationic liposomes: ex vivo study. Jpn. J. Cancer Res. **88**(7), 630–632 (1997)
13. Mosbach, K., Anderson, L.: Magnetic ferrofluids for preparation of magnetic polymers and their application in affinity chromatography. Nature **270**, 259 (1997)
14. Jianhua, C., Naru, Y.: Present situation of cancer hyperthermia. Mater. J. Chin. Ceram. Soc. **29**, 238–244 (2001)
15. Shliomis, M.I.: Magnetic fluids. Sov. Phys. Usp. **17**, 153–184 (1963)
16. Hergt, R., Andrä, W., D'ambly, C.G., Hilger, I., Kaiser, W.A., Richter, U., Schmidt, H.G.: Physical limits of hyperthermia using magnetite fine particles. IEEE Trans. Magn. **34**, 3745–3754 (1998)
17. Alcaide, M., Ramirez, S.C., Feito, M.J., De La Concepci, N., Matesanz, M., Ruiz, E.H., Arcos, D., Vallet, R.M., Portolos, M.T. In vitro evaluation of glass–glass ceramic thermoseed-induced hyperthermia on human osteosarcoma cell line. J. Biomed. Mater. Res. A **100A**, 64–71 (2012)
18. Hildebrandt, B., Wust, P., Ahlers, O., Dieing, A., Sreenivasa, G., Kerner, T., Felix, R., Riess, H.: The cellular and molecular basis of hyperthermia. Crit. Rev. Oncol. Hematol. **43**, 33–56 (2002)
19. Clavel, C.M., Nowak-Sliwinska, P., Paunescu, E., Dyson, P.J.: Thermoresponsive fluorinated small-molecule drugs: a new concept for efficient localized chemotherapy. Med. Chem. Commun. **6**, 2054–2062 (2015)
20. Overgaard, J.: Effect of hyperthermia on malignant cells in vivo: a review and a hypothesis. Cancer **39**, 2637–2646 (1977)

21. Jordan, A., Scholz, R., Wust, P., Fähling, H., Felix, R.: Magnetic fluid hyperthermia (MFH): cancer treatment with AC magnetic field induced excitation of biocompatible superparamagnetic nanoparticles. J. Magn. Magn. Mater. **201**, 413–419 (1999)
22. American Cancer Society. www.cancer.org. Accessed 31 March 2016
23. Williamson, J.F.: Brachytherapy technology and physics practice since 1950: a half-century of progress. Phys. Med. Biol. **51**(13), R303–R325 (2006)
24. Li, G., Feng, S., Shou, D.: Magnetic bioactive glass ceramic in the system $CaO–P_2O_5–SiO_2–MgO–CaF_2–MnO_2–Fe_2O_3$ for hyperthermia treatment of bone tumor. J. Mater. Sci. Mater. Med. **22**, 2197–2206 (2011)
25. Pereira, M.M., Clark, A.E., Hench, L.L.: Calcium phosphate formation on sol–gel derived bioactive glasses in vitro. J. Biomed. Mater. Res. **28**, 693–698 (1994)
26. Vallet-Regí, M., Arcos, D., Pariente, J.: Evolution of porosity during in vitro hydroxycarbonate apatite growth in sol–gel glasses. J. Biomed. Mater. Res. **51**, 23–28 (2000)
27. Hench, L.L.: Bioceramics: from concept to clinic. J. Am. Ceram. Soc. **74**, 1487–1510 (1991)
28. Balas, F., Arcos, D., Perez-Pariente, J., Vallet-Regí, M.: Textural properties of $SiO_2·CaO·P_2O_5$ glasses prepared by the sol–gel method. J. Mater. Res. **6**, 1345–1348 (2001)
29. Baeza, A., Arcos, D., Vallet-Regí, M.: Thermoseeds for interstitial magnetic hyperthermia: from bioceramics to nanoparticles. J. Phys.: Condens. Matter **25**, 11 (2013)
30. Wang, H., Zhao, S., Zhou, J., Zhu, K., Cui, X., Huang, W., Rahman, M.N., Zhang, C., Wang, D. Biocompatibility and osteogenic capacity of borosilicate bioactive glass scaffolds loaded with Fe_3O_4 magnetic nanoparticles. J. Mater. Chem. **3**, 4377–4387 (2015)
31. Kokubo, T.: Bioactive glass ceramics: properties and applications. Biomaterials **12**(2), 155–163 (1991)
32. Da Li, G., Zhou, D.L., Lin, Y., Pan, T.H., Chen, G.S., Yin, Q.D.: Synthesis and characterization of magnetic bioactive glass-ceramics containing Mg ferrite for hyperthermia. Mater. Sci. Eng. C **30**, 148–153 (2010)
33. Eniu, D., Cacaina, D., Coldea, M., Valeanu, M., Simon, S.: Structural and magnetic properties of $CaO–P_2O_5–SiO_2–Fe_2O_3$ glass–ceramics for hyperthermia. J. Magn. Magn. Mater. **293**, 310–313 (2005)
34. Singh, R.K., Kothiyal, G.P., Srinivasan, A.: Magnetic and structural properties of $CaO–SiO_2–P_2O_5–Na_2O–Fe_2O_3$ glass ceramics. J. Magn. Magn. Mater. **320**, 1352–1356 (2008)
35. Bretcanu, O., Verné, E., Cöisso, M., Tiberto, P., Allia, P.: Magnetic properties of the ferrimagnetic glass-ceramics for hyperthermia. J. Magn. Magn. Mater. **305**(2), 529–533 (2006)
36. Jayalekshmi, A.C., Victor, S.P., Sharma, C.P.: Colloids Surf. B **101**, 196–204 (2013)
37. Boccaccini, A.R., Erol, M., Stark, W.J., Mohn, D., Hong, Z., Mano, J.F.: Polymer/bioactive glass nanocomposites for biomedical applications: a review. Compos. Sci. Technol. **70**, 1764–1776 (2010)
38. Roberto, S., Magalhães, M.: Analysis of bioactive glasses obtained by sol–gel processing for radioactive implants. Mater. Res. **6**, 123–127 (2003)
39. Roberto, W.S., Pereira, M.M., Campos, T.P.R.: Dosimetric analysis and characterization of radioactive seeds produced by the sol–gel method. Key Eng. Mater. **242**, 579–582 (2003)
40. Roberto, W.S., Pereira, M.M., Campos, T.P.R.: Structure and dosimetric analysis of biodegradable glasses for prostate cancer treatment. Artif. Organs **27**, 432–436 (2003)
41. Campos, T.P.R., Andrade, J.P.L., Costa, I.T., Silva, C.H.T.: Study of the Sm-153 seeds degradation and evaluation of the absorbed dose in rabbit's liver implants. Prog. Nucl. Energy **50**, 757–766 (2008)
42. Nogueira, L.B., Campos, T.R.P. Nuclear characterization of radioactive bioglass seed for brachytherapy studies. International Conference on Mathematics and Computational Methods Applied to Nuclear Science and Engineering, pp. 1–9 (2011)
43. El-Kady, A.M., Ali, A.F., Rizk, R.A., Ahmed, M.M.: Synthesis, characterization and microbiological response of silver doped bioactive glass nanoparticles. Ceram. Int. **38**, 177–188 (2012)

44. Sadeghi, M., Taghdiri, F., Hosseini, S.H., et al.: Monte Carlo calculated TG-60 dosimetry parameters for the β-emitter S 153 m brachytherapy source Monte Carlo calculated TG-60 dosimetry parameters for the Sm emitter brachytherapy source (2010)
45. Hosseini, S.H., Enferadi, M., Sadeghi, M.: Dosimetric aspects of Ho brachytherapy biodegradable glass seed. Appl. Radiat. Isot. **73**, 109–115 (2013)
46. Khorshidi, A., Ahmadinejad, M., Hosseini, S.H., N-particle, C.: Evaluation of a proposed biodegradable 188 Re source for brachytherapy application a review of dosimetric parameters. Medicine **94**, 1–7 (2015)
47. Amols, H., Coffey, C., Duggan, D., et al.: Intravascular brachytherapy physics : Report of the AAPM Radiation Therapy Committee Task Group No. 60. Med. Phys. **26**, 119–152 (1999). doi:10.1118/1.598496
48. Christie, J.K., Malik, J., Tilocca, A.: Bioactive glasses as potential radioisotope vectors for in situ cancer therapy: investigating the structural effects of yttrium. Phys. Chem. Chem. Phys. **13**, 17749–17755 (2011)
49. Chem, J.M., Christie, J.K., Tilocca, A.: Integrating biological activity into radioisotope vectors: molecular dynamics models of yttrium-doped bioactive glasses. 12023–12031 (2012)

Glasses for Treatment of Liver Cancer by Radioembolization

Oana Bretcanu and Iain Evans

Abstract This chapter presents an overview of existing commercial and potential (non-commercially available) glasses used for the treatment of liver cancer by radioembolization therapy. The chapter explains how radioembolization works and the required properties of the glass particles used for radioembolization. A short description of the properties and method of synthesis for commercial glasses, TheraSpheres®, together with their clinical benefits, risks and limitations are reported. Two non-commercial glasses were considered: phosphate glasses containing ^{32}P radioisotope and borate glasses containing ^{186}Re and ^{188}Re radioisotopes. Their fabrication methods and properties were compared to those of the commercial glass.

Keywords Glass · Liver cancer · Radioembolization · Radioactive microspheres · Radioisotopes

1 Introduction

According to the World Health Organization cancer is among the leading cause of death with 8.2 million cancer-related deaths and 14 million new cancer cases worldwide in 2012. The estimated number of new cancer cases could rise to 22 million within the next two decades. More than 60 % of new cancer cases occur in Africa, Asia, and Central and South America. These regions currently represent approximately 70 % of the cancer deaths worldwide. It is estimated that in 2016 nearly 0.6 million people will die from cancer and approximately 1.7 million new cases of cancer will be diagnosed in the United States alone [1, 2].

O. Bretcanu (✉) · I. Evans
School of Mechanical and Systems Engineering, Newcastle University,
Newcastle upon Tyne, UK
e-mail: oana.bretcanu@newcastle.ac.uk

J. Marchi (ed.), *Biocompatible Glasses*, Advanced Structured Materials 53,
DOI 10.1007/978-3-319-44249-5_11

Liver cancer is one of the most common forms of cancer. The American Cancer Society estimates that in 2016, more than 27,000 people (4.6 % of all cancers) will die from liver cancer in the United States and in excess of 39,000 new cases of liver cancer (about 2.3 % of all cancers) will be diagnosed [3].

Patients with early stage liver cancer, and without cirrhosis, having tumours smaller than 50 mm can be treated successfully by tumour resection (partial hepatectomy). Only 15–30 % of liver cancer patients can undergo partial hepatectomy and within 5 years of liver resection, cancer will recur in approximately 75 % of these [4]. Liver transplantation may be an option for patients with hepatocellular carcinoma, but there is a limited supply of suitable donor organs. Other treatments include radiofrequency ablation (local use of small electrodes that generate heat and destroy the tumour), arterial chemotherapy (local delivery of anticancer drug via the artery) or embolization (blocking blood flow to the tumour) [4]. In the last two decades radioembolization, the process of delivering internal radiation therapy to a deliberately occluded blood vessel, has been used for the treatment of a number of life-threatening forms of liver cancer to extend the lives of patients with inoperable tumours or without the possibility of liver transplant. These include primary hepatocellular carcinoma which originates in the liver and metastatic liver cancer which had spread to the liver from another part of the body. Radioembolization is a minimally invasive procedure that combines embolization (deliberate occlusion of the blood vessel) and radiation therapy. Conventional radiotherapy uses X-rays to irradiate tumours externally and often causes damage to adjacent healthy tissues. Radioembolization uses small particles containing radioisotopes that irradiate the

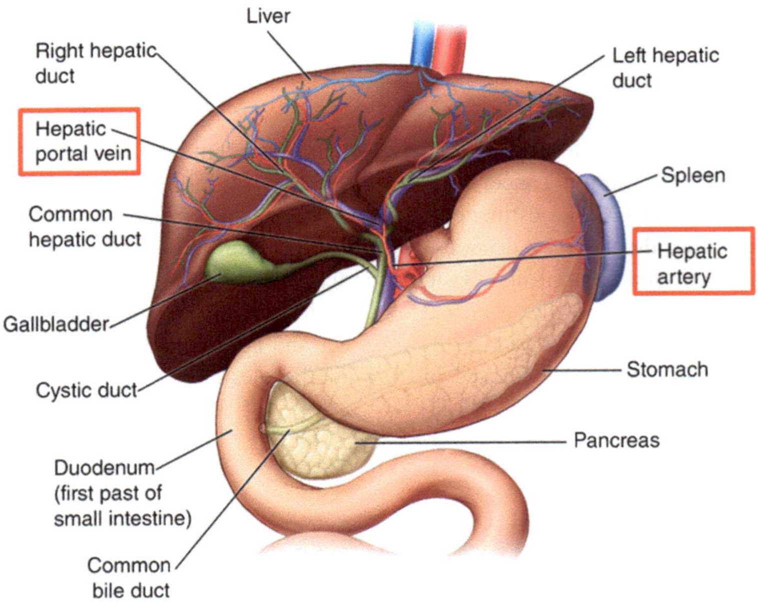

Fig. 1 Liver anatomy (adapted from [7])

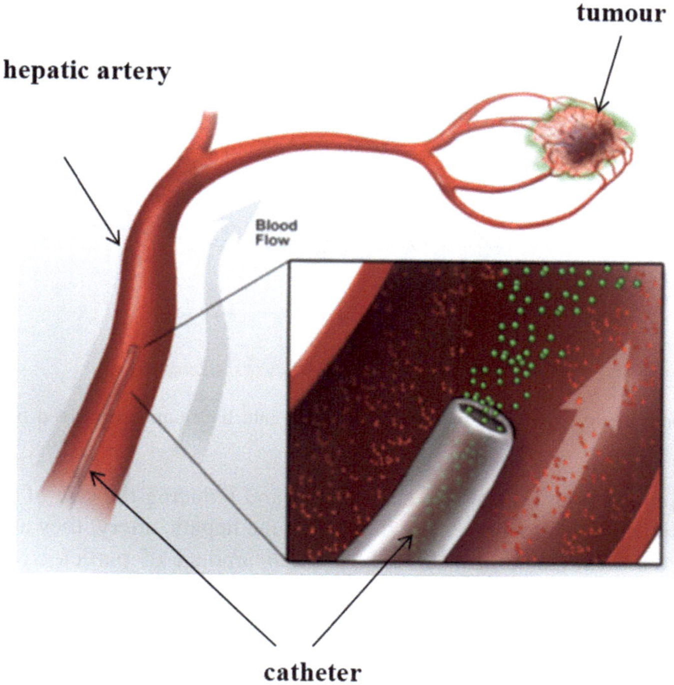

Fig. 2 Introduction of microspheres in the hepatic artery (adapted from [5])

target tumour area locally, minimising damage to healthy tissue. The maximum dose of radiation that can be safely applied in external radiotherapy is much lower than that used for internal radiation and hence external radiation treatment is less efficient than radioembolization.

There are two primary blood vessels involved in the supply of blood to the liver, the hepatic portal vein and the hepatic artery (Fig. 1). Normal liver tissue (healthy tissue) receives more than 80 % of its blood supply from the portal vein and up to 20 % from the hepatic artery. Tumoural liver tissue is often more vascular than the surrounding normal tissue and receives most of its blood supply from the hepatic artery [5].

During radioembolization treatment, radioactive microspheres with particles sizes of 20–30 μm are introduced to the hepatic artery via a catheter (Fig. 2). These microspheres can pass through the hepatic artery but are too large to pass through the small tumour capillaries, which have a diameter of 8–10 μm, and hence preferentially accumulate in the tumour. Tumour nodules have a higher concentration of blood vessels compared to the surrounding healthy tissue, enabling up to 20 times more particles to be deposited in the malignant tissue [6]. The microspheres block or decrease the blood flow inside the tumour, inhibiting the delivery of oxygen and nutrients to the tumour and thus impeding the tumour growth. Once the microspheres are trapped inside the tumour site, they deliver a high dose of radiation

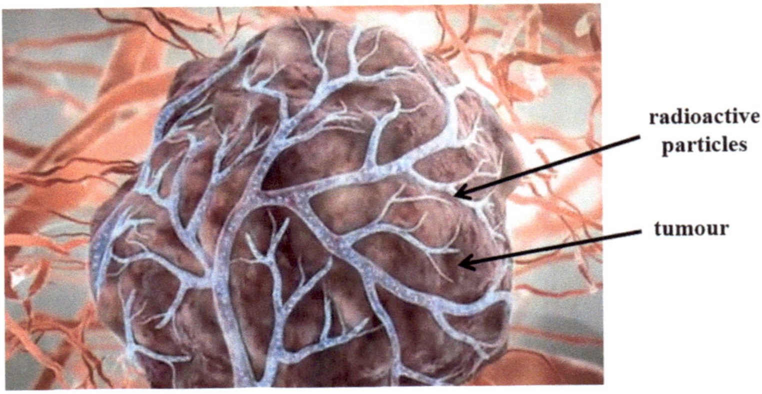

Fig. 3 Simulation of radioactive particles distribution into liver tumour (adapted from [8])

directly to the tumour, killing the cancer cells and reducing the size of the tumour. As the radioactive microspheres are injected in the hepatic artery, they are primarily transported into the tumour with only a small amount of particles reaching the healthy liver tissue. Even if the hepatic artery is blocked during radioembolization, the healthy liver cells will continue to receive blood from the hepatic portal vein and thus maintain the supply of oxygen and nutrients to the healthy tissue.

Hepatic artery injection allows preferential delivery of radioactive particles into the tumour. In clinical practice, millions of microspheres with diameters below 30 μm incorporating an active radioisotope are distributed via an arterial catheter to the tumour (Fig. 3).

Many elements have multiple isotopes, some of which may be radioactive. Radioactive isotopes are characterized by a constant rate of decay, forming other elements or isotopes. During radioactive decay, the unstable radioisotopes emit radiation (alpha, beta or gamma radiation) and become more stable. As each radioisotope is characterised by a specific time for decay, the parameter used in practice is the half-life which is a measure of the amount of time that the isotope's radioactivity takes to decay to half of its initial value. Thus, the half-life of a radioisotope indicates how fast an unstable radioisotope undergoes radioactive decay. Isotopes with shorter half-life decay faster. Radioisotopes could be generated by neutron irradiation of non-radioactive isotopes in a nuclear reactor. Examples of radioisotopes activated after neutron bombardment are given in Table 1, while the half-life and decay energy of some radioisotopes is shown in Table 2. Some radioisotopes such as ^{12}B can have a very short half-life (20.2 ms), while the others such ^{238}U have an extremely long half-life (4,470,000,000 years).

The isotopes used in clinical studies generally emit beta radiation which can penetrate the cell membrane and hence have the potential to destroy the cells. These radioisotopes can be incorporated into a glass network and delivered into the blood vessels that feed the tumour in the form of glass microspheres as noted earlier (Fig. 4). These glass microspheres can irradiate the surrounding malignant tissue up

Table 1 Examples of elements with stable isotopes that forms radioisotopes after neutron activation in a nuclear reactor

Element	Most stable isotope	Natural abundance (%)	Radioisotopes
B	^{11}B	80.1	^{12}B
	^{10}B	19.9	–
O	^{16}O	99.8	–
Na	^{23}Na	100	^{24}Na
Mg	^{24}Mg	79	–
	^{25}Mg	10	–
	^{26}Mg	11	^{27}Mg
Al	^{27}Al	100	^{28}Al
Si	^{28}Si	92.2	–
	^{29}Si	4.7	–
	^{30}Si	3.1	^{31}Si
P	^{31}P	100	^{32}P
K	^{39}K	93.3	^{40}K
	^{41}K	6.7	^{42}K
Ca	^{40}Ca	96.9	^{41}Ca
	^{44}Ca	2.1	^{45}Ca
Y	^{89}Y	100	^{90}Y
Re	^{185}Re	37.4	^{186}Re
	^{187}Re	62.6	^{188}Re
U	^{238}U	99.3	^{239}U

to a distance of 12 mm, depending on the isotope's radioactivity [9]. They can deliver a high dose of localised radiation directly into the tumour without causing significant damage to healthy cells.

The maximum amount of radiation that glass microspheres can safely deliver to the liver (or other target organ) depends on the mass and volume of the organ, type of radiation emitted during radioisotope decay and the microspheres' radioactivity at the time of injection.

2 Required Properties of Glass Particles

Glass microspheres used for radioembolization should have the following general characteristics:

- be biocompatible and non-toxic for human body
- have high chemical durability and high corrosion resistance in body fluids at different pH
- have a composition that will produce only radioisotopes with short half-life after neutron activation

Table 2 Examples of half-life, decay mode and decay energy of some radioisotopes

Radioisotope	Half-life	Decay mode	Decay energy (MeV)	Decay product
^{12}B	20.2 ms	β−	13.37	^{12}C
^{24}Na	14.96 h	β−	5.52	^{24}Mg
^{27}Mg	9.46 min	β−	2.61	^{27}Al
^{28}Al	2.24 min	β−	4.64	^{28}Si
^{31}Si	2.62 h	β−	1.49	^{31}P
^{32}P	14.26 days	β−	1.71	^{32}S
^{40}K	1.25×10^9 years	β−	1.31	^{40}Ca
		β+	0.48	^{40}Ar
^{42}K	12.36 h	β−	3.5	^{42}Ca
^{41}Ca	1.02×10^5 years	EC	0.42	^{41}K
^{45}Ca	162.7 days	β−	0.26	^{45}Sc
^{90}Y	2.67 days	β−	2.28	^{90}Zr
^{186}Re	3.72 days	β−	1.07	^{186}Os
		γ	0.136	
		EC	0.58	^{186}W
^{188}Re	17 h	β−	2.12	^{188}Os
		γ	0.155	
^{238}U	4.47×10^9 years	α	4.27	^{234}Th
^{239}U	23.45 min	β−	1.26	^{239}Np

EC = electron capture, α = alpha particles, β− = beta minus particles (electron emission), β+ = beta plus particles (positron emission)

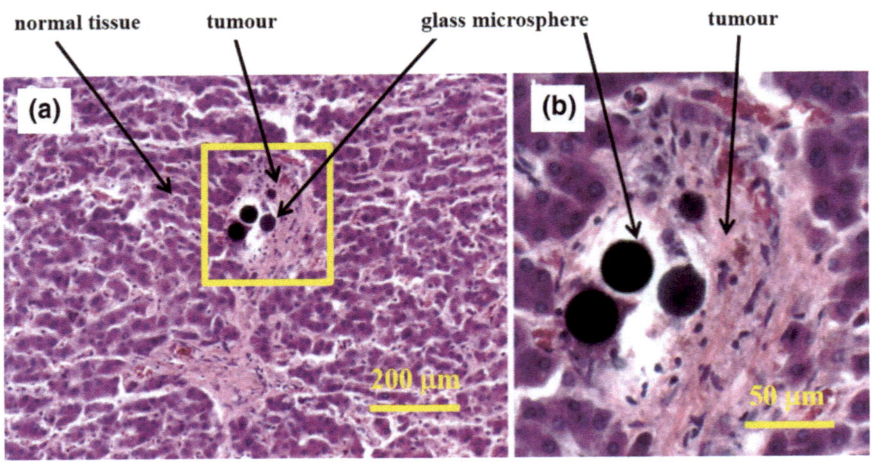

Fig. 4 Optical microscope images of a stained human liver with glass microspheres at the periphery of the tumour; *inset* **b** shows a higher magnification of the region marked in *yellow* in **a** (adapted from [5])

- do not contain any element that could form long half-life radioisotopes during neutron activation
- contain a radioactive isotope with appropriate level of radioactivity at the time of injection (to allow local administration of higher doses of radioactivity directly to the target organ)
- be spherical in shape
- have thermal properties that enable the glass particles to be spheroidized
- have appropriate particles size to embolize (occlude) the blood vessels of the target tissue
- have appropriate density to be carried by the blood flow into the target tissue and to not deposit on the blood vessel wall before reaching the tumour.

The chemical composition of the glass plays an important role in selecting appropriate materials for radioembolization. Many chemical elements became radioactive after neutron activation (see Table 1), so care should be taken to avoid elements that form long half-life radioisotopes, such as Ca and K (Table 2). Biocompatible silicate glasses could contain Ca and K ions, and their presence in the glass composition should be avoided. Similarly, the raw materials utilised for the synthesis of the glass should be of high purity to avoid the activation of unwanted radioisotopes (present in some impurities) after neutron bombardment. Glass containing radioisotopes with a shorter half-life are safer for patients and their relatives, medical staff and environment. If the radioisotopes remain active in the patient's body for a long time after the treatment, the patient needs to avoid close contact with family members. Most isotopes in Table 2 produce β radiation which is an ionising radiation that can penetrate a couple of centimetres into the skin. After radioembolization treatment, β radiation will be contained in the patient's body so the patient will not need to be kept in an isolation room until the radioisotopes become inactive. The patient is allowed to go home with a minimum risk of radiation exposure to family members.

The glass should have high chemical durability and high corrosion resistance, to avoid leaching of the radioisotopes entrapped in the glass structure while they are still radioactive. The pH value of human body fluid is about 7 under normal condition but it can have lower values in tumours. Thus, the glass should have high chemical durability even under acidic conditions and should not release active radioisotopes into normal tissue.

The glass particles should have a smooth spherical shape to minimise micro-lacerations or similar effects which might irritate the blood vessels when they are injected into the blood stream. The particles size should be small enough to flow through the hepatic artery and stop in the liver capillaries.

3 Commercial Glass Particles

TheraSpheres® are commercial glass microspheres that contain ^{90}Y radioisotope. They have been used since 1990 in the USA and Canada for the treatment of liver, kidney and spleen cancers [10, 11]. These glass particles have a diameter of 20–30 μm and can be delivered into the tumour by hepatic artery injection. TheraSphere® treatment is not curative but it can reduce the size of the tumour (Fig. 5), allowing the patients to have other curative treatment options such as surgery, liver transplant, chemotherapy, etc. Clinical studies showed that TheraSpheres® are generally well tolerated and 70–90 % of the patients improved after treatment, with an increase in the survival rate. Histological studies showed that the distribution of microspheres is heterogeneous, the ratio of particles concentration into tumour to normal tissue being 2–50:1. Hence, the majority of targeted microspheres are accumulated in the tumour as described earlier.

3.1 Glass Synthesis and Properties

The nominal glass composition of TheraSpheres® is $17Y_2O_3$–$19Al_2O_3$–$64SiO_2$ mol % (YAS glass). Non-radioactive YAS glass contains ^{89}Y isotope and it is prepared by melting homogeneous mixtures of high purity Al_2O_3, Y_2O_3 and SiO_2 powders in a platinum crucible at 1600–1650 °C [12]. As noted earlier, high purity of raw materials is required to avoid the generation of undesirable radioisotopes during subsequent neutron activation.

After grinding, the glass powders are sieved to select suitably sized solid YAS glass particles. These are irregular in shape and they are formed into regular microspheres with 20–30 μm particles size by spheroidizing the glass particles in

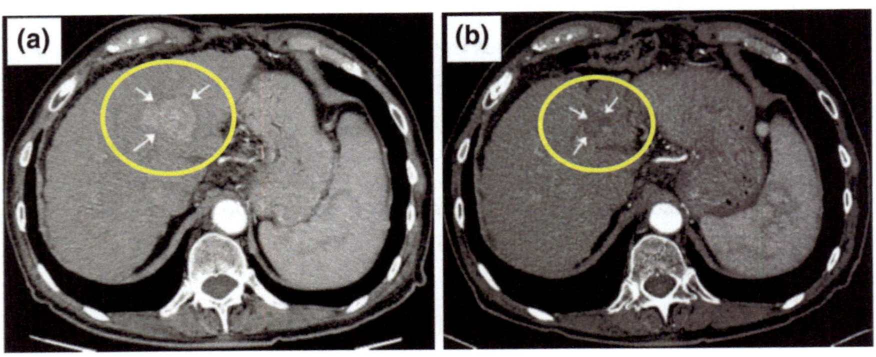

Fig. 5 X-ray computed tomography of hepatocellular cancer (*yellow circles*). **a** Before Theraspheres® treatment; **b** 2 years after Theraspheres® treatment, showing the tumour size reduction (adapted from [9])

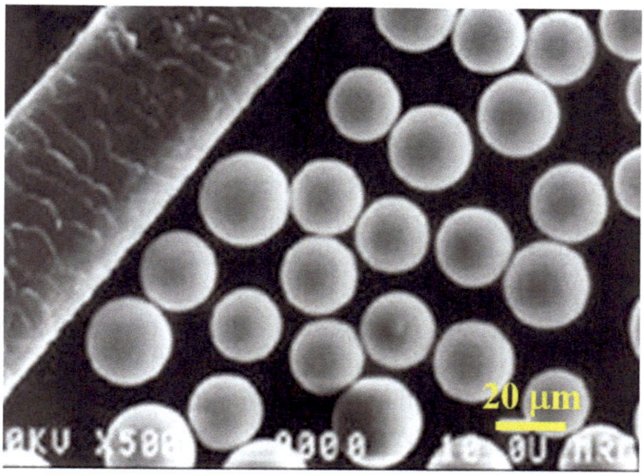

Fig. 6 SEM image of glass microspheres and a human hair (adapted from [15])

an acetylene/oxygen flame. During the spheroidizing process the glass softens, decreasing its viscosity, and the glass particles become spherical due to surface tension. The temperature and timing of this process are carefully controlled to avoid glass crystallization. After cooling, the glass microspheres are sieved once again to select the desired range of sizes.

A scanning electron microscope (SEM) image of the glass microspheres particles compared to a human hair is illustrated in Fig. 6. The YAS glass density is 3.2 g/cm^3.

The non-radioactive YAS microspheres are transformed into radioactive microspheres in a nuclear reactor where the ^{89}Y isotope is activated to form the β-emitting ^{90}Y isotope. As can be seen in Table 1, ^{89}Y is the stable isotope of Y and it has 100 % natural abundance. It can be activated to ^{90}Y (half-life of 2.67 days) during neutron bombardment. Even if ^{27}Al (100 % natural abundance) and ^{30}Si (3.1 % natural abundance) could be activated to ^{28}Al and respectively ^{31}Si during neutron bombardment, the half-lives of these isotopes are very short, being only 2.24 min for ^{28}Al and 2.62 h for ^{31}Si (Table 2). Other isotopes of Si (^{28}Si and ^{29}Si) and O (^{16}O) are not activated by neutron bombardment.

^{90}Y decays to stable ^{90}Zr by emission of β-radiation with a corresponding decay energy of 2.28 MeV (Table 2). The emission of β particles generates a high local radiation dose at the site of glass microsphere deposition, producing tumour shrinkage by cell necrosis whilst having minimal impact on the surrounding healthy liver tissue. β-radiation emitted by ^{90}Y has a maximum penetration range of 12 mm [13] and about 95 % of the radiation is delivered in 12 days. Radiation levels become negligible within a few weeks after TheraSphere® treatment [9, 14]. Due to short half-life of ^{90}Y, the patient does not present a significant radiation risk after treatment and is allowed to go home.

3.2 TheraSphere® Treatment

A preliminary examination of the blood vessels (angiogram) is required before TheraSphere® therapy to determine if the patient can be treated with the glass particles. During the angiogram a catheter is inserted through the femoral artery into the hepatic artery of the liver and non-radioactive spheres with diameters similar to TheraSpheres® are injected into the catheter for diagnostic imaging [14]. The spheres contain albumin protein labelled with a contrast agent which highlights the blood vessels to be examined. These diagnostic imaging spheres provide information about the distribution of blood flow inside the liver and their accumulation in the liver and other organs (lung, stomach, duodenum, gallbladder). For some patients the blood vessels that feed the stomach and duodenum will be blocked with small coils or wires to prevent the formation of ulcers due to accumulation of microspheres in these areas.

As only a small number of blood vessels in the liver nodules have diameters greater than 30 μm, a low percentage of microspheres will be able to pass through the liver and potentially accumulate in the lungs or other organs. Liver vasculature mapping helps to identify the blood vessels that feed the tumour. The estimation of the percentage of spheres accumulated in liver relative to the other organs is used to establish if the patient can have the TheraSphere® treatment and the correct dose. If the amount of particles accumulated in the lungs is higher than 15 %, a significant dose reduction is applied to avoid pulmonary fibrosis [6, 14]. The treatment takes place within 2 weeks of the preliminary angiogram. The glass microspheres are injected slowly in the catheter through a 10 ml disposable syringe which can deliver 1.2–8 millions spheres per injection, depending on the required dose size (Fig. 7). Immediately after treatment the patients are scanned using computed tomography to map the location of the microspheres. Liver function is monitored every few weeks after TheraSphere® treatment [6, 14].

3.3 TheraSphere® Clinical Benefits

TheraSphere® particles are generally used for the treatment of hepatocellular carcinoma and metastatic liver cancer, being successfully used for unresectable cancers. This treatment improved the survival rate of terminal patients (life expectancy of 5–7 months) to 12–24 months. For unresectable cancers, intra-arterial administration of radioactive microspheres can reduce the tumour size. Clinical studies reported a significant shrinkage of tumours, allowing a follow-up treatment such as surgery (surgical resection), transplant or chemotherapy [16, 17].

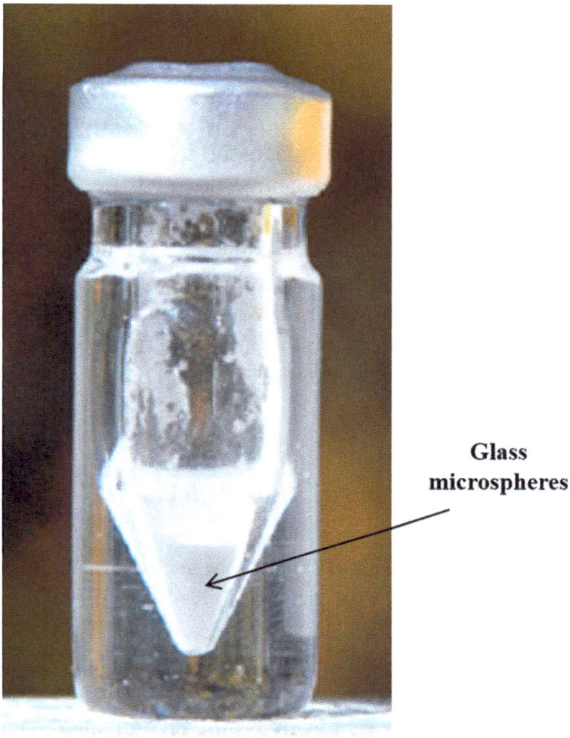

Fig. 7 A typical treatment vial containing white glass microspheres at the bottom of the vial (adapted from [5])

Therefore, the main advantages of TheraSpheres® are:

- can be used for unresectable cancers
- can be used for hepatocellular carcinomas
- can be used for metastatic cancers
- can extend the lives of the patients with inoperable tumours from months to years
- can produce significant shrinkage of large tumours, allowing alternative curing techniques such as surgery, transplant or chemotherapy
- is a minimally invasive technique, as only a small incision is made
- can deliver a higher radiation dose directly to the tumour, being more efficient than external radiotherapy
- has lower toxicity than external radiotherapy
- has fewer side effects than external radiotherapy
- has a fast recovery rate of patients

TheraSphere® treatment is not a cure. Clinical studies showed that approximately 70–95 % of the patients improved after this treatment and about 95 % of the patients with colorectal metastases increased their survival rate [17].

3.4 TheraSphere® Clinical Risks

There are few clinical risks associated with the use of this treatment. The main risks are infection, allergy, ulcers in the stomach or duodenum, bleeding at the incision site and blood vessel damage due to insertion of catheters.

Patients need to take antibiotics after treatment to avoid infection with 0.1 % patients acquiring a related infection after radioembolization. Intra-arterial administration of radioactive microspheres via catheters could damage the blood vessels, producing bleeding and bruising. There is also a low risk of allergic reactions to the contrast agent administrated during angiography. Approximately 2 % of patients may develop ulcers in the stomach or duodenum due to accumulation of the radioactive particles in these areas [17].

3.5 TheraSphere® Side Effects and Limitations

Typical side effects of TheraSphere® treatment include mild to moderate fatigue, fever, abdominal pain, nausea, loss of appetite, vomiting and temporary changes in liver blood tests. These side effects could last for approximately 1 week. Rarely, acute adverse events may occur, such as chronic pain, gastric ulcer, cholecystitis, loss of liver function [8].

TheraSphere® treatment is not recommended for severe liver or kidney dysfunction, or for patients with abnormal blood clotting or bile duct blockage [17]. The particles should not be administered to pregnant women. Theraspheres® have a shelf life of 12 days [8].

4 Non-commercial Glass Particles

In order to compare the properties, benefits and limitations of non-commercial glasses with Theraspheres® two further formulations were examined.

4.1 Glass Particles Containing ^{32}P

^{31}P has 100 % natural abundance (Table 1) and can be activated into the ^{32}P radioisotope by neutron irradiation in a nuclear reactor. As can be seen in Table 2, the half life of ^{32}P is approximately 14.3 days which is almost five times longer than ^{90}Y. However, the released energy is lower (the decay energy of ^{32}P is 1.71 MeV compared to 2.28 MeV for ^{90}Y), so the radiation dose of ^{32}P needs to be

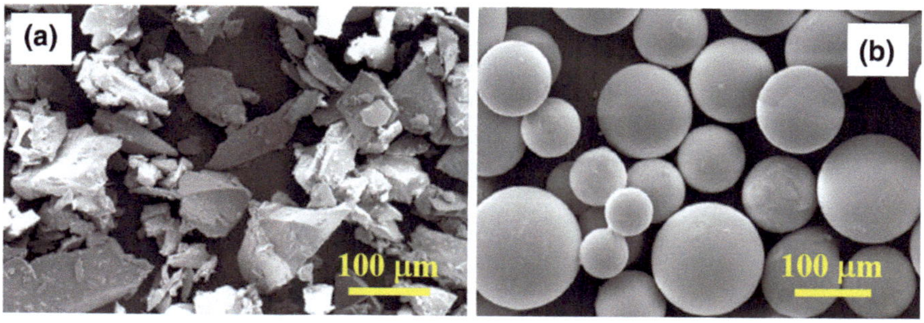

Fig. 8 Phosphate glass particles **a** before and **b** after spheroidizing (adapted from [18])

Table 3 Examples of nominal glass compositions used for radioembolization and their active radioisotope

Glass type	Radio-isotope	Composition (wt%)					
		Y_2O_3	P_2O_5	Al_2O_3	SiO_2	MgO	B_2O_3
YAS (Theraspheres®)	^{32}Y	40	–	20	40	–	–
Phosphate glass	^{32}P	–	42	10	4	44	
Borate glass	–	–	–	32		25	43

Table 4 Process conditions for the preparation of YAS, phosphate and borate glasses

Properties	YAS[a]	Phosphate glass[a]	Borate glass[b]
Density (g/cm^3)	3.2	3.1	2.9
Melting temperature (°C)	1600–1650	1250–1550	1350
Melting time (min)	120	120	15
Crucible	Platinum	Alumina	Platinum
Sintering treatment	–	–	1050 °C/10 min

[a]One step fabrication process; [b]two-steps fabrication process

higher than that used for ^{90}Y. Phosphate glasses containing ^{31}P could be used for radioembolization therapy if they satisfy all the requirements noted in Sect. 2.

In order to increase the chemical durability of phosphate glasses, Al, Mg and Si ions are added to the glass structure. Similar to ^{90}Y glasses, during neutron bombardment ^{27}Al, ^{26}Mg and ^{30}Si are activated to ^{28}Al, ^{27}Mg and ^{31}Si, having half-lives of 2.24 min (^{28}Al), 9.46 min (^{27}Mg) and respectively 2.62 h (^{31}Si) (Table 2). Other isotopes of Si (^{28}Si and ^{29}Si), Mg (^{24}Mg and ^{25}Mg) and O (^{16}O) are not activated by neutron bombardment.

Phosphate glasses containing ^{31}P and belonging to the system P_2O_5–Al_2O_3–SiO_2–MgO can be obtained by melting ammonium phosphate salts (such as $(NH_4)_2HPO_4$), Al_2O_3, SiO_2 and MgO at temperature between 1250 and 1550 °C for 2 hours. After grinding and sieving the glass particles are spheroidized to obtain

Table 5 Summary of the ^{90}Y, ^{32}P, ^{186}Re and ^{188}Re radioisotopes properties

Property	Radioisotopes			
	^{90}Y	^{32}P	^{186}Re	^{188}Re
Half-life (hours)	64.1	342.2	89.3	17
Maximum beta energy (MeV)	2.28	1.71	1.07	2.12
Gamma emission energy (keV)	–	–	136	155
Maximum tissue penetration (mm)	12	9	5	11

50–100 μm size microspheres (Fig. 8) [18]. An example of phosphate glass formulation is given in Table 3. This glass has good chemical durability, good cellular viability, high mechanical resistance and good blood corrosion resistance [19]. A summary of the process conditions for the synthesis of phosphate glass is presented in Table 4. The glass has a density of 3.1 g/cm^3, similar to the density of YAS glasses (3.2 g/cm^3). The melting temperature is lower than the one for YAS glasses, but an alumina crucible should be used to avoid corrosion of platinum crucible by the phosphate groups.

The nuclear properties of the ^{31}P radioisotope are summarized in Table 5. ^{31}P has a maximum tissue penetration of 9 mm, slightly lower than ^{90}Y radioisotope (12 mm).

4.2 Borate Glass Particles Containing Rhenium

A $MgO–Al_2O_3–B_2O_3$ glass containing rhenium (Re) provides another glass developed for radioembolization. Natural Re has two isotopes: ^{185}Re, with a natural abundance of 37.4 % and ^{187}Re, with a natural abundance of 62.6 % (Table 1). These isotopes can be activated into ^{186}Re and ^{188}Re radioisotope by neutron irradiation. ^{186}Re has a half-life of 89.3 h, while ^{188}Re has a shorter half-life of 17 h (Table 2). During the radioactive decay, ^{186}Re and ^{188}Re radioisotopes emit both beta and gamma radiation [20]. One main advantage of gamma emission is that it can be easily monitored by using a gamma camera immediately after particle injection. The nuclear properties of the ^{186}Re and ^{188}Re radioisotopes are summarized in Table 5. The maximum tissue penetration is 11 mm (^{188}Re), slightly lower than that for ^{90}Y radioisotope (12 mm). The decay energy of ^{188}Re is similar to ^{90}Y. Dose calculation of Re-containing glass particles is more complex as two radioisotopes must be considered, each of them emitting both beta and gamma radiation.

During neutron bombardment ^{27}Al, ^{26}Mg and ^{11}B are activated to ^{28}Al, ^{27}Mg and ^{12}B, having half-lives of 2.24 min (^{28}Al), 9.46 min (^{27}Mg) and 20.2 ms (^{12}B) (Table 2). The other isotopes (^{24}Mg, ^{25}Mg, ^{10}B and ^{16}O) are not activated by neutron bombardment.

$MgO–Al_2O_3–B_2O_3$ borate glass with the composition given in Table 3 can be formed by melting MgO, Al_2O_3 and H_3BO_3 in a platinum crucible at 1350 °C for

15 minutes. The glass is ground and sieved. The resultant borate glass powder with particles size below 45 μm is mixed with 15 wt% of ReO_2 powder, having an average particles size of 8.5 μm. Mixing is carried out in a ball mill with ethanol for approximately 12 h. The mixture is dried at 50 °C, placed in a platinum crucible with a lid, and then heated at 1050 °C for 10 minutes for sintering. The lid is used to avoid volatilisation of ReO_2 powder at high temperatures. After sintering, the mixture is ground and sieved below 45 μm. The resultant powder is spheroidized using a propane/air flame and sieved again to select spheres between 25 and 32 μm [21]. A sintering process was selected as ReO_2 powder decomposes at temperatures above 1000 °C. If ReO_2 is added to the initial glass composition, the melting temperature of the glass would have been too high (probably between 1250 and 1350 °C) and ReO_2 would become volatile. Therefore, borate glass containing Re is produced by a two-step process. In the first step the borate glass powder is produced by melting, while the second step consists of sintering a mixture of ReO_2 powder and borate glass powder for a short period of time (10 minutes) at a temperature at which ReO_2 volatilization is not rapid (1050 °C) [21]. A summary of the process conditions for the synthesis of Re-containing borate glass is presented in Table 4. The glass has a density of 2.9 g/cm^3, slightly lower than the YAS and phosphate glasses, so it would be carried more effectively by the blood flow.

The X-ray diffraction (XRD) data shows that the only crystalline phase is metallic Re in a glassy matrix. Re was produced by decomposition of ReO_2 during sintering and spheroidizing (flame temperature above 1200 °C). SEM images of the glass particles before and after spheroidizing are presented in Fig. 9. These glasses satisfy the requirements presented in Sect. 2, so they could be used for radioembolization. The glasses have good chemical corrosion resistance in phosphate buffered saline solution at 37 °C.

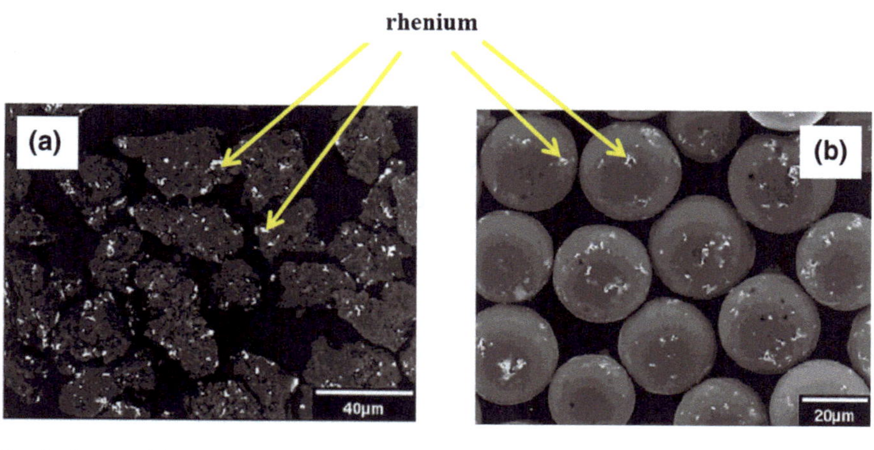

Fig. 9 Re-containing borate glass particles **a** before and **b** after spheroidizing (adapted from [21]) (The *bright white regions* contain high concentrations of rhenium)

5 Summary

Liver cancer is one of the most common cancers worldwide. Radioembolization is one of the therapies used for the treatment of primary hepatocellular carcinoma and metastatic liver cancers that consists of reducing the size of tumours by using radioactive microparticles. These microparticles (20–30 μm in diameter) are preferentially accumulated in the tumour and can deliver a high dose of β-radiation directly to the targeted cancer tissue, killing the tumoural cells. β-radiation is highly localised and thus, a high dose of radiation can be safely delivered to patients, without major damage of the adjacent healthy tissue.

The commercial microparticles, TheraSpheres®, contain ^{90}Y radioisotope in a glass matrix (YAS yttria-alumina-silicate glass). They have been used since 1990 in the USA and Canada for the treatment of liver, kidney and spleen cancers. The glass is prepared by melting using non-radioactive Y_2O_3 that is activated into ^{90}Y radioisotope via neutron bombardment in a nuclear reactor. ^{90}Y has a half-life of 2.67 days and a maximum depth of penetration of 12 mm.

TheraSphere® treatment is not a cure for cancer; it can reduce the size of the tumour, allowing the patients to have other curative treatment options such as surgery, liver transplant, chemotherapy, etc.

Different formulations of phosphate and borate glasses containing P and respectively Re radioisotopes have been developed for radioembolization, but they have lower chemical durability compared to YAS glasses. ^{32}P has a half-live of about 14.3 days which is almost five times longer than that of ^{90}Y, so ^{32}P could be more effective than ^{90}Y if the same dose is administered. Rhenium radioisotopes ^{186}Re and ^{188}Re can emit both beta and gamma radiation during the radioactive decay. Gamma emission can be easily imaged using a gamma camera immediately after particles injection. As both ^{186}Re and ^{188}Re are activated in the nuclear reactor, the calculation of the radiation dose is more complex and it should consider both beta and gamma emissions. Forming suitable glasses containing Rhnium is a two steps process, while the YAS and phosphate glasses require only one step for glass manufacturing.

Currently, TheraSphere® glass microspheres are the only commercial glasses used for radioembolization. TheraSphere® treatment has been demonstrated to extend the lives of patients with inoperable tumours or without possibility of liver transplant.

References

1. Cancer Fact Sheet 297. World Health Organisation. http://www.who.int/mediacentre/factsheets/fs297/en. Accessed 18 Sept 2016
2. https://cancerstatisticscenter.cancer.org/?_ga=1.35387425.1655096634.1455333684#/. Accessed 18 Sept 2016

3. http://www.cancer.org/cancer/livercancer/detailedguide/liver-cancer-what-is-key-statistics. Accessed 18 Sept 2016
4. http://emedicine.medscape.com/article/197319-treatment#d10. Accessed 18 Sept 2016
5. Kennedy, A.S., Dezarn, W.A., McNeillie, P.: Chapter 1: 90Y microspheres: Concepts and Principles. In: Bilbao, J.I, Reiser, M.F. (eds.) Liver Radioembolization with 90Y Microspheres, pp. 1–10. Springer, Berlin, Heidelberg (2013)
6. Kennedy, A.S.: Radioactive microspheres for liver cancers. US Oncol. Rev. **1**(1), p25–p28 (2005)
7. https://www.urmc.rochester.edu/encyclopedia/content.aspx?ContentTypeID=85&ContentID=P00676. Accessed 18 Sept 2016
8. https://www.btg-im.com/Therasphere/RoW. Accessed 18 Sept 2016
9. Murthy, R., Kamat, P., Nunez, R., Salem, R.: Radioembolization of Yttrium-90 microspheres for hepatic malignancy. Semin. Interv. Radiol. **25**(1), 48–57 (2008)
10. Kawashita, M., Shineha, R., Kim, H.-M., Kokubo, T., Inoue, Y., Araki, N., Nagata, Y., Hiraoka, M., Sawada, Y.: Preparation of ceramic microspheres for in situ radiotherapy of deep-seated cancer. Biomaterials **24**, 2955–2963 (2003)
11. Kovziridze, Z., Khorava, P., Mitskevich, N.: Controlled local hyperthermia and magnetic hyperthermia of surface (skin) cancer diseases. J. Cancer Ther. **4**, 1262–1271 (2013)
12. Erbe, E.M., Day, D.E.: Chemical durability of Y_2O_3–Al_2O_3–SiO_2 glasses for the in vivo delivery of beta radiation. J. Biomed. Mater. Res. **27**(10), 1301–1308 (1993)
13. Welsh, J.S.: Beta radiation. Oncologist **11**, 181–183 (2006)
14. https://www.btgim.com/Therasphere/RoW/Products/About-TheraSphere. Accessed 18 Sept 2016
15. https://www.urmc.rochester.edu/news/story/2879/medical-center-launches-new-treatment-for-liver-cancer.aspx. Accessed 18 Sept 2016
16. Georgiades, C.S., Salem, R., Geschwind, J.-F.: Radioactive microspheres for the treatment of HCC. In: Golzarian, J., Sun, S., Sharafuddin M.J. (eds.) Vascular Embolotherapy, pp. 141–148. Springer, Berlin, Heidelberg (2006)
17. http://www.radiologyinfo.org/en/pdf/radioembol.pdf. Accessed 18 Sept 2016
18. Sene, F.F., José, R.: Phosphate glass microspheres for radiotherapy applications. J. Non-cryst. Solids **354**, 4887–4893 (2008)
19. Guimarães, C.C., Moralles, M., Sene, F.F., Martinelli, J.R.: Dose-rate distribution of ^{32}P-glass microspheres for intra-arterial brachytherapy. Med. Phys. **37**(2), 532–539 (2010)
20. Argyrou, M., Valassi, A., Andreou, M., Lyra, M.: Rhenium-188 production in hospitals, by W-188/Re-188 generator, for easy use in radionuclide therapy. Int. J. Mol. Imaging. **2013**, 290750 (2013)
21. Conzone, S.D., Hafeli, U.O., Day, D.E., Ehrhardt, G.J.: Preparation and properties of radioactive rhenium glass microspheres intended for in vivo radioembolization therapy. J. Biomed. Mater. Res. **42**(4), 617–625 (1998)

Biocompatible Glasses for Controlled Release Technology

Roger Borges, Karen Cristina Kai and Juliana Marchi

Abstract In order to treat, relief or prevent diseases, new drugs and alternative procedures have been continuously developed. Recently, the introduction of concepts involving controlled release technology brought new perspectives for the development of drug systems. These systems aim to diminish drugs side effects and, at the same time, to increase their efficacy. In this sense, bioactive glasses have been used as new carrier systems to delivery ions, bioactive molecules (including drugs) and even cells. In this chapter, it was covered most of the main characteristics of bioactive glasses that must be take into account during the development of new carrier systems: glass composition, morphology and its interaction with the chosen drug. A relevant discussion about composites consisted of polymer/bioactive glasses was also included along the chapter. Finally, some of the most recent pharmacological breakthroughs using bioactive glasses are reviewed, such as applications in bone regeneration, osteomyelitis and cancer treatment.

1 Drugs and Controlled Release: Basic Concepts

Drugs are chemical compounds developed to promote, to treat, or to relief diseases. In order to understand how drugs work, first it is need to know how cells communicate to each other in the human body. This communication is known as cell signaling. In this process, a cell release a signaling molecule that will interact with receptor placed in the target cell membrane. Signaling molecules can belong to several chemical classes, such as lipids, amino acids, proteins, glycoproteins, other biomolecules, gases and ions. In addition, these molecules, in many cases, interact with other molecules before interacting with the target cell receptor, establishing a complex mechanism that can interfere on more than one tissue or organ, and then, integrating the human organism [1].

R. Borges · K.C. Kai · J. Marchi (✉)
Center for Natural Science and Humanities (CCNH), Federal University of ABC (UFABC), Santo André, SP, Brazil
e-mail: juliana.marchi@ufabc.edu.br

J. Marchi (ed.), *Biocompatible Glasses*, Advanced Structured Materials 53,
DOI 10.1007/978-3-319-44249-5_12

The effects of drugs are related to the interaction between drugs and the mechanism involving cell signaling. Briefly, this happens when a drug establishes intermolecular interactions with the target receptor. Thus, drugs usually mimic these specific signaling molecules, and can lead to the same response as the endogenous molecule (agonist), or block the response of these receptors (antagonist) [2–4]. Based on the desired effect, drugs may be classified into analgesics, antibiotics, anti-inflammatory, chemotherapies, muscles relaxing, among other [3].

If on the one hand, drugs' interactions explain their mechanism, on the other, pharmacokinetics and pharmacodynamics explain their performance. Pharmacokinetics and pharmacodynamics are stages involving drugs after administration. Pharmacokinetics is the study of drug concentration and kinetics in the bloodstream, also including the evaluation of some parameters, such as drug absorption, distribution, metabolism and excretion. Complementarily, pharmacodynamics is related to the evaluation of the drug effect in the body, establishing relationships between the dose taken and the time after administration [5–7]. One of the most important concepts of pharmacodynamics is the therapeutic window. The therapeutic window (Fig. 1) is a range between a minimum toxic concentration (MTC) and a maximum effective concentration (MEC), in which the drug concentration in the target tissue produces the intended effects for a specific treatment [8].

An ideal system should keep drug within the therapeutic window, however burst release or biotransformation process may lead to concentration peaks. Eventually, these peaks can exceed the MTC, and posteriorly decrease under the MEC along the time. In order to maintain the drug concentration within the therapeutic window, it is needed a maintained release and materials with suitable properties to allow a proper delivery [9, 10]. Therefore, drugs are mixed with other chemical substances for bringing the intended medicinal effect, and then, these substances are able to deliver the drug on a controlled manner, being it the principle of controlled release

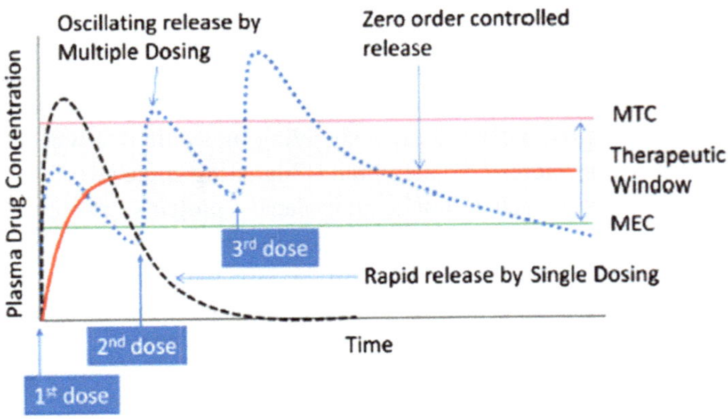

Fig. 1 Plasma drug concentration profiles obtained by single dosing (*short dashed line*), multiple dosing (*dotted line*), and zero order controlled release (*solid line*). The range between the minimum toxic concentration (MTC) and the maximum effective concentration (MEC) displays the therapeutic window, where drug is effective without displaying toxicity [9]

[11, 12]. Controlled release is a term that refer to compounds released in a time dependent manner. This term was firstly intended to define a drug release concept, but with the time, this term changed to controlled release technology, having a more comprehensive definition, and being not only applied to delivery of drugs, but also of molecules, cells and ions.

Different substances, also as known as vehicles, can be used to deliver drugs into the organism, such as polymers, ceramics and organic molecules. Once these materials interact with a living organism, they are considered as biomaterials (you can review the definition of biomaterials on the chapter "Bioactive Materials: Definitions and Application in Tissue Engineering and Regeneration Therapy"). In a similar way, the same approach is used to carrier biomolecules (proteins, DNA, grow factors, hormones) that act as cell signaling. As simplification, since the same approach is used to carrier drugs and biomolecules, and they play a similar role on biological systems, we shall generalize them as bioactive molecules [13, 14]. As an alternative definition, the association of a vehicle (biomaterial) with a bioactive molecule (BM) is called as system. In this chapter, we will consider a system the use of one or more biomaterials to carrier one or more bioactive molecules.

Studies involving materials suitable for controlled release systems have been done since 1950 through the development of oral devices for once-a-day or twice-a-day release, or transdermal adhesives devices for once-a-day or once-a-week release, which were also as know as first generation devices (1G). The second generation (2G) established between 1980 and 2010 was characterized by zero-order delivery systems, which means a constant drug concentration in the bloodstream. The 2G delivery systems were responsible for the development of smart polymers and hydrogels, which are sensitive to changes in pH, temperature, as well as other physical chemistry variations at the inserted environment. Besides the smart polymeric materials, other materials were also developed during the 2G generation, such as biodegradable microparticles, solids implants with in situ gelation and nanoparticles, which all of them aimed the delivery of either peptides, proteins, genes or cancer drugs [15, 16]. In 1990, the first 2G delivery system was approved by FDA (Food and Drugs Administration, USA), and was made of liposomal amphotericin B. Since then, other materials have been developed, approved and applied to different purposes, as showed in the Fig. 2 [17].

The current generation, 3G, was started in 2010, and highlighted with the continuous development of nanotechnology for controlled release by nanoparticles, dendrimers, liposomes, micelles, and nanotubes mostly inclined to cancer treatment applications [18, 19]. Some of these applications can be seen in the Fig. 3, which shows some controlled release systems approved by FDA over the last 25 years.

Controlled release systems are more complex than the traditional routes of administration due to more factors to be taken into account, such as the release environment, the system composition and physical-chemical properties, the drug-carrier interaction, and the carrier surface functionalization [16, 20–22]. Such variables are responsible to alter the BM release kinetic, because they determine the mechanism involved to release the BMs. The BM release kinetic can be classified into three different profiles (Fig. 4), according to different kinetics approaches (Eqs. 1–3):

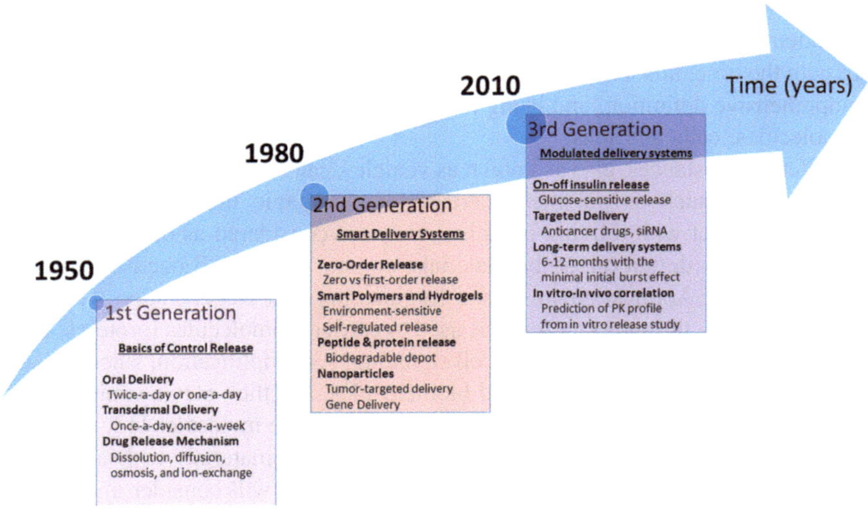

Fig. 2 Historic development of controlled release technologies [17]

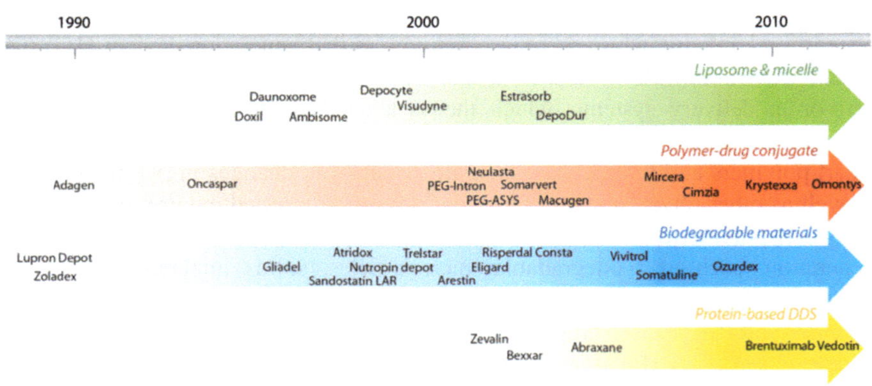

Fig. 3 Timeline showing FDA approved controlled release systems in the market [17]

$$\text{Zero order: } D_t = D_0 + k_0 t \tag{1}$$

$$\text{First order: } \ln D_t = \ln D_0 + k_1 t \tag{2}$$

$$\text{Higuchi: } D_t = D_0 + k_h t^{1/2} \tag{3}$$

where, D_t tis the amount of released drug at the time t, D_0 is the initial amount of released drug (burst effect), K_0 is the zero order constant, K_1 is the first order constant, and K_h is the Higuchi constant.

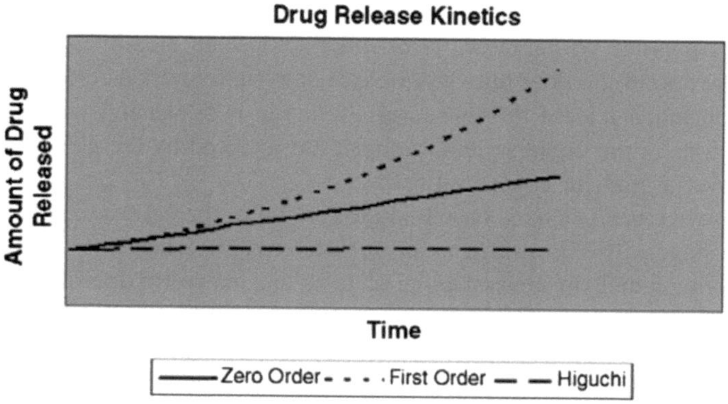

Fig. 4 Drug release profiles from zero order, first order, and Higuchi kinetics [10]

The drugs administrated under conventional routes usually follow a first order kinetics. In contrast, the formulations for controlled release shows a Higuchi release profile, and sometimes are close to zero order kinetics [10]. Figure 4 shows the difference between a first order, zero order and Higuchi model release. Note that zero order and Higuchi models are those that allow a most sustained release.

The zero order kinetics was already considered as the ideal release kinetics. However, a suitable release kinetics not only depends on the kinetics order, but also on the drug therapeutic window related to the drug released by the delivery system, as previously reported. Regardless of the kinetics order, controlled systems that increase the therapeutic index of a drug are able to improve the drug delivery, once they can reduce the side effects related to drug release, and maximize the efficiency through maintaining the drug concentration within the therapeutic window [8].

Even though there is no clear delivery mechanism for controlled release systems, some models have been proposed, such as those based on controlled diffusion, osmosis, ionic exchange and erosion [4]. These mechanisms are used to explain why the release profile fits in one of the three models mentioned above. Bellow, there are some examples of these models:

- The *drug controlled diffusion* mechanism occurs through interconnected pores of the system carrier modulated by water in the system. In this model, the kinetic release depends if the systems are monolithic or reservoir. In most cases, monolithic systems are associated with biodegradable materials, and its limiting factor is whether the drug concentration is higher or lower than the system solubility limit. If the drug concentration is lower, the drug will diffuse quicker through the system, otherwise it will diffuse slower. On the other side, a reservoir system is associated with systems containing a coated layer that controls the release kinetics, and is characterized by an initial burst or delay, depending on the system, followed by zero order kinetics.

- Another mechanism is the *controlled osmosis*, which the drug is released by the osmotic pressure within the carrier. Under a constant rate, this pressure leads to the diffusion of the drug outward the carrier system under a zero order kinetics.
- The controlled release *through ionic exchange* is associated with ionic drugs, which ions in the organism environment are replaced by the electronic charged drug over a gradient concentration.
- The *erosion mechanism* is based on the erosion of the carrier matrix that occurs at two stages. The first stage is the surface erosion, where the matrix is superficially degraded, in general quicker than the matrix hydration, leading to a weight loss at the surface. This superficial degradation is easier to control, allowing a zero-order release kinetics, and protecting drugs sensitives to early degradation. The second stage is the bulk degradation, where the hydration is faster than the matrix degradation, leading to the system degradation with time.

Other mechanisms include dissolution, swelling, stimuli-responsive, among others [23–28]. It is important to note that these release mechanisms are strictly associated with the controlled release systems properties, which, in turn, is related to the biomaterial used as vehicle. In this context, new biomaterials have been explored to improve the controlled release technologies. Among these biomaterials, biocompatible glasses have been used to achieve the requirements of the new generation of carriers, as we will see in the next section.

2 Biocompatible Glasses for Controlled Release Technology

Biocompatible glasses have been applied to controlled release purposes, but they are not only limited to deliver drugs. Due to their glass structure, these glasses can be doped with other chemical elements from periodic table, and delivery therapeutic ions as well. In addition, biomolecules can be also used to cause a desired effect in a specific tissue. Therefore, this chapter will cover all of these possible delivery systems in separated, because of their complexity and specificity.

2.1 Release of Ions

Bioinorganic chemistry is an interdisciplinary field of study that involves both chemistry and biology concepts. In general, bioinorganic chemistry studies the role of inorganic elements in biochemical process. These processes are well known by using metallic elements, as shown in Table 1, and are related to molecular conformation through electrostatic interactions, or acting as cofactors in either enzymatic or catalytic processes. Currently, the strategy used by chemists consists of using these metallic elements to trigger biochemical responses, including the

Table 1 Examples of inorganic ions associated with biomolecules and biochemical process [29]

Functional biomolecule	Example of biomolecules	Associated inorganic ions
Metalloenzymes	Oxidoreductases	Fe, Cu, Mn, Mo, Ni, V
	Hydrolases	Zn, Mg, Ca, Fe
Nonenzymatic metalloproteins	Hemoglobin	Fe
VItamins	Vitamin B_{12}	Co
Nucleic acids	$DNA^{n-}(M^{+})_n$	M = Na, K
Hormones	Thyroxine	I
Antibiotics	Ionophores, valinomycin	K
Biominerals	Bones, teeth	Ca, Si, P

enhancement or blockage of biochemical reactions in an organism. In this sense, these metallic elements are known as therapeutic inorganic ions, since they are used for therapeutic purposes, such as treatment of cancer, enhancement of osteogenesis, angiogenesis, anti-inflammatory process, nerve regeneration, among other features [29].

In addition, therapeutic inorganic ions show interesting advantages compared to organic biomolecules—e.g. grow factors, genes, or drugs composed by organic elements—such as chemical stability, effortless processing and obtainment, and easy interaction with other compounds [30]. Since these therapeutic ions need to be placed into the tissue where a specific treatment is required, carriers are used to deliver them into the application site.

Biomaterials are used to carrier therapeutic inorganic ions into a specific organism. Regarding the field of bioceramics, in specific, there are two possibilities: the use of crystalline ceramics (e.g., hydroxyapatite, tricalcium phosphate, alumina) or non-crystalline ceramics (bioactive glass or glass ceramic). In crystalline materials, these ions are integrated in the material's lattice in a limited weight percentage. Otherwise, they may lead to the nucleation of undesired phases. As an alternative to the usage of crystalline ceramics, the use of non-crystalline solids should be taken into account as a way to overcome this obstacle. The greater advantage of using glasses for loading therapeutic inorganic ions is the fact that almost all the chemical elements of the periodic table can be incorporated into the glass structure without forming secondary crystalline phases [31]. The most common ions added in the bioactive glass structure are shown in Table 2.

These ions are related to enhancement of bone regeneration, angiogenesis, or bactericidal effect, as shown in the Fig. 5. Further information regarding the applications of these ions is found in the final of this chapter, in the section "Examples of bioactive glasses applications in controlled release technology".

After being doped with a specific ion, the bioactive glass (BG) becomes bifunctional, i.e., the glass has a biocompatible matrix with a specific treatment effect. Thus, the material may be placed in different tissues where the therapeutic effect is required without leading to inflammatory damage responses [30]. However, these two functions have influence on one another. Considering that mostly of the bioactive glasses' compositions are based on either the SiO_2–Na_2O–CaO–P_2O_5

Table 2 Effects of ions derived from BG on biological responses

Ion	Biological response
Si	– Essential for metabolic processes, formation and calcification of bone tissue – Dietary intake of Si increases bone mineral density – Aqueous Si induces hydroxyapatite precipitation – SI(OH)4 stimulates collagen I formation and osteoblastic differentiation
Ca	– Favors osteoblast proliferation, differentiation and extracellular matrix mineralization – Activates Ca-sensing receptors in osteoblast cells, increases expression of growth factor, e.g., IGF-I or IGF-II
P	– Stimulates expression of matrix 1a protein, a key regulator in bone formation
Zn	– Shows anti-inflammatory effect and stimulates bone formation in vitro by activation protein synthesis in osteoblasts – Increases ATPase activity, regulates transcription of osteoblastic differentiation genes, e.g. collagen 1, ALP, osteopontin and osteocalcin
Mg	– Stimulates new bone formation – Increases bone cell adhesion and stability (probably due to interactions with integrins)
Sr	– Shows beneficial effects on bone cells and bone formation in vivo
Cu	– Significant amounts of cellular Cu are found in human endothelial cells when undergoing angiogenesis – Promotes synergetic stimulating effects on angiogenesis when associated with angiogenic growth factor FGF-2 – Stimulates proliferation of mesenchymal cells towards the osteogenic linage
B	– Stimulates RNA synthesis in fibroblast cells – Dietary boron stimulates bone formation

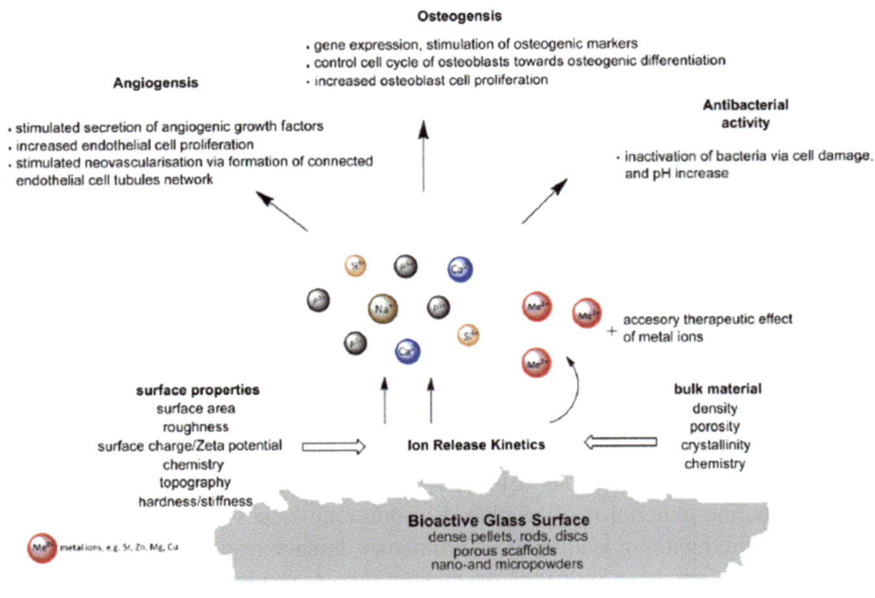

Fig. 5 Schematic illustration about the effect of therapeutic ions derived from bioactive glasses [30]

quaternary system or SiO_2–CaO–P_2O_5 tertiary system, which exhibit high bioactivity, when additional ions are integrated into the glass structure, they may decrease the glass' ability to nucleate a hydroxyapatite layer on its surface, and trigger a loss of biocompatibility.

This phenomenon was well verified in the work of Shruti et al. [32] that evaluated the bioactivity of mesoporous bioactive glasses (MBG) containing two different concentrations of cerium, gallium or zinc. Cerium stimulates the mineralization of primary osteoblasts, while zinc and gallium have antimicrobial activity, and act in the maintenance of bone formation and as inhibiter of osteoclast activity, respectively. The bioactivity test was performed in simulated body fluid solution at 37 °C up to 7 days. The results showed that doped mesoporous bioactive glasses had a loss of bioactivity ability with the enhanced concentration of these therapeutic ions in the glass structure. These results were confirmed through XDR patterns of the glass surface after the bioactivity teste (Fig. 6), mainly because of the absence or diminishment of hydroxyapatite peaks at 32° and 25.8° (2θ). A further accentuated bioactivity inhibition was observed in the compositions doped with 4 % of zinc due to the formation of zinc phosphate into the solution before the nucleation of calcium phosphate. Similar results can be found in the literature [32].

Furthermore, the effect of therapeutic ions in the glass behavior is not only limited to inhibit the biocompatibility, but also to change the glass dissolution profile, and consequently to change the therapeutic ion delivery and its effectiveness. This effect was demonstrated by El-Kady et al. [33] that studied the effect of the Ag_2O on BG nanoparticles, aiming antibacterial applications triggered by ions Ag^+. In this study, bioactive glasses were produced by sol-gel method, and replacing CaO by up to 10 wt% of Ag_2O. The glass dissolution behavior was

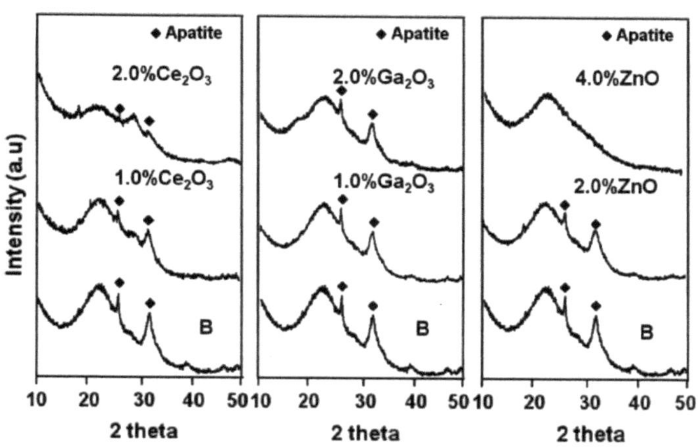

Fig. 6 XRD patterns after 7 days of SBF soaking of the B (not doped), Ce, Ga and Zn mesoporous bioactive glass [32]

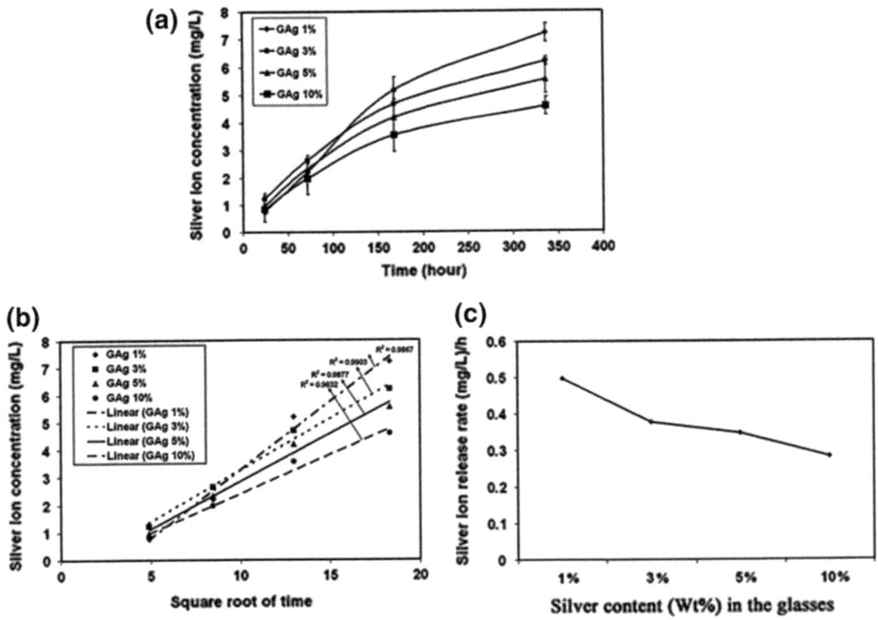

Fig. 7 Silver ion concentration in SBF solution, with time (**a**) and square root of time (**b**). Silver ion release rate in function of silver content (wt%) in the glasses [33]

evaluated by immersion in SBF solution up to 336 h at 37 °C. The results suggested glass dissolution was directly affected by silver oxide content in the glass composition. The higher the amount of Ag_2O, the slower the glass dissolution (Fig. 7). The authors associated the results with two main factors: glass connectivity and electronegativity. Regarding glass connectivity, Ca^{2+} ions are able to bond to two non-bridging oxygen, while Ag^+ ions are only able to bond to one. Hence, it is needed the double amount of Ag^+ ions to connect to the same quantity of non-bridging oxygen, which means that the substitution of CaO by Ag_2O lead to a more connected glass structure. On the other hand, in relation to the electronegativity effect, Ag^+ ions are more electronegative than Ca^{2+} ions (1.93 and 1 Pauling Unit, respectively). Then, a Ag–O bond is stronger and more covalent than Ca–O. Both of these factors are the responsible for changing the glass dissolution behavior and consequent silver delivery behavior as well.

Note that a specific ion in a glass structure has an influence on, but not limited to, the two main properties of a bioactive glass, that is, its bioactivity and specific therapeutic property. In this way, the influence over other properties, such as surface, morphology, mechanical, texture, among other properties, should be taken into consideration in order to understand the role of these ions on the glass properties as a whole.

2.2 *Release of Bioactive Molecules*

Systems based on either bioactive glasses or composites made of polymers/bioactive glasses have been used to carrier bioactive molecules into different tissues. The advantage of using systems based on bioactive glasses is the fact that either the bioactive molecule or the glass effect can be further stimulated in the presence of one another. Specifically, the use of bioactive glass or glass composites to carrier drugs into different tissues makes possible in situ applications, which means the avoidance of processes like biotransformation, excretion by renal filtration, and improvement of the pharmacokinetics and biodistribution performance. Likewise, the use of bioactive molecules can enhance the biocompatibility and biofunctionality of bioactive glasses through cell signaling, surface functionalization, increasing gene expression, and other ways that synergistically work together with bioactive glasses [3, 13, 34].

In this section, we shall further cover the facts that influence on the biomolecules' release, while in the next two sections will be better discuss the effect of glass morphology on the BMs delivery, and the effect of BMs on the BG's properties.

Below are listed the main factors that influence on the BM release:

- How the BM is bonded to the carrier system
- The glass composition and morphology;
- The concentration of BG in the polymer matrix, in the case of composites materials.

2.2.1 BM–BG Bond

A BM can be bounded to glass surface through two mechanism: electrostatic interactions or functionalization. Regarding electrostatic interactions, hydroxyl groups (–OH) are founded on BG surface because of Si–OH and P–OH functional groups, resulting in a superficial partial negative charge. Then, BMs that have partial positive charges can electrostatically bound to glassy surface, or even being bounded through hydrogen bond interactions. The Fig. 8 shown the interaction between gentamicin, which is used as an antibiotic, and a mesoporous BG surface through hydrogen bound interactions of amino (–NH_2) and hydroxyl groups. Note that the bounds between them is not limited to the BG external surface, but also includes bound placed in the internal surface of the pores. Furthermore, these bounds are sensitive to pH changes, because of the chemical equilibrium stablished in aqueous solution (Eq. 4). It is well known that over the bioactivity process the pH is supposed to fluctuate, and therefore interfere on the chemical equilibrium and in the BM release [35].

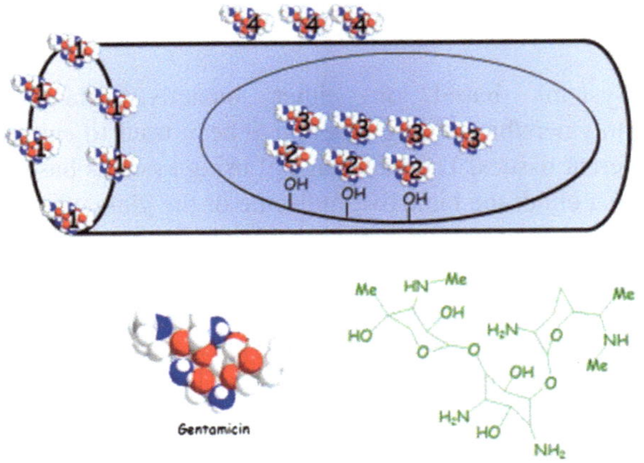

Fig. 8 Interactions between gentamicin and mesoporous bioactive glass through electrostatic and hydrogen bound interactions [3]

$$\mathrm{Si{-}O{-}H} + \mathrm{BM} \rightleftarrows \mathrm{Si{-}O} \cdots \mathrm{BM} + \mathrm{H}^+ \tag{4}$$

Although functional groups are naturally found on the BG surface, sometimes they are not always effective to stablish bonds with BMs, being required a functionalization process. Moreover, functionalization does not only is used to increase hydroxyl groups, but also to bind to intermediary molecules, which are bounded to the interested BM. The organosilane (aminopropyl)triethoxysilane (APTES) is the intermediary molecule most used for functionalization purposes onto silicon based materials. APTES is able to bond to both silanol groups through non-bridge oxygen bonds, and to a biomolecule through a remained amine group in the opposite side.

The main benefits of using a functionalization approach are both the possibility of increasing the interaction of the BM and the glass surface, and preventing a burst effect, immediate release of the drug provided by a more stable surface interaction. On the other hand, functionalization can also bring disadvantages: the loss of bioactivity caused by the modification of the surface in which change the surface charge, and decreases the phosphate and calcium precipitation. The Fig. 9 shown different possibilities in which BM can be bound to glass surface [3].

2.2.2 Chemical Composition and Morphology

In overall, the chemical composition by itself plays an important role on the electrostatic interaction between the BM and BG. However, chemical composition can also lead to morphologic changes, and then change the BM release process. Shruti et al. [32] studied the effect of different ions (Ce, Ga, Zn) on the ability of mesoporous bioactive glass to delivery curcumin, a drug used in cancer treatment applications. The authors suggested acid-basic interactions of the drugs and the ions probably changed the release profile. Since curcumin is a hard Lewis base, it has more affinity towards hard acids like Ga^{3+} and Ce^{3+}. As a positive point, these ions

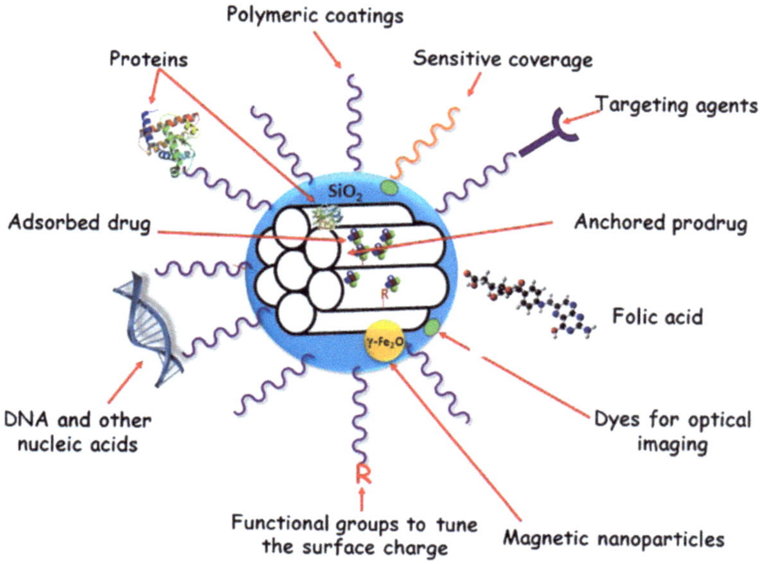

Fig. 9 Representation of a mesoporous bioactive glass with different possibilities of functionalization using bioactive molecules (e.g. DNA, proteins, polymers, antibodies, carbohydrates and drugs). Observe that most of the BMs are bounded in an intermediary molecule connected to glass surface [3]

support a higher drug loading within and surround the mesoporous structure; however the chemical strong interaction between the drug and the ions lead to a negative impact on the drug release, as showed in the Fig. 10a. Similar results were also founded by Zhu et al. [36] after evaluating the release profile of mesoporous calcium silicate doped with strontium (Sr) and loaded with gentamicin, an antibactericidal drug that was used as model. The author observed a slight lower gentamicin release in the glasses doped with Sr, which they associated with a slower chemical durability of the doped glasses. However, gentamicin is a strong base and Sr is a strong acid, then the same theory could also be applied for the observed mechanism.

Furthermore, the influence of ions is not only limited to the chemical interactions, but also includes morphological changes that influences on the release profile. Regarding mesoporous bioactive glasses (MBGs), the addition of doping components usually lead to the decrease of the porous structure, and it inhibit the loading capacity of the glass, affecting the release profile [36]. The Fig. 10b shows the result of pore size analysis of a Copper-containing mesoporous bioactive glass through the distribution curve of N_2 absorption method following the Barrett-Joinned-Helenda method. The higher the amount of Cu, the smaller is the porous size. We shall cover further details about the influence of the glass morphology in the section *Glass Morphology in Controlled Release Technology*.

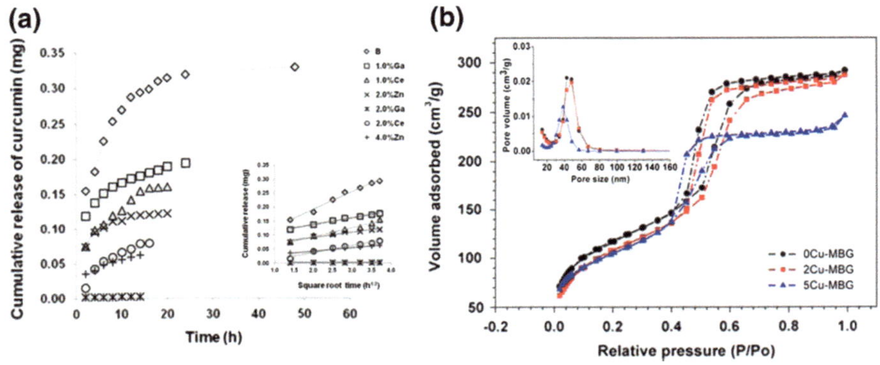

Fig. 10 The influence of glass composition on the release of BM. **a** The release of curcumin in MBG doped with Zn, Ga and Ce. The results shows that the Lewis acid-basic interaction of curcumin and Ga and Ce influences on the curcumin release [32]. **b** Pore size analysis of MBG doped with Cu. The higher the amount of Cu, the smaller are the pores; as consequence, less amount of drug can be loaded within the MBG porous structure [37]

2.2.3 Concentration of BG Within Polymer Matrixes

Despite the fact that BGs are able to bond to BM, and become suitable control release systems, this ability is further improved when BGs are associated with polymer matrixes. Composites carrier systems made of bioceramic and polymers have been comprehensively explored in the last decade, mainly because of the union of the osteoconductivity ability of bioceramics (e.g. tricalcium phosphates, hydroxyapatite and bioactive glasses) and the suitable carrier properties of polymers (e.g. hydrogels, chitosan, alginates, collagen, PLA, PGA, PLGA, etc.). Polymers are able to load drugs within their structure, and they are degraded releasing their monomers that are either biocompatible or non-toxic in the human tissue. Moreover, the BM loading is also improved, because both the BG and the polymer are able to load the BM. Figure 11 is an illustration of the ability of BG-polymer systems load BM, which used an antibacterial Ag-doped borate BG as example. In this example, it is possible to explore the synergetic effect of a therapeutic ion, a drug, and the polymer loading ability though using BG-polymer systems [38].

Furthermore, the further addition of BGs into the polymer matrix also influences on either the dissolution profile or the BM delivery. In general, the BM delivery is proportional to the BG percentage in the polymer matrix; however it is not normative for all the contexts. In a study carried out by Kouhi and collaborators [39], regarding the drug delivery ability of nanofibers made of poly (e-caprolactone) (PCL) incorporated with BGs nanoparticles, using simvastatin (a statin drug used for inhibiting the bone resorption). Comparing the different amount (up to 20 wt%) of BGs in the nanofiber matrix, it was observed the higher the amount of BG, the higher was the nanofiber degradation and the drug release. Due to the fact that PCL is a hydrophobic polyester, and its drug delivery ability is due to its hydrolytic

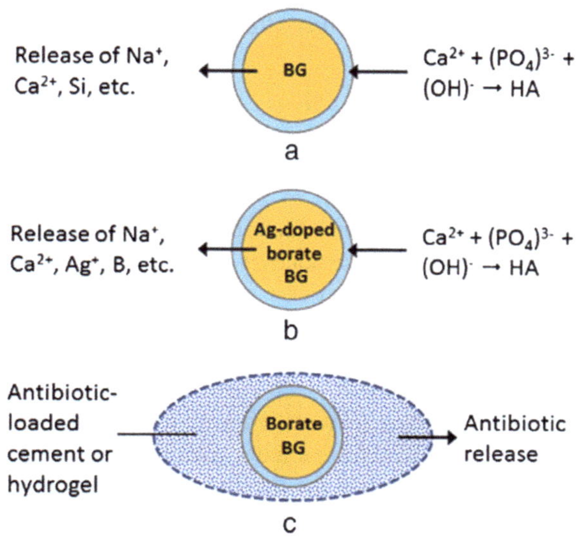

Fig. 11 The BM ability of a BG-polymer system used to load antibiotic drugs. Note that despite the glass being within the polymer structure, its ability to nucleate a biocompatible surface of hydroxyapatite-like layer is not influenced by this incorporation. In this example, the drug is loaded within the polymer matrix, however, considering MBG, the drug could be either loaded in within mesoporous structure or the polymer matrix [38]

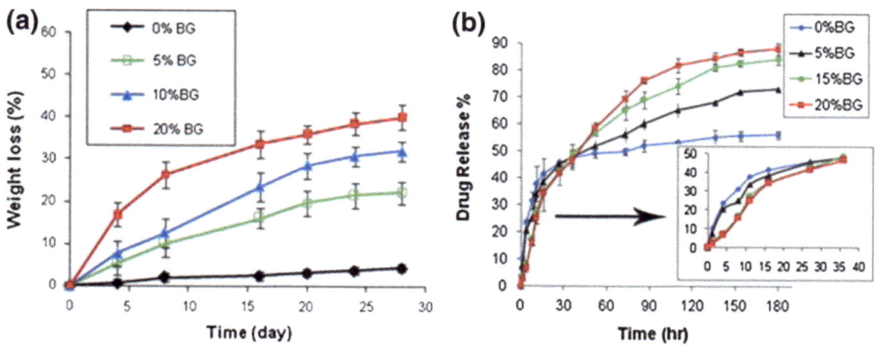

Fig. 12 Dissolution behavior of nanofibers made of PCL and different percentages of BG nanoparticles: **a** the weight loss (%) during 20 days of experiment; **b** the drug released (%) after 180 h of experiment. The results show the percentage of BG in the polymer matrix structure plays an important role on the dissolution and delivery behavior. In the proposed mechanism, BGs increase the PCL hydrophilicity, and facilitate hydrolysis reactions that, consequently, lead to the polymer degradation [39]

degradation, which creates channels that allows the drug delivery, the addition of BG was related to an increased hydrophilic ability of the composite nanofiber. Hence, the BG addition allowed a more intense hydrolytic attack, and a consequent weight loss and more drug release, as showed in the Fig. 12.

2.3 Glass Morphology in Controlled Release Technology

In controlled release technology, the delivery kinetics plays an important role, since it can change pharmacokinetics and pharmacodynamics processes, which, in turn, change the intended beneficial effect. For this reason, new glass morphologies (Fig. 13) have been explored in order to achieve better delivery kinetics, mostly changing the chemical interactions in which the BMs are loaded. As time went by, nanotechnology principles and techniques were applied on the bioactive glass synthesis, and materials like nanoparticles, mesoporous and nanofibers structures were gaining prominence. Nowadays, either bioactive glasses nanoparticles (nBGs) or microparticles are mostly used as disperse particles in polymeric matrixes, like composite materials containing BMs. Such materials are produced as scaffolds and membranes, and mostly applied to bone regeneration. On the other hand, mesoporous bioactive glasses (MBGs) have a more comprehensive usage, because these materials are able to load drugs onto the porous' surface. Recently, bioactive glass nanofibers have also been studies as prominent candidates to load drugs in their hollows, acting in the same ways as the MBGs.

2.4 Particulate Bioactive Glass Used as Composite Materials

The use of BGs as BMs carrier within a composite structure comes from the needed of replacing PMMA cements for more appropriated biomaterials. PMMA cements

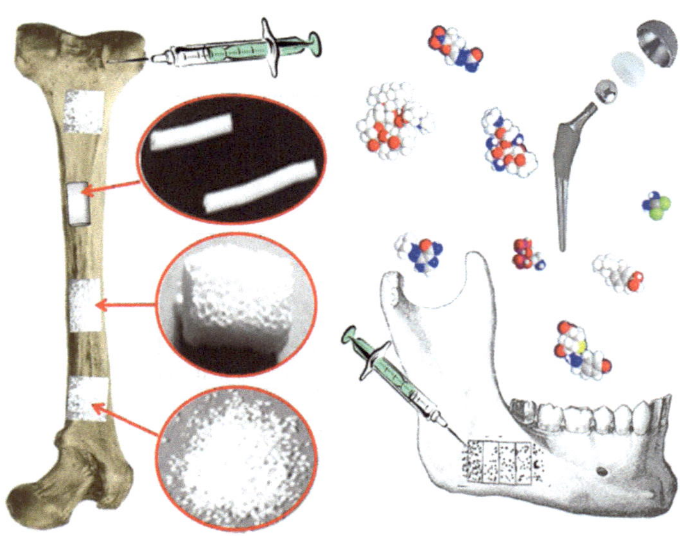

Fig. 13 Schematic representation showing the different forms in which BGs may be used for bone regeneration purposes, such as—from the top to the bottom—injectable, membrane, 3D scaffolds or particulate materials [40]

have been used as bone graft materials for bone reconstruction, and as drug delivery carrier of either antibiotic or analgesic drugs in order to minimize post-surgery infections and pains, respectively. Nevertheless, PMMA cements have the disadvantage of being bioinert, and then those cements are unable to bonds to bone tissue [41]. Therefore, new biomaterials have been developed to create bioactive biomaterials able to promote osseointegration. Among these new biomaterials, BGs composites with polymer matrix have been explored as promise candidate to replace PMMA cements. Polymers are suitable for drug delivery applications because they are able to release BMs in a constant and controlled rate, which, in turn, will influence on the pharmacokinetic and pharmacodynamics. Additionally, BGs can promote the expected osseointegration with bone tissues through their bioactivity property. Taken together, these composite materials seem to have more appropriate properties for bone graft applications, and can also be applied to tissue engineering purposes, since BGs are also osteoinductor.

Polymer based scaffolds can be made of bioresorbable or biodegradable polymers, and then when placed in a host tissue, there is no need for a second surgery to remove them, as usually happen with metallic based implants. Furthermore, polymers can be shaped in the format of the intended tissue to be replaced, improving their biofunctionality. However, such materials do not have adequate mechanical competence, and are unable to bond to living tissues by their own. Then, the addition of BGs brings the benefits of better mechanical properties and osseointegration [42–44].

An ideal scaffold should be degradable, and promote cell attachment, proliferation, migration, differentiation, as well as extracellular matrix deposition. In order to reach all of these requirements, porous scaffolds have been indicated as better microenvironment to promote the migration of cells, and to allow them to resemble a new bone structure within the scaffold. In the literature, it is possible to find different scaffold morphologies that allow the production of porous structure, trapping BMs in either the polymer or BG structure.

Li and collaborators [44] produced scaffolds made of porous BGs coated with PHBV microsphere. In this case, the strategy adopted was to trap the BM within the microsphere structure. As first step, PHBV microspheres containing vancomycin was produced by the water/oil/water method, allowing the drug to be trapped within the PHBV microsphere. PHBV was chosen because its biocompatibility and ability to sustained release of drugs, while vancomycin was chosen as model of bactericidal drug. Then, as second step, BG porous scaffold was prepared using the replication method, which consists of sintering particulate BG (Fig. 14a). Finally, the scaffold was coated with PHBV microspheres (Fig. 14b). The results showed PHBV microsphere coated scaffold has a further sustained release of vancomycin than the free microsphere (Fig. 14c), as well as better mechanical properties, and the bioactivity of the BG scaffold was not committed due to coating. Similar results were found for BG scaffolds coated with poly(D,L-lactide-co-glycolide) and poly (n-isopropylacrylamide-co-acrylic acid) microgels loaded with vancomycin [42].

Besides the production of BG scaffolds coated with BMs trapped within polymers microspheres, there is another alternative of preparing injectable scaffolds

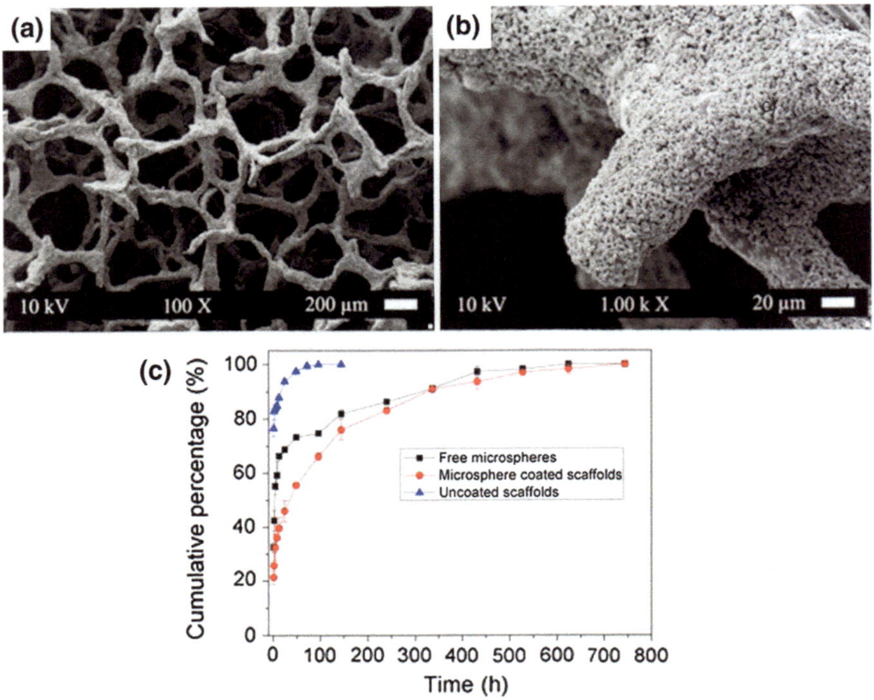

Fig. 14 SEM images of BG scaffold **a** before and **b** after coating. And **c** the cumultative release of vancomycin from free microspheres (*black*), PHBV microsphere coated scaffolds (*red*) and uncoated scaffolds (*blue*) [43]

using collagen-based matrix that works like bone graft cements. Such injectable biomaterials are prepared through mixing BG powder plus a BM, and adding the mixture into a solution made of chitosan, citric acid and glucose. The obtained final material is a dense biocompatible collagen structure with dispersed BG and BM. Borate bioactive glass/chitosan composites loaded with antibiotic have been evaluated as a prominent substitute for bone graft cements, such as calcium sulfate materials. Studies [45] have shown gentamicin sulfate-loaded borate BG/chitosan composite has further sustained release of gentamicin and higher compression strength than gentamicin sulfate-loaded calcium sulfate. Moreover, the borate BG based scaffold maintained a compression strength near to 10 MPa even after 14 days soaked in PBS solution, while the calcium sulfate cement is completely instable after 8 days soaked in the same solution [45]. In another study, borate BG/chitosan composite was used as delivery vehicle of vancomycin for treating osteomyelitis. In vivo studies were performed through inducing osteomyelitis in the tibia of healthy rabbits. The induction of osteomyelitis was done using methicillin-resistant Staphylococcus Aureus. In overall, when compared with the control group treated with commercial-like calcium sulfate cement, the borate BG/chitosan scaffold had the same ability to eradicate osteomyelitis, but both of them showed to be more effective than intravenous injection of vancomycin. Furthermore, unlikely calcium sulfate cement, borate BG/chitosan injectable scaffold was more osteoconductive as demonstrated in the radiography evaluation [46].

BG/collagen composites can be also used as membranes for guided bone regeneration, which consists of using growth factors to induce bone regeneration. This application is further appreciated in dentistry techniques, where a thin membrane is placed in a defective region of the periodontal pockets in order to prevent the growth of fibrous tissue, securing the growth of the intended cells, as well as allowing osteoinductive events. Hong et al. [47] developed a BG/collagen membrane containing fibroblast growth factor 2 (FGF2). In this study, a BG nanofibrous mesh structure was reached by electrospinning method, soaked into a collagen solution, centrifuged, and then soaked again in a FGF2 solution (Fig. 15a). The growth factor was loaded within the membrane's surface. The osteoinductive ability of the FGF2 loaded membrane was evaluated in vivo applying it in rat calvarium (Fig. 15b, c). The group that was treated with FGF2 loaded membrane showed a higher bone formation percentage than the groups treated with an unloaded

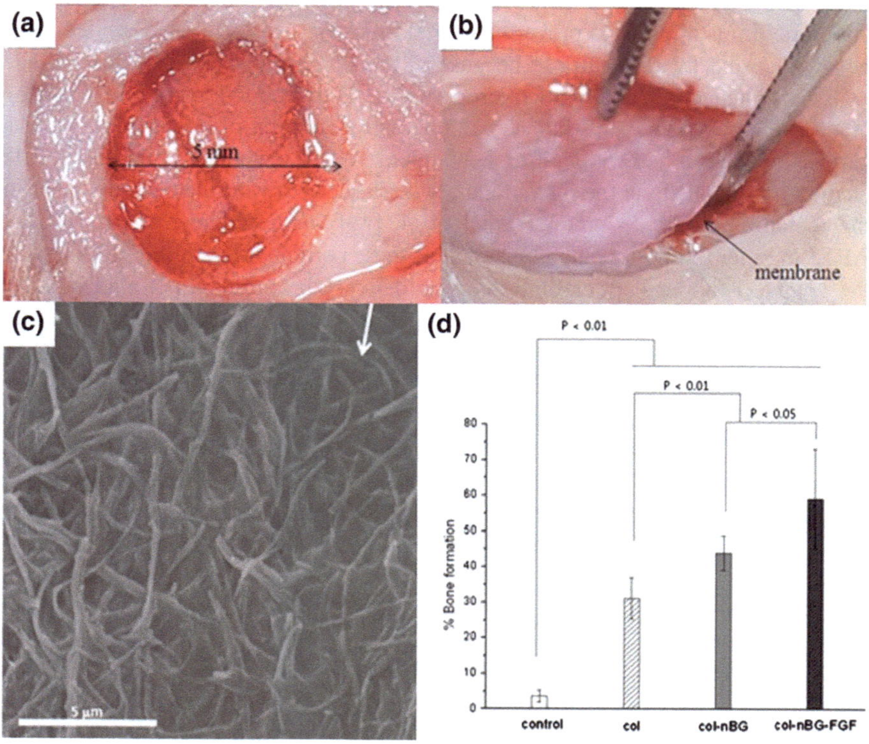

Fig. 15 Photography of in vivo experiment, showing the use of collagen-BG-FGF membrane (**a**, **b**). SEM of this membrane (**c**), and a graph showing the percentage of bone formation after an in vivo experiment using this membrane and comparing with the use of collagen and collagen-BG composite [47]

membrane or the group only treated with collagen (Fig. 15d). Thus, the results suggested synergetic osteoinductive effect of the BG, collagen and FGF2.

In another study, Rivadeneira et al. [48] developed an antimicrobial nano-BG/collagen membranes containing tetracycline hydrochloride (THC) using a different approach. Instead of coating BG with collagen, the scientists did the opposite; they coated a bovine-derived collagen using a solution of isopropanol containing nano-BG, which was subsequently dried. The THC was trapped in the membrane through the co-precipitation method, which consists in incubating the BG/collagen membrane in a SBF solution containing THC. Then, when calcium and phosphate precipitates, the THC was trapped within the amorphous layer of apatite. The use of nano-sized BG promoted a higher biocompatible environment, contributing to a higher deposition of apatite. The antimicrobial efficacy tests using Staphylococcus Aureus showed that membranes are able to inhibit cell proliferation up to a concentration of 10^6 CFU ml^{-1}, and the amount of THC released with time is out of the range of cytotoxic effects.

Aiming to improve the biocompatibility of metallic implants, BG/collagen composites have also been used for surface modification, mainly through using the electrophoretic deposition method [49–51]. These coatings were loaded with antibiotic drugs in order to prevent bacterial infections. In addition, nano-BGs have been suggested for this purpose because of their higher dispersity within collagen matrices when compared with microparticles. The production of this coating is made using a metallic substrate as cathode and a solution of collagen, BG and an antibiotic, such as vancomycin or gentamicin. When a voltage is applied, all the elements that constitute the membrane are dislocated forward the cathode, covering the metallic substrate structure. Patel et al. [49] suggested recovering BG with APTS in order to improve the movement of these particle forward the cathode when the voltage is applied. Regarding the drug delivery profile, it was found in all the results of the literature that this kind of coating containing antibiotics has a burst release of the drug, followed by a sustained release. Furthermore, it has been observed coatings containing BGs allow a higher uptake of antibiotic than those made of only collagen [50]. On the face of it, BG/collagen composite coating has seemed to be an effective and improved procedure to bring bioactivity properties to metallic implants, allowing them to bond to living tissues through the apatite layer nucleated on the coating surface, besides the possibility of loading antibiotics that avoid and/or prevent infection post-surgery.

2.5 *Mesoporous and Nanofibers Bioactive Glass*

Silica mesoporous materials are ordered porous structures of SiO_2, characterized by high pore volume and large surface area [52]. The first time that such materials were used as biomaterials happened in 2001, when it was proposed to use them for drug delivery applications in bone tissue due to their good biocompatibility. Since that time, SiO_2-ordered structure like MCM-41, MCM-48 and SBA-15 have been

Table 3 The requirements for an ideal drug delivery system and the reasons in which MBGs meet these criteria

Requirement	Reason
Biocompatibility of the carrier material	The biocompatible chemical composition similar to BG
High load and protection capability of desired drug molecules	Molecules are protected and loaded within the pores structure
Zero premature release of drug molecules before reaching its target	MBGs can be stimuli responsive, allowing the drug release only after reaching the target tissue
Cell type or tissue specific and endosomal escape; efficient cellular uptake; effective local concentration	MBGs can be functionalized using biomolecules that will either interact with cell membrane structure or to mimic an body structure or to avoid a foreign body reaction, as well as it will enabling a very specific cellular delivery

suggested as potential local drug delivery systems to be implanted in bone [3]. Despite the fact that such materials show a minimum bioactivity behavior, the kinetics of apatite formation is too slow to consider them as bone-bonding materials, which worked as an effort to the development of multicomponent mesoporous materials based on the same ternary system as BGs (SiO_2–CaO–P_2O_5) [53, 54]. As time went by, mesoporous bioactive glasses (MBG) were seen as one of the most promising carriers and platforms to build smart delivery devices, since they meet most of the requirements for an ideal drug delivery system, in accordance with Arcos and Vallet-Regí [3], as shown in Table 3.

The concept of zero premature release comes from the principle that an ideal drug delivery system should avoid burst release of drug, and have a sustained release since the time “zero” instead. In order to develop MBGs with zero premature release, new stimuli-responsive mesoporous carriers have been made. These materials are able to trap a BM within the mesoporous structure, and just allow it to be released after chemical, biological or physical stimuli, such as pH, light, redox potential, enzymes, antigens, or even the combination of more than one stimulus. The Fig. 16 illustrate some of these stimuli-responsive MBG.

Regarding pH-sensitive materials, the pore structure of MBG can be functionalized with polymers sensitive to pH, as well as the pores can be filled with drugs, as indicated in the Fig. 16a, b. As the pH changes in a body under pathological condition, it is possible to choose polymers that will have a morphological modification under the pathological pH, allowing the drug to be released when the functionalized MBG reach the damaged host tissue. In a similar way, enzyme-sensitive MBGs can be used as an approach due to the fact that pathologic tissues usually shows higher enzymatic activity, making the drug to be specifically released. In this case, the pores of the MBG can be coated with an enzyme-responsive pH, while the drugs are placed within the pores. Therefore, the drug will be released when the MBG reach the pathologic tissue [3].

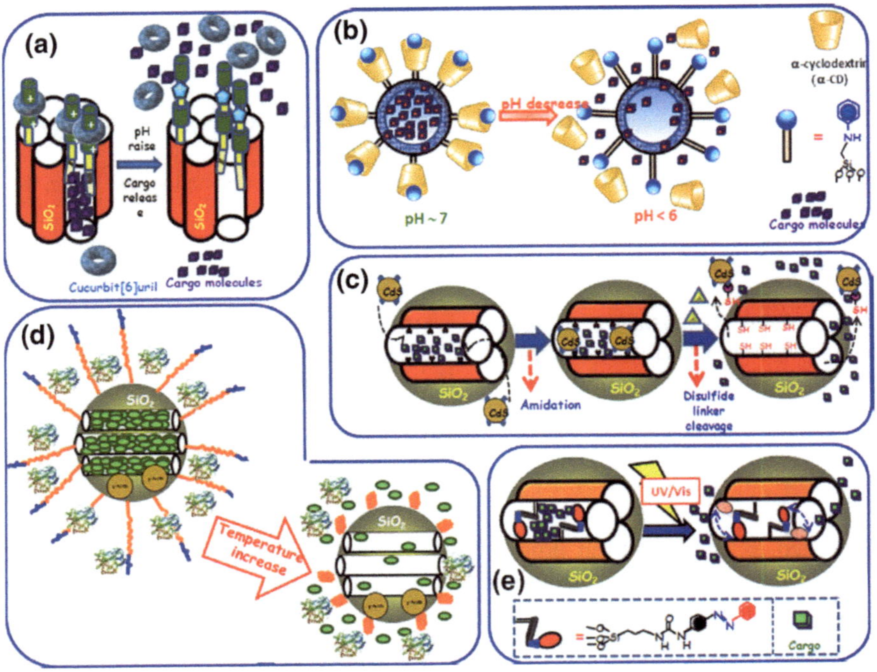

Fig. 16 Illustrative figure showing pH-sensitive (**a**, **b**), thermo-sensitive (**c**) and light-sensitive systems [3]

The approach used in light-sensitive MBG is also similar to those pH-sensitive ones. In this case, the MBGs are filled with the intended drug, and then the pores are blocked through a subsequent functionalization with a light-sensitive polymer. Thus, the pH-sensitive polymer works as a nanogates, mainly because the structural conformational modification of the polymer after interacting with light is usually reversible, and it is the responsible to allow the loaded drugs to go out of the pores, as shown in the Fig. 13e. The advantage of using light-sensitive composites is due to the possibility of improving the drug delivery through making the release at the local of the disease and damaged tissue, because it is possible to make the light cross over the living tissues and reach a specific location. Therefore, unlike pH or enzyme sensitive composites, which the stimuli is internal (the body), for light-sensitive MBGs the stimuli is from outside of the body that may be consider as a better way to manage the drug delivery.

Other stimuli-responsive composites use local physical or chemical changes in an organism in order to deliver the drug. For example, cells exhibit different intracellular and extracellular redox potential. In this sense, new MBGs have been developed using redoxpotential-sensitive polymers, which can only delivery the drug after the composite pass thought the extracellular membrane, and reach the cytoplasm.

3 Examples of Bioactive Glasses Applications in Controlled Release Technology

Bone regeneration was the first motivation for the development of bioactive glasses by Larry L. Hench. However, together with the development of BGs with new morphologies, properties and compositions, it was found broad applications for these glasses. Many of these new approaches, such as treatment of osteoporosis and osteomyelitis, are still related to bone applications, but other implementations are also possible, such as cancer treatment. In this section, all of these approaches will be highlighted under the light of new possibilities of BGs applications using controlled release techniques.

3.1 Bone Regeneration and Osteoporosis

The approaches used in applications of BGs for bone regeneration include the delivery of ions, genes and biomolecules (such as specifics drugs). Regarding the delivery of ions, a long review has been published by Hoppe and collaborators [30] about BG doped with therapeutic ions for bone regenerations purposes, where more details about these applications can be found. In this section we will discuss some new breakthroughs regarding therapeutic ions.

Boron has been used as a therapeutic ion to induce angiogenesis and osteogenesis. Haro Durand et al. [55] have shown 45S5 BGs doped with 2 wt% of B promotes new vascularization process through expressing angiogenic cytokines like IL-6 and bFGF. In additions, the authors showed human umbilical vein endothelial cells have a further migration, proliferation and vascularization ability when in contact with ionic degradation products of BGs doped with B, even when compared with cells cultivated in a medium supplemented with bFGF. Taken together, these results confirm an alternative material that can induce bone and vascular regeneration at the same time. The need of angiogenetic materials for bone regeneration comes from the need of vascularization process within scaffolds that are able to transport nutrients to cells, making possible their proliferation, migration and differentiation. Other elements like zinc, strontium and magnesium have also been used for improve bone regeneration ability, and have also shown improved osteoconductivity-related responses [29, 56]. Studies carried out by Zhang et al. [57] shows MBGs doped with Sr can be used for treatment of osteoporotic bone due to the anti-osteoporotic response of Sr. Their results showed MBG doped up to 5 wt% of Sr promotes a better bone regeneration in osteoporotic bone defects using rat models, besides a further proliferations and differentiation of bone marrow stem cells into osteoblast-like cells in a concentration-dependent manner.

Regarding the applications of biomolecules for bone regeneration, it has been noticed the usage of molecules that allow guided bone regeneration, associating angiogenetic strategies when it is appropriated and possible. Usually, the production of scaffolds made of polymers and BGs has been seen as synergic combination in order to reproduce a bone-similar environment for cell growth, as well as trap the biomolecules within the scaffold structure. In relation to osteogenic biomolecules, the use of fibroblast growth factor 2 (FGF-2) [47], osteogenic growth peptide (OGP) [58] and osteoactivin gene [59] have been seen as potential candidates. However, due to the need of scaffolds that lead to both new vascularization and bone regeneration, other biomolecules has also been proposed, such as vascular endothelial growth factor (EGF) [60] and dimethyloxallyl glycine (DMOG) [61].

The delivery of pre-osteoblast M3CT3-E1 cells has been seen as a promisor procedure to improve bone regeneration. Perez et al. [62] studied the biological properties of BG microspheres containing FGF and loaded with pre-osteoblast MC3T3-E1 cells. Through using rat subcutaneous tissue model, the authors showed these microspheres are able to gathering and grow fibroblastic cells around the microspheres due to the interaction of both the pre-osteoblast cells and the FGF on the surrounding host tissue. In another study, Zeng et al. [63] developed BG-Alginate hydrogels containing pre-osteoblast MC3T3-E1 cells, and showed that these hydrogels were able to induce the osteoblastic differentiation of the pre-osteoblast cells, as well as stimulated the proliferation and differentiation of rat bone marrow mesenchymal stem cells, and promoted the formation of tubules-like structure using HUVECs. In overall, the encapsulation of pre-osteoblast cells seems to be an interesting and effective procedure to obtain improved bone regeneration process associated with angiogenesis.

3.2 Cancer Treatment

Using the advantage that BGs are biocompatible, and do not lead to severe immunological response, particulate BG has been used to load anti-cancer drugs, and used as drug delivery system. Wu et al. [64] studied the efficacy of MBGs nanospheres loaded with doxorubicin (DOX). In their results, they showed the drug did not influences on the biomineralization of MBGs, and the material loaded with (DOX) decreased the cellular viability of osteosarcoma cells. In another work, Zhang et al. [65] developed a composite of poloxamer 123/MBGs/Fe_2O_3 containing DOX. The addition of iron oxide was due to its magnetic property suitable for hyperthermia applications. Therefore, this composite ally the anti-drug effect of DOX with hyperthermia. The results of this works suggests the composite has suitable biocompatibility, and the magnetic property of iron oxide was not interfered by the composite. In addition, although no culture cell test with osteosarcoma was performed, the drug release profile suggests the composite has promise properties for cancer treatment.

An interesting experiment done by Lin and collaborators [66] compared the anti-drug effect of folate-modified MBG containing camptothecin (CPT). The MBG was functionalized with folic acid, because it interacts with folate receptors in cancer cells, and works as endocytosis intermediate. Then, once the interface of cell surface-materials surface is improved, the drug can have an improved effect as well. In order to evaluate the material, HeLa and fibroblast cultures were interacted with the functionalized MBG particles containing CPT. Results showed the uptake drug in HeLa cells was higher than the fibroblast cells due to the folate-intermediate endocytosis. This result contributes to new thoughts about how to design new materials for treatment of cancer.

3.3 Bactericidal Properties and Osteomyelitis

The development of bioactive glasses with bactericidal properties has been increased in the last years, mainly due to the need of materials that avoid post-operatory complications because of bacterial infection. In this sense, BGs with bactericidal properties have been broadly used for coating of metallic implants, mainly because the surgery of those implants are sometimes very invasive, and exposes the host tissue to the external environment that can lead to bacterial infections [50]. Another interesting application is in osteomyelitis. BGs with bactericidal properties are promise materials for treatment of osteomyelitis because they can bring together the bactericidal properties needed to kill the bacteria in the bone tissue with the osteogenesis properties needed to induce the regeneration of the damaged tissue [38].

BGs doped with silver (Ag) have been widely explored as an alternative material that exhibit bactericidal properties. The broad spectrum antibacterial properties of Ag make this element an effective ion to inhibit bacteria colonization, which can be related to a biomaterial infection. Ag-BGs have showed effective against bacteria colonies like Escherichia coli (*E. coli*), Pseudomonas Aeruginosa (*P. aeruginosa*) and S. Aureus. Moreover, biological characterizations of BGs containing Ag using pre-osteoblast MC3T3-E1 cells and L929 fibroblast demonstrated BGs doped with up to 1 wt% of Ag do not upset the glass biocompatibility, as well as maintain antibacterial properties [38]. Another interesting ion that can be used for the same purpose is gallium (Ga), which also has broad spectrum properties, being effective against *P. Aeruginosa*, Methicillin Resistant S. Aureus and C. Difficile. The mechanism of the antibacterial properties of Ga is related to the competition with Fe ions whose are responsible for redox intracellular environment in the bacteria. When Ga goes towards the intracellular site in the bacteria, it does not induce the supposed redox environment, leading to more vulnerable bacteria. Mouriño et al. [67] studied the properties of Ga-crosslinked alginate/NBGs films, and conclude this composite is suitable for bone engineering in applications that requires antibacterial properties, despite the slight reduction on the cell proliferation and small increase in cell death.

BG-based composite materials have been powerful tools for the development of drug carriers. Several drugs have been combined with BGs or BGs-based composites in order to reach new alternatives for the need of bactericidal materials or treatment of osteomyelitis. Among the drugs combined with BGs-based composites, we can cite tetracyclin, vancomycin, teicoplanin, gentamicin, gatifloxacin, ciprofloxacin, ampicillin and carbenicillin, being the first four one used for osteomyelitis.

Ampicillin has been incorporated into calcium-silicate-based glasses and mesoporous structures [68], while carbenecillin has been used to modify the surface of BGs [69]. So far, for both drugs, the results from the literature have shown they are effective against bacteria colonization without having influence on either bone-like cells behavior or biomineralization. Similar results were found for MBG functionalized with ciprofloxacin, however a study carried out by Ehlert et al. [70] showed that a previous MBG surface modification with bis(trimethoxysilyl)hexane or dioctyltetramethyldisilazane can lead to more controlled release of ciprofloxacin. This drug was also incorporated into the structure of polyvinyl-alcohol/BGs composites [71], and the results shows this composite was able to release the drug up to more than 12 days, being suitable for either antibacterial purposes or osteomyelitis treatment, despite no antibactericidal test was done.

Regarding BGs for osteomyelitis treatment, either BGs or BGs-composites have also been used. Borate glass scaffolds loaded with vancomycin were studied by Liu et al. [72], who showed through in vivo studies, using rabbit tibia infected with osteomyelitis model, which more than 80 % of the rabbits treated with the scaffolds showed bone regeneration, angiogenesis and antimicrobial activity. Similar results from the literature, using rabbit tibia with osteomyelitis model, have shown that pellets composites of chitosan/borate glass containing teicoplanin are able to treat osteomyelitis, and convert to hydroxyapatite-like structure within 4 months [73, 74]. Other results using chitosan/borate glasses containing gentamicin are even more surprising. In a study carried out by Xie et al. [75], pellets of chitosan/borate glasses containing gentamicin were implanted in rabbit tibia infected with osteomyelitis using *E. Coli* as model. The results showed the composite eradicated the osteomyelitis condition and regenerated the bone within 6 weeks (one and a half month), being a better results when compared with chitosan/borate glasses containing teicoplanin.

4 Concluding Remarks

The development of glass-based controlled release systems is still a new feature, which has not been entirely explored. There are many drugs that can exhibit better physical chemical properties to interact with BGs, and then, lead to an improved sustained release in relation to the current evaluated drugs. Indeed, it is needed a better understanding of the intermolecular interactions stablished between the drugs and the glass-based carriers. The lack of tools to predict such interactions is the main cause of a hard experimental work that makes researchers to spend a lot of time evaluating whether new compositions and systems will lead to better sustained release. With the advance of computational simulations for materials development, the use of this technology should be taken into account to predict intermolecular interactions, and to the best of our knowledge such theoretical approach has not been employed when glass-based systems were developed. Furthermore, considering that new glasses have been developed at the same time that better drugs have been also researched, new and more effective treatments and other applications will be explored in a near future.

References

1. Alberts, B., et al.: General principles of cell communication. In: NCBI Bookshelf. Molecular Biology of the Cell, 4th edn. Garland Science, New York (2002)
2. Wilson, C.G.: The need for drugs and drug delivery systems. In: Siepmann, J., et al. (eds.) Fundamentals and Applications of Controlled Release Drug Delivery. Advances in Delivery Science and Technology, pp. 3–18 (2012). doi:10.1007/978-1-4614-0881-9_9
3. Arcos, D., Vallet-Regí, M.: Bioceramics for drug delivery. Acta Mater. **61**, 890–911 (2013). doi:10.1016/j.actamat.2012.10.039
4. Yun, Y.H., Lee, B.K., Park, K.: Controlled drug delivery: historical perspective for the next generation. J. Controlled Release **219**, 2–7 (2015). doi:10.1016/j.jconrel.2015.10.005
5. Mager, D.E.: Quantitative structure–pharmacokinetic/pharmacodynamic relationships. Adv. Drug Deliv. Rev. **58**, 1326–1356 (2006). doi:10.1016/j.addr.2006.08.002
6. Gabrielsson, J., Green, A.R.: Quantitative pharmacology or pharmacokinetic pharmacodynamic integration should be a vital component in integrative pharmacology. J. Pharmacol. Exp. Ther. **331**, 767–774 (2009). doi:10.1124/jpet.109.157172
7. Asín-Prieto, E., Rodríguez-Gascón, A., Isla, A.: Applications of the pharmacokinetic/pharmacodynamic (PK/PD) analysis of antimicrobial agents. J. Infect. Chemother. **21**, 319–329 (2015). doi:10.1016/j.jiac.2015.02.001
8. Acharya, G., Park, K.: Mechanisms of controlled drug release from drug-eluting stents. Adv. Drug Deliv. Rev. **58**, 387–401 (2006). doi:10.1016/j.addr.2006.01.016
9. Lee, J.H., Yeo, Y.: Controlled drug release from pharmaceutical nanocarriers. Chem. Eng. Sci. **125**, 75–84 (2015). doi:10.1016/j.ces.2014.08.046
10. Hughes, G.A.: Nanostructure-mediated drug delivery. Nanomed. Nanotechnol. Biol. Med. **1**, 22–30 (2005). doi:10.1016/j.nano.2004.11.009
11. Tiwari, G., et al.: Drug delivery systems: an updated review. Int. J. Pharm. Investig. **2**, 2–11 (2012). doi:10.4103/2230-973X.96920
12. Reddy, L.H., Bazile, D.: Drug delivery design for intravenous route with integrated physicochemistry, pharmacokinetics and pharmacodynamics: illustration with the case of taxane therapeutics. Adv. Drug Deliv. Rev. **71**, 34–57 (2014). doi:10.1016/j.addr.2013.10.007
13. Hum, J., Boccaccini, A.R.: Bioactive glasses as carriers for bioactive molecules and therapeutic drugs: a review. J. Mater. Sci. Mater. Med. **23**, 2317–2333 (2012). doi:10.1007/s10856-012-4580-z
14. Wu, C., Chang, J.: Mesoporous bioactive glasses: structure characteristics, drug/growth factor delivery and bone regeneration application. Interface Focus **2**, 292–306 (2012). doi:10.1098/rsfs.2011.0121
15. Park, K.: Facing the truth about nanotechnology in drug delivery. ACS Nano **7**, 7442–7447 (2013). doi:10.1021/nn404501g
16. Park, K.: Drug delivery of the future: controlled drug delivery systems: past forward and future back. J. Controlled Release **190**, 3–8 (2014). doi:10.1016/j.jconrel.2014.03.054
17. Zhang, Y., Chan, H.F., Leong, K.W.: Advanced materials and processing for drug delivery: the past and the future. Adv. Drug Deliv. Rev. **65**, 104–120 (2013). doi:10.1016/j.addr.2012.10.003

18. Safari, J., Zarnegar, Z.: Advanced drug delivery systems: nanotechnology of health design: a review. J. Saudi Chem. Soc. **18**, 85–99 (2014). doi:10.1016/j.jscs.2012.12.009
19. Park, K.: Drug delivery of the future: chasing the invisible gorilla. J. Controlled Release (2015). doi:10.1016/j.jconrel.2015.10.048
20. Xia, Y., Pack, D.W.: Uniform biodegradable microparticle systems for controlled release. Chem. Eng. Sci. **125**, 129–143 (2015). doi:10.1016/j.ces.2014.06.049
21. Torchilin, V.: Multifunctional and stimuli-sensitive pharmaceutical nanocarriers. Eur. J. Pharm. Biopharm. **71**, 431–444 (2009). doi:10.1016/j.ejpb.2008.09.026
22. Sarkhel, S., et al.: High-throughput in vitro drug release and pharmacokinetic simulation as a tool for drug delivery system development: application to intravitreal ocular administration. Int. J. Pharm. **477**, 469–475 (2014). doi:10.1016/j.ijpharm.2014.10.062
23. Tongwen, X., Binglin, H.: Mechanism of sustained drug release in diffusion-controlled polymer matrix-application of percolation theory. Int. J. Pharm. **170**, 139–149 (1998). doi:10.1016/S0378-5173(97)00402-X
24. Siepmann, J., Siepmann, S.: Mathematical modeling of drug delivery. Int. J. Pharm. **364**, 328–343 (2008). doi:10.1016/j.ijpharm.2008.09.004
25. Fu, Y., Kao, W.J.: Drug release kinetics and transport mechanisms of nondegradable and degradable polymeric delivery systems. Expert Opin. Drug Deliv. **7**, 429–444 (2010). doi:10.1517/17425241003602259
26. Raval, A., Parikh, J., Engineer, C.: Mechanism of controlled release kinetics from medical devices. Braz. J. Chem. Eng. **27**, 211–225 (2010). doi:10.1590/S0104-66322010000200001
27. Mönkäre, J., et al.: Characterization of internal structure, polymer erosion and drug release mechanisms of biodegradable poly(ester anhydride)s by X-ray microtomography. Eur. J. Pharm. Sci. **47**, 170–178 (2012). doi:10.1016/j.ejps.2012.05.013
28. Cheng, W., Gu, L., Ren, W., Liu, Y.: Stimuli-responsive polymers for anti-cancer drug delivery. Mater. Sci. Eng. C **45**, 600–608 (2014). doi:10.1016/j.msec.2014.05.050
29. Kaim, W., Schwederski, B., Klein, A.: Bioinorganic chemisitry—inorganic elements in the chemistry of life: an introduction and guide. In: Kaim, W., Schwederski, B., Klein, A. (eds.), 1st edn. John Wiley and Sons, Chichester (2013). ISBN: 9780470975237
30. Hoppe, A., Mourino, V., Boccaccini, A.R.: Therapeutic inorganic ions in bioactive glasses to enhance bone formation and beyond. Biomater. Sci. **1**, 254–256 (2013). doi:10.1039/c2bm00116k
31. Zanotto, E.D., Coutinho, F.A.B.: How many non-crystalline solids can be made from all the elements of the periodic table? J. Non Cryst. Solids **347**, 285–288 (2004). doi:10.1016/j.jnoncrysol.2004.07.081
32. Shruti, S., Salinas, A.J., Ferrari, E., et al.: Curcumin release from cerium, gallium and zinc containing mesoporous bioactive glasses. Microporous Mesoporous Mater. **180**, 92–101 (2013). doi:10.1016/j.micromeso.2013.06.014
33. El-Kady, A.M., Ali, A.F., Rizk, R.A., Ahmed, M.M.: Synthesis, characterization and microbiological response of silver doped bioactive glass nanoparticles. Ceram. Int. **38**, 177–188 (2012). doi:10.1016/j.ceramint.2011.05.158
34. Wu, C., Chang, J.: Multifunctional mesoporous bioactive glasses for effective delivery of therapeutic ions and drug/growth factors. J. Control Release **193**, 1–14 (2014). doi:10.1016/j.jconrel.2014.04.026
35. Xia, W., Chang, J.: Well-ordered mesoporous bioactive glasses (MBG): a promising bioactive drug delivery system. J. Control Release **110**, 522–530 (2006). doi:10.1016/j.jconrel.2005.11.002
36. Zhu, Y., Zhu, M., He, X., et al.: Substitutions of strontium in mesoporous calcium silicate and their physicochemical and biological properties. Acta Biomater. **9**, 6723–6731 (2013). doi:10.1016/j.actbio.2013.01.021
37. Ye, J., He, J., Wang, C., et al.: Copper-containing mesoporous bioactive glass coatings on orbital implants for improving drug delivery capacity and antibacterial activity. Biotechnol. Lett. **36**, 961–968 (2014). doi:10.1007/s10529-014-1465-x

38. Rahaman, M.N., Bal, B.S., Huang, W.: Review: emerging developments in the use of bioactive glasses for treating infected prosthetic joints. Mater. Sci. Eng. C **41**, 224–231 (2014). doi:10.1016/j.msec.2014.04.055
39. Kouhi, M., Morshed, M., Varshosaz, J., Fathi, M.H.: Poly (ε-caprolactone) incorporated bioactive glass nanoparticles and simvastatin nanocomposite nanofibers: preparation, characterization and in vitro drug release for bone regeneration applications. Chem. Eng. J. **228**, 1057–1065 (2013). doi:10.1016/j.cej.2013.05.091
40. Manzano, M., Vallet-Regi, M.: Revising bioceramics: bone regenerative and local drug delivery systems. Prog. Solid State Chem. **40**, 17–30 (2012). doi:10.1016/j.progsolidstchem.2012.05.001
41. Provenzano, M.J., Murphy, K.P.J., Riley, L.H.: Bone cements: review of their physiochemical and biochemical properties in percutaneous vertebroplasty. Am. J. Neuroradiol. **25**, 1286–1290 (2004)
42. Olalde, B., Garmendia, N., Sáez-Martínez, V., et al.: Multifunctional bioactive glass scaffolds coated with layers of poly(d, l-lactide-co-glycolide) and poly(n-isopropylacrylamide-co-acrylic acid) microgels loaded with vancomycin. Mater. Sci. Eng. C **33**, 3760–3767 (2013). doi:10.1016/j.msec.2013.05.002
43. Li, W., Ding, Y., Rai, R., et al.: Preparation and characterization of PHBV microsphere/45S5 bioactive glass composite scaffolds with vancomycin releasing function. Mater. Sci. Eng. C **41**, 320–328 (2014). doi:10.1016/j.msec.2014.04.052
44. Li, W., Nooeaid, P., Roether, J.A., et al.: Preparation and characterization of vancomycin releasing PHBV coated 45S5 Bioglass??-based glass-ceramic scaffolds for bone tissue engineering. J. Eur. Ceram. Soc. **34**, 505–514 (2014). doi:10.1016/j.jeurceramsoc.2013.08.032
45. Cui, X., Gu, Y., Li, L., et al.: In vitro bioactivity, cytocompatibility, and antibiotic release profile of gentamicin sulfate-loaded borate bioactive glass/chitosan composites. J. Mater. Sci. Mater. Med. **24**, 2391–2403 (2013). doi:10.1007/s10856-013-4996-0
46. Ding, H., Zhao, C.J., Cui, X., et al.: A novel injectable borate bioactive glass cement as an antibiotic delivery vehicle for treating osteomyelitis. PLoS ONE **9**, 1–9 (2014). doi:10.1371/journal.pone.0085472
47. Hong, K.S., Kim, E.C., Bang, S.H., et al.: Bone regeneration by bioactive hybrid membrane containing FGF2 within rat calvarium. J. Biomed. Mater. Res., Part A **94**, 1187–1194 (2010). doi:10.1002/jbm.a.32799
48. Rivadeneira, J., et al.: Novel antibacterial bioactive glass nanocomposite functionalized wuth tetracycline hydrochloride. Biomed. Glasses **1**, 128–135 (2015). doi:10.1515/bglass-2015-0012
49. Patel, K.D., El-Fiqi, A., Lee, H.-Y., et al.: Chitosan–nanobioactive glass electrophoretic coatings with bone regenerative and drug delivering potential. J. Mater. Chem. **22**, 24945–24956 (2012). doi:10.1039/c2jm33830k
50. Ordikhani, F., Simchi, A.: Long-term antibiotic delivery by chitosan-based composite coatings with bone regenerative potential. Appl. Surf. Sci. **317**, 56–66 (2014). doi:10.1016/j.apsusc.2014.07.197
51. Pishbin, F., Mouriño, V., Flor, S., et al.: Electrophoretic deposition of gentamicin-loaded bioactive glass/chitosan composite coatings for orthopaedic implants. ACS Appl. Mater. Interfaces **6**, 8796–8806 (2014). doi:10.1021/am5014166
52. Kresge, C.T., Leonowicz, M.E., Roth, W.J., et al.: Ordered mesoporous molecular sieves synthesized by a liquid-crystal template mechanism. Nature **359**, 710–712 (1992)
53. Yan, X., Yu, C., Zhou, X., et al.: Highly ordered mesoporous bioactive glasses with superior in vitro bone-forming bioactivities. Angew. Chem. Int. Ed. **43**, 5980–5984 (2004). doi:10.1002/anie.200460598
54. Yan, X., Huang, X., Yu, C., et al.: The in-vitro bioactivity of mesoporous bioactive glasses. Biomaterials **27**, 3396–3403 (2006). doi:10.1016/j.biomaterials.2006.01.043

55. Haro Durand, L.A., Góngora, A., Porto López, J.M., et al.: In vitro endothelial cell response to ionic dissolution products from boron-doped bioactive glass in the SiO_2–CaO–P_2O_5–Na_2O system. J. Mater. Chem. B **2**, 7620–7630 (2014). doi:10.1039/C4TB01043D
56. Hoppe, A., Güldal, N.S., Boccaccini, A.R.: Biomaterials A review of the biological response to ionic dissolution products from bioactive glasses and glass-ceramics. Biomaterials **32**, 2757–2774 (2011). doi:10.1016/j.biomaterials.2011.01.004
57. Zhang, Y., Wei, L., Chang, J., et al.: Strontium-incorporated mesoporous bioactive glass scaffolds stimulating in vitro proliferation and differentiation of bone marrow stromal cells and in vivo regeneration of osteoporotic bone defects. J. Mater. Chem. B **1**, 5711 (2013). doi:10.1039/c3tb21047b
58. Mendes, L.S., Saska, S., Martines, M.A.U., Marchetto, R.: Nanostructured materials based on mesoporous silica and mesoporous silica/apatite as osteogenic growth peptide carriers. Mater. Sci. Eng. C Mater. Biol. Appl. **33**, 4427–4434 (2013). doi:10.1016/j.msec.2013.06.040
59. Li, X., Chen, X., Miao, G., et al.: Synthesis of radial mesoporous bioactive glass particles to deliver osteoactivin gene. J. Mater. Chem. B **2**, 7045–7054 (2014). doi:10.1039/C4TB00883A
60. Wu, C., Fan, W., Chang, J., Xiao, Y.: Mesoporous bioactive glass scaffolds for efficient delivery of vascular endothelial growth factor. J. Biomater. Appl. **28**, 367–374 (2013). doi:10.1177/0885328212453635
61. Wu, C., Zhou, Y., Chang, J., Xiao, Y.: Delivery of dimethyloxallyl glycine in mesoporous bioactive glass scaffolds to improve angiogenesis and osteogenesis of human bone marrow stromal cells. Acta Biomater. **9**, 9159–9168 (2013). doi:10.1016/j.actbio.2013.06.026
62. Perez, R., El-Fiqi, A., Park, J.-H., et al.: Therapeutic bioactive microcarriers: co-delivery of growth factors and stem cells for bone tissue engineering. Acta Biomater. **10**, 520–530 (2014). doi:10.1016/j.actbio.2013.09.042
63. Zeng, Q., Han, Y., Li, H., Chang, J.: Bioglass/alginate composite hydrogel beads as cell carriers for bone regeneration. J. Biomed. Mater. Res. Part B Appl. Biomater. **102**, 42–51 (2014). doi:10.1002/jbm.b.32978
64. Wu, C., Fan, W., Chang, J.: Functional mesoporous bioactive glass nanospheres: synthesis, high loading efficiency, controllable delivery of doxorubicin and inhibitory effect on bone cancer cells. J. Mater. Chem. B **1**, 2710 (2013). doi:10.1039/c3tb20275e
65. Zhang, J., Zhao, S., Zhu, M., et al.: 3D-printed magnetic Fe 3 O 4/MBG/PCL composite scaffolds with multifunctionality of bone regeneration, local anticancer drug delivery and hyperthermia. J. Mater. Chem. B **2**, 7583–7595 (2014). doi:10.1039/C4TB01063A
66. Lin, H.-M., Lin, H.-Y., Chan, M.-H.: Preparation, characterization, and in vitro evaluation of folate-modified mesoporous bioactive glass for targeted anticancer drug carriers. J. Mater. Chem. B **1**, 6147 (2013). doi:10.1039/c3tb20867b
67. Mouriño, V., Newby, P., Pishbin, F., et al.: Physicochemical, biological and drug-release properties of gallium crosslinked alginate/nanoparticulate bioactive glass composite films. Soft Matter **7**, 6705 (2011). doi:10.1039/c1sm05331k
68. Chengtie, Wu, Chang, Jiang, Fan, Wei: Bioactive mesoporous calcium-silicate nanoparticles with excellent mineralization ability, osteostimulation, drug-delivery and antibacterial properties for filling apex roots of teeth. J. Mater. Chem. **22**, 16801–16809 (2012). doi:10.1039/c2jm33387b
69. Miola, M., Vitale-Brovarone, C., Mattu, C., Verné, E.: Antibiotic loading on bioactive glasses and glass-ceramics: an approach to surface modification. J. Biomater. Appl. **28**, 308–319 (2013). doi:10.1177/0885328212447665
70. Ehlert, N., Badar, M., Christel, A., et al.: Mesoporous silica coatings for controlled release of the antibiotic ciprofloxacin from implants. J. Mater. Chem. **21**, 752 (2011). doi:10.1039/c0jm01487g
71. Mabrouk, M., Mostafa, A.A., Oudadesse, H., et al.: Effect of ciprofloxacin incorporation in PVA and PVA bioactive glass composite scaffolds. Ceram. Int. **40**, 4833–4845 (2014). doi:10.1016/j.ceramint.2013.09.033

72. Liu, X., Xie, Z., Zhang, C., et al.: Bioactive borate glass scaffolds: in vitro and in vivo evaluation for use as a drug delivery system in the treatment of bone infection. J. Mater. Sci. Mater. Med. **21**, 575–582 (2010). doi:10.1007/s10856-009-3897-8
73. Jia, W.T., Zhang, X., Luo, S.H., et al.: Novel borate glass/chitosan composite as a delivery vehicle for teicoplanin in the treatment of chronic osteomyelitis. Acta Biomater. **6**, 812–819 (2010). doi:10.1016/j.actbio.2009.09.011
74. Zhang, X., Jia, W., Gu, Y., et al.: Teicoplanin-loaded borate bioactive glass implants for treating chronic bone infection in a rabbit tibia osteomyelitis model. Biomaterials **31**, 5865–5874 (2010). doi:10.1016/j.biomaterials.2010.04.005
75. Xie, Z., Cui, X., Zhao, C., et al.: Gentamicin-loaded borate bioactive glass eradicates osteomyelitis due to Escherichia coli in a rabbit model. Antimicrob. Agents Chemother. **57**, 3293–3298 (2013). doi:10.1128/AAC.00284-13

Future Applications of Bioglass

Vidya Krishnan

1 Introduction

Summing up the applications of Bioglass[1], its versatility and lack of adverse effects have been proved, but studies are still underway for its more prospective applications more so with clinical usages.

Due to painful multiple surgeries and less graft supply, autologous replacements are getting replaced by synthetic biocompatible materials. Immunological issues deterred allografts and xenografts. Thus silica based bioactive materials have become vital in replacement and augmentation of hard and soft tissues. The most initial and successful trials of bioceramics had been as replacement material, due to its most important advantage of being osteogenic. This has received tremendous results in orthopaedic and dental applications. This unique biocompatibility is due to the biologically active hydroxyapatite layer formed by the bioglass in the interface of itself and the human tissue. Latest research accepts that HCA (Hydroxy carbonate apatite) layer, to be important, but the more crucial is the ionic dissolution which may be the trigger to activate the gene responsible for the osteoprogenitor cells to cause bone regeneration.

Production of bioglass can be of conventional melt derived or of Sol–Gel technique. Either way they posess the same qualities of reaction, of HCA layer

This Chapter is dedicated to my husband S. Shanmugham, for being everything to me, and My children Sharan Vidash and Mithil Vidash for giving purpose to my deeds.

[1]Please consult the Editor's note in order to clarify the usage of the terms bioglass, bioactive glass and biocompatible glasses

V. Krishnan (✉)
Department of Oral Medicine and Radiology, SRM Kattankulathur
Dental College and Hospitals, Chennai, India
e-mail: vidyashanmugam@yahoo.com

J. Marchi (ed.), *Biocompatible Glasses*, Advanced Structured Materials 53,
DOI 10.1007/978-3-319-44249-5_13

formation–dissolution and ion release–cellular reactions–gene expression–activation of osteo progenitor cell-accelerated bone formation. In Sol gel derived bioglass, more surface and composition area, increased soluble silica, easier doping of chemicals maybe advantageous compared to the traditional melt and quench method derived bioglass. Sol–gel derived bioglass—58S nanopowders have been synthesized and investigated by immersion of bioglass powder discs in simulated body fluids. The SEM and XRD patterns proved formation of hydroxyapatite, and presence of silicate bonds. With aging time carbonates decreased. TEM pictures showed an increase of grain sizes with aging time from 50 to 200 nm. pH value increased consistently for the first 7 days in simulated body fluid confirming the possibility of accelerated reactions, in turn improving bioactivity [1].

The Bioglass can be made user specific depending on their composition, morphology, and inclusion of doping elements, like fluorine, magnesium, strontium, iron, silver, boron, potassium or zinc [2]. Their uses include replacement of large bone defects, regeneration of vascularized bone, coating of orthopedic and dental implants, healing of wounds, delivery of drugs and repairing of soft tissue [3]. Trials are on for the replacement of vertebrae, ear, nose, head and neck region and complete tooth root [4].

Strontium doping of bioactive glass enhances osteogenesis. When calcium was substituted [5] completely by strontium, in bioglass, their in vitro effect on osteoblast was anabolic, on osteoclast it was anti-catabolic. Osteoclast inhibition was due to decreased acid phosphatase and calcium phosphate. Osteoblasts had showed increased alkaline phosphatise activity. Along with bioglass's controlled delivery, strontium substituted bioglass would be making a mark in bone regeneration.

2 Bone Tissue Engineering and Regenerative Medicine

In order to overcome restrictions associated with autologous grafts, alloplastic materials were used. Local infection following membrane exposure hindered bone formation, and along with adverse immune responses and increased incidence of disease transmission reduced the widespread usage of these grafts.

Thus biomaterials became the choice in regenerative medicine. When using bioengineered materials, optimization like combining bioceramics with biodegradable polymers became significant. Commonly used biomaterials were calcium phosphates, Hydroxyapatite (HA), bioactive glasses, and modified composite materials. Bioglass react with living tissue, releasing soluble ions such as Si, Ca, P and Na ions. These ions at critical concentrations, trigger gene expression to induce osteoprogenior cells to promote rapid bone formation.

In Tissue engineering, biodegradable scaffolds impregnated with functional cells are of great use in restoring damaged tissue. This scaffold needed to be biocompatible as well as argumentive. The mimicking of this extracellular matrix was a huge hurdle in bone tissue engineering, which was overcome with scaffolds built with biocomposite nanofibres. These were porous naturally, facilitating excellent cell occupancy, increased blood supply along with easy movement of both nutrients and metabolic waste. This improved adherence of human foetal osteoblasts, which in turn migrated, proliferated and mineralized into bone.

Biomaterials have been used in bone tissue regeneration, exploiting its osteoinductive capacity. The electro spinning of a sol–gel derived material into nano sized fibers has shown excellent attachment, proliferation and differentiation into bone forming cells than melt driven nanofibers. Following this, filament bundles, membranes, adjunct with biopolymers, three dimensional scaffoldings are becoming viable futuristic regeneration material.

Conventionally melt driven bioglasses had been used as granule and whole forms, but nanofibers are able to act as bases and provide support mechanically. Adjunct with polymers, it helped in retaining the shape. Electro spinning makes it a cost effective process, in producing micro diameter fibers. This size minimizing makes way for the possibility for bioactive sensors, catalysts and membranes in the future. The osteogenic capacity of the cells grown on the nanofibers, were assessed by staining the cells for ALP (alkaline phosphatase) enzyme. It was significantly high when compared to bulk glasses. The improved osteogenicity was suggested to be because of increased surface area, abundant ion release and morphological roughness, proving nanofibres's superiority over bulk forms.

Nanofibers have good mechanical strength, osteogenic potential, versatility of being able to be made into bundles and compacting, nanofibre sheets can be compressed into 3D membranes. In hard tissue regeneration this nanocomposite with polymers are prospective [6].

Nanoscaled bioactive glass [7] along with gelatin and alginate dialdehyde in combination, provide exceptional bioactivity in the form of cell adhesion, proliferation, differentiation and prompt degradation. Covalent cross linking of alginate and gelatin helps in overcoming the few limitations.

2.1 *Prospective Improvisations*

Main issues to be improved on scaffolds are

- Mechanical strength
- Controlled degradation
- Vascularization
- Function
- Sterilization

2.2 Mechanical Strength

As far as mechanical properties of porous glass composites or polymer composites are concerned, they are weaker than cancellous bone, nevertheless lots more weaker than cortical bone. Reasons for this maybe due to

- Microstructural properties
- Inadequate particle–matrix bonding
- These are best tackled by addition of bioglass as fillers in polymer composite scaffolds. Studies highlighting the interrelation between the morphology of composites, their pore size, distribution, orientation, inter connection affecting the mechanical integrity of the composites are required. Strengthening of composites is best achieved by improving the quality of bonding in the interface of filler and matrix for load bearing and uniform distribution of particles in the matrix.

2.3 Vascularity

In synthetic grafts, absence of innate vascularity proves to be a great disadvantage. So the scaffold should possess good topographical, mechanical and biological properties to regenerate huge bone defects as well as tolerate heavy loads. To improve and accelerate these qualities, growth factors in the form of active biomolecules can be incorporated into the scaffolds. But, possible toxicity due to quick disintegration and uncontrolled release of factors restricts this method. May be using bioglass as filler, to induce the controlled expression of markers (ALP), to accelerate osteogenesis could be an alternative.

2.4 Function

Surface modification helps enhance function of the scaffold. Scaffolds which are more compatible, with provision of functional groups to increase improved cell attachment are necessary. This provision of incorporating functional groups is made possible through controlling of specific and non specific protein adsorption, enzyme grafting or plasma treatment.

More light needs to be thrown on biodegradation, angiogenic stimuli and on, ion release mechanisms.

2.5 Ion Release

The ionic dissolution products of bioglass i.e., soluble calcium and silica ions are critical in causing bone formation by way of gene expression in inducing osteo progenitor cells. These osteogenic cells in turn, cause osteoblast differentiation and proliferation. The proposed mechanisms by which gene expression maybe triggered are by

- Surface interaction.
- Topography.
- Quantity and quality of dissolution ions released.
- Shear stress at interface [8].

The concentration and composition of bioglass at which the ions maybe released, needs to be quantitatively analysed.

2.6 Sterilization

The effect of sterilization of these systems on the physical characteristics viz crystallinity and glass transition temperature, mechanical characteristics like fracture toughness and compressive strength, and its cellular toxicity need to be critically evaluated. It is of greater importance in systems with biopolymers. Along with optimizing of scaffold designs, importance for sterilization is due, as conventional sterilizing techniques of exposure to ethylene oxide gas, gamma radiation etc. have proved that the polymers lose a molecular weight factor of 2–3.

More in vivo studies are mandatory to evidence the potential of these scaffolds. Scaffolds made of amorphous silicate or partially crystallised systems along with biodegradable polymers maybe widely used with further improvisations. Stem cell incorporation into these scaffolds maybe of greater value. Bioresorbable polymers with bioglass, nanoparticles of glass ceramics and carbon nanotubes may be of value addition for increased cellular attachment and proliferation, improving angiogenic and osteogenic potential of the scaffold. Toxicity related to carbon nanotubes and nanoparticles needs to be further investigated [2].

Polymer scaffolds are going to be a stay in tissue engineering. Biological polymers are better compared to synthetic polymers. These scaffolds can be made to control the biological system both physically and chemically. Though lot of improvements, have been done related to their porosity, biological activity and mechanical properties, more limitations need to be eliminated. Futuristic changes, need to concentrate on fabricating scaffolds with importance given to mechanical properties, surface topography, assembling the polymer, structure-both macro and nano, cell function, compatibility, degradation and induction to produce natural tissue [9].

Nanoparticles of Bioactive glass with gelatin, in scaffolds is one another on-trial investigation. The in vitro properties and bone forming ability on rabbit ulna bone, was evaluated using Fourier infrared spectroscopy, SEM, X-Ray diffraction analysis. No cytotoxicity was reported. Bone formation was adequate [10].

Lanthanides doped bioglass has shown improved cell adhesion, proliferation indicating sufficient bioactivity. This study synthesized the new $10CaF_2$-$10Na_2CO_3$–15CaO–$59P_2O_5$–$5SiO_2$ glass doped with lanthanum oxide and cerium. Morphology being smooth, glassy with absence of contamination and increased biological behaviour makes it a, prospective applicant in bone tissue engineering [11].

3 Angiogenesis

Maintaining of Skeletal integrity depends on the interconnection between the blood vessels and osteo cells. The high vascularity of the bone needs to be preserved for healing and regeneration. To overcome the disadvantage of lack of innate vascular supply in artificial templates, pre vascularized scaffolds in vitro have been tried. Alternates, are to have bioglass with controlled release of genes to stimulate in vivo osteogenesis and angiogenesis.

Very few studies have focused on the angiogenic potential of bioglass. Of these studies, bioglass when used as fillers showed promising angiogenic characteristics, when compared to scaffolds of polymer without bioglass fillers. There was more tissue infiltration and forming of blood vessels [12]. Interestingly, physical morphology such as size, orientation of pores, their interconnectivity also seem to influence the blood vessel forming ability of the scaffolds.

This hypothesis that geometry and morphology of scaffold being significant, has been supported and confirmed by an in vivo study using 45S5 bioglass impregnated collagen sponges in rats to treat calvarial defects. Bioglass has been seen to promote vascularization [12–14].

Composite structures like microspheres and foams are lesser angiogenic, than impregnated sponges, meshes, tubes and porous scaffolds. However in vivo and in vitro results are not synchronized. Further clarifications needs to be carried out [2].

Studies have proved dose dependant influence of bioglass on stimulation of fibroblasts to secrete angiogenic growth factors, endothelial cell proliferation and endothelial tubule formation.

In Indian medicine system of siddha, Alum or potash alum ($KAl(SO_4)_2 \cdot 12(H_2O)$) has been widely used as an antimicrobial and a haemostat in wound healing [13, 15]. The astringent effect of alum in combination with nano sized bioglass of 100 nm seems to have a synergistic effect on angiogenesis [16]. The study had tried bioglass doped with alum and only bioglass. Cell viability on Osteoblast cell line was 50–60 % [17].

Surface area, abundant silanol group and soluble silica seem to be the cause for increased osteogenesis [18].

The artificial scaffolds must have the capability to trigger formation of mature blood vessels, capable of differentiating into arteries and veins, thus promoting functional ability of the scaffold. Bioglass, in appropriate levels when used as fillers in scaffolds has the potency to regulate the release of growth factors required for this differentiation to improve angiogenesis. This enhances vascularization in the man-made graft and subsequently prevents failure [2].

4 Stimulation and Interaction with Human Mesenchymal Stem Cells

Certain studies have concluded that bone marrow cells can be provoked to form bone in presence of bioglasses. Following this, submicron bioglasses have been synthesized. Their cellular activity, effect on human mesenchymal cells, related to cellular viability, proliferative capability, osteogenic potential and cytotoxicity were evaluated. There was no cytotoxicity in any of the concentrations of bioglass in 1–4 days. A decrease in the cell proliferation and metabolic activity of mesenchymal cells, were noted after 7 days. Cell cytoplasm and endosomes were localised with bioglass. This attribute of localization can help in using bioglass as injectables, and also possible incorporation into porous polymer scaffolds. Sol–gel process produced bioglass, was more porous with additional surface area, increasing the solubility and bioactivity.

The reason for dissolution of bioglass inside the endosomes, seem to raise the silica and calcium levels. These levels could cause the cytotoxicity, decreased metabolism and response to inflammation. The concentration of 150 and 200 umg/ml showed decreased metabolic activity, making them useful in regeneration [19].

5 Cytotoxicity of Silica, for Prospective Use in Cancer

Nanoparticles enter systems and cells through different mechanisms. Detailed understanding of these mechanisms help us to design and modulate these areas for inter cellular imaging, diagnostic accuracy and other treatment modalities.

The nanoparticles enter cells through endocytosis [20]. Specifically pinocytosis, through its four mechanisms viz macropinocytosis, clathrin-mediated endocytosis, caveolae- mediated endocytosis, and clathrin-caveolae and dynamin-independent endocytosis [21]. Depending on the surface charge it can be specific or non specific cellular uptake. Size, shape and surface charge determine the non specific uptake of nanoparticles.

Crystalline silica (Min-u-sil 5) being the control, SiO_2nanoparticles of size 15 and 46 nm were analysed for 48 h in the dosage of 10 and 100 μg/ml on bronchoalveolar carcinoma-derived cells. SiO_2 was seen to be more cytotoxic, with reduced cell viability.

Indicators for oxidative stress and cytotoxicity viz total reactive oxidative species (ROS), glutathione (GSH), malondialdehyde (MDA) lactate dehydrogenase (LDH) were assessed. SiO_2 showed increase of ROS, and decrease of glutathione.

15 nm SiO_2 exposure produces oxidative stress in cells as exhibited by the decrease in GSH levels and increase of MDA and LDH suggestive of lipid peroxidation and membrane damage. The ROS generation is not clear. Crystalline silica has been evidenced to produce ROS, like hydroxyl free radical by fenton reaction on silica's surface. Crystalline silica's content of metal impurities maybe the evidenced cause, but on the contrary SiO_2 nanoparticles contain ultra low levels of metal impurities.

The cell viability decrease maybe from the penetration of particles into nucleus of cells. Protein aggregation and topoisomerase 1 inhibits replication, transcription and cell proliferation.

Genes also seem to be sensitive to ROS during transcription. The genes affected are MAP Kinase signaling, DNA damage, cAmp/Ca^{2+} signaling, NFKB signaling, P13-AKT signaling and apoptosis [22, 23]. Studies are underway for the signaling pathways in which these genes are expressed, on exposure to SiO_2 nanoparticles.

This shows the dose dependant and time dependant effect of 15 nm and 46 nm SiO_2 nanoparticles in dosages of 10–100 μg/ml on cell viability of bronchoalveolar carcinoma-derived cells [24].

When the biomaterials act at the cellular levels, their therapeutic value increases manifold. Hydroxy nanoparticles in specific sizes exert cell toxicity and apoptosis in cancer cells. Study on Human hepatoma cells have displayed significant results in the particle cell size range of 20–80 nm, promising hydroxyl apatite nano particles based, therapeutic systems. These nanoparticles activated caspase-3 and 9, increased Bax and Bid levels and decreased Bcl-2 protein. Cytochrome c got released into cytoplasm from mitochondria.

These cellular changes and internal localization, maybe largely responsible for the apoptosis protein levels and cellular toxicity in HepG2 cells. The size of the hydroxyl apatite was found to be the crux for this activity. The most efficient size being from 45 nm. There was efficacy decline in the sequence of 45 nm > 26 nm > 78 nm > 175 nm. The size efficacy needs to be further evaluated [25].

The changes in the efficacy related to particle size, raised interest in studies to further investigate whether shape of the particles, in any way affected the cellular function. Shape of the nanoparticles seems to affect the systemic distribution. Magnetic worm shaped nanoparticles, improved imaging and targeting of tumors in vivo, for better therapeutic delivery in view of their multipoint attachment, longer half lie in blood and increased surface area [26].

Mesoporous silica are proven agents for medical applications in lieu of their better surface area, uniform pores with increased volume, in vivo degradation and unique biocompatibility [27]. Therapeutic agent carrying has been already proved.

Non spherical nanoparticles, specifically rod shaped mesoporous nanoparticles have demonstrated great promise in cell monitoring, metastatis of cancer cells, DNA or drug delivery [28].

Particles of same size, composition and surface charge, but three various shaped mesoporous silica nanoparticles with aspect ratio of 1, 2, and 4 were chosen to be studied on A375 human melanoma cells.. Results showed larger ARs were absorbed in higher amounts and had increased rate of internalization. The particles had greater effect on cell functions like proliferation, migration, cytotoxicity, adhesion and cytoskeleton production. Thus inferring that biomaterials need to be viewed not only as drug carriers, but also as efficient therapeutic systems to mediate and modulate biological functions, by way of engaging molecular processes. The environmental fate of nanoparticles have to be evaluated [29].

Glass ceramics doped with Mg ferrite, to form Wollastonite-flouroapatite containing glass-ceramics. Improved adherence of osteoblast like ROS 17/2.8 cells, makes this material possible to be used as thermoseeds in hyperthermia [30].

Ferrimagnetic $ZnFe_2O_4$ containing glass ceramics are bioactive and useful in treating hyperthermia [31]. Reason may be the way the cations are dispersed. Rapid cooling and effects of $ZnFe_2O_4$ caused haphazard distribution of cations Zn^{2+} and Fe^{3+}.

Bioglass has been evaluated in therapeutics of irradiated tissues. Irradiation induced osteoporosis in rat models were in vitro assessed on osteoblast cells using curcumin covered chitosan-bioglass. The rats were exposed to CO gamma rays, then grafted with CUR-BG-CH. After 3 days of exposure to bioglass, viability of cells improved by 164 %. Activated partial thromboplastin time and prothrombin time were seen to be prolonged. Pyridinoline to dihydroxylsinonorleucine cross links ratio were normal. An increase of superoxide dismutase, catalase, Glutathione Peroxidase and decrease of thiobarbituric acid-reactive substance in oxidative stress analysis was significant in CUR-BG-CH group. The treatment with CUR-BG-CH increased Young's modulus and femoral stiffness. Callus formation and highest anticoagulant effect were significant findings. This study opens therapeutic avenues, for bioglass especially in osteoporosis [32].

6 Dental Applications

Collagen fibrils are the building blocks in the chemical reaction of bioglass with bone, connective tissue and tubules in dentin. Basically made of layered fibrils of protein-amino acids viz glycine, proline, hydroxyproline and arginine. The microfibrils are interlinked with each other by literal crystalline bonds. Glycine being a small protein without side chains, plays a very important role in the collagen structure being able to get arranged in many forms.

Aggregates of collagen or fibrils get stacked in multiple forms, the arrangement unique to each tissue. In bone, triple helices are arranged parallel to each other, with nucleation points in bone allowing HA crystals to fill in the ends of tropocollagen subunits. Crack filling and subsequent bone toughening is obvious [33].

Dentin forms the base matrix framework for support of enamel. Dentin is formed by proteins like phosphoproteins, proteoglycans, phospholipids and 90 % fibrous collagen [33].

6.1 Graft Material [12, 13]

As is already known, synthetic bone grafting especially bioactive glass overcedes open debridement in periodontal osseous defects and intrabony defects. Extraordinary tissue response was elicited. Bone support is vital for dental treatment modalities be it prostheses fabrication or implant placements. Trials for improving the bone height by raising the schneiderian membrane, in posterior maxilla along with graft material placement to stimulate bone regeneration is being carried out.

One such study, a single step surgery has been tried successfully, using adipose tissue as the graft, source for mesenchymal stem cells. Trials need to be carried out using bioglass as the scaffold, for better adherence of stem cells, proliferation and differentiation of osteo progenitor cells. Proper addition of growth factors like BMP-2 of 10 ng/ml with short incubation would evade the dose dependant complications [34].

6.2 Endosseous Implants

In post dental extraction, loss of stimulation to the alveolar bone, and pressure caused by dentures increase bone resorption. This rate of resorption varies from individual to individual and also at varying degrees in the same individual.

Augmentation modes have been many, after autogenous bone grafting, natural root replantation faced failure due its resorption, pocket formation and ankylosis.

Dehiscence was the problem when bio ceramics was used to augment. Thus, then cone shaped Bioglass was tried with success as endosseous implants, Bioglass ankylosed with direct deposition of graded mineralized bone reducing from outward to inward, providing periodontal ligament like mechanical compliance [35–39].

Titanium dental implants are in use for replacement prostheses in dentistry, for quite sometime now. The titanium implant when coated with an osteoinductive material like bioglass should be favourable in providing mechanical compliance. Such a study was conducted to compare titanium alloy (Ti6Al4v) human jaw bone implants, coated with bioglass and Hydroxyapatite. Bioglass particle size used were 0.2–20 um, and HA size was 0.1–10 um. Cytotoxicity was nil for both. An uneventful healing period was noted for both kinds of implants. A 6 month postoperative follow up was carried out. Radiographic assessment showed good bone formation in both implants. Periodontal status remained same.

The failed HA coated implants showed resorption of the HA coating on entire surface with mobility of tooth, but no bioglass coated implant showed resorption of bioglass. In case of bioglass coated implant, the alkaline environment created by the dissolution ions along with the germicidal effect maybe the reason for non resorption and nil infection. On the contrary, the acidic medium would be the reason for resorption and infection. Concluding that bioglass would be a better choice in case of dental implants [40].

6.3 Demineralizing Agent

Bioglass incorporated in oral dentrifices replacing abrasive silica part proved to be an excellent vehicle in treatment of dentinal hypersensitivity [41]. Bioactive glass S53P4 in comparison to commercial glass released more silica treating dentinal hypersensitivity better [42].

Melt driven Bioglass particles formed more adherent and continuous apatite layer with particle formation [43]. Bioerodible gel films in delivery of remineralizing agents have been proved to be useful [44].

In vitro studies, for the desensitizer's efficiency in varied oral environment was carried out. 1 min exposure to bioglass, followed by 30 s water rinse proved rapid and continuous dentin dentrifice occlusion. More than 3 % concentration as single application either as dentrifice or prophylactic paste closed 75 % dentinal tubules. A 95 % closure in many cases was also noted [45]. Single applications were able to resist the regular acid challenges. On repeated use, continuous and persistent blockage was present even in the presence of repeated acid attacks [46]. Clinical studies have proved the greater efficiency with which bioglass eases hypersensitivity within the 6 week point, on comparison with other products [47–49].

6.4 Antibacterial Activity

Bioglass in aqueous environment causes osseointegration. Has caused considerable decrease in antibacterial viability, proving to be a good antibacterial agent, because of its alkaline nature [50].

6.5 Periodontal Tissue Engineering

Ions especially Li ions help in being mood stabilizers, used in bipolar depressive disorders. These ions promote remyelination of neural cells. Proliferation of neural progenitor cells and retinoblastoma cells are stimulated via the wnt/β-catenin signaling pathway.

Subsequently this has been verified on human periodontal ligament-derived cells. Li ions on mesoporous bioglass scaffolds had caused differentiation of cementum, through activation of wnt/β-catenin signalling pathway. The Li-mesoporous Bioglass scaffolds need to be having huge and (300–500 mm), and orderly placed mesopores (5 nm). The scaffolds had Li ions replacing part of calcium ions. These Li ions released from the bioactive scaffold act via wnt and SHH signalling pathway in stimulating proliferation and differentiation of cementum from human periodontal ligament-derived cells [51].

6.6 Bioglass in Glass Ionomer Cement

Conventional GIC, with modifications can be of multidisiplinary use. In its conventional form, it is a fluoroaluminasilicate powder-inorganic glass particles in calcium aluminium hydrogel matrix. The release of aluminium ions causing restriction of bone mineralization and neurotoxicity limited the GIC's use in repair of skull defects and cerebrospinal fluid fistulas. Kamitakahara et al. [52] modified glass ionomer without aluminium, adding polyacrylic acid and water, but this cement was not bioactive. Removal of aluminium, reducing size of particles, doping with strontium, compositional increase of SiO_2 were tried. Later, GIC from iron oxide powder containing Fe_2O_3 to the minimum of at least 10 % were made, but again trivalent cations had to be used for the setting.

The later bioactive compositions, contained 49–54 % SiO_2, P_2O_5-1.5 %, CaO-7–10 %, SrO-8–19 %, Na_2-0–7 %, ZnO-3 % and MgO-10–20 %. Trivalent cations were substituted with divalent cations like Sr^{2+}, Zn^{2+}, Mg^{2+}. Since Mg ions may reduce bioactivity [53], compositions of polyacid and free from trivalent cations and Mg ions were produced.

The novel bioglass, which was produced contained SiO_2 42–62, Na_2O 20–29, CaO 11–28, P_2O_5 Oz-5–5.5, in molar percentages, with preference of sodium oxide and calcium oxide to be minimum of 35 mol% to the total amount. Strontium could replace calcium oxide in 1–.13.5 molar percent to a maximum of up to 50 mol%. Optimum particle size of 45 μm or lesser, these submicron levels are best achieved by bar milling, then deposited into deionised water. Preferred polymer is polyacrylic acid, with setting modifier like Maleic acid, itaconic acid or phosphoric acid to extend working time.

Value addition by addition of antibiotics, bioactive molecules like proteins or chlorhexidine. With respect to the changes the GIC can be put to use in drug delivery. This new cement is made available as two parts kit of bioactive glass and polyacid. Also made available as pre set GIC in granule form and moulded shapes like spheres, blocks and customised shapes. These different forms of bioglass can be put to u e in otology, bone repair to stop CSF leak, bone stimulation in periodontal conditions, filling of bone sockets and bony defects, orthopaedic bone graft substitutes, osteoporotic vertebrae reinforcement, application on devices to promote bone integration. Structural stability was excellent thus justifying the novel GIC-bioglass's multifaceted use [54].

7 Gene Therapy Applications

In Nanotechnology, carriers to deliver genes could possibly help in curing brain pathologies, modulate its regeneration and healing capabilities. There are specific regions in the adult brain, with the capacity for neurogenesis. Subventricular zone of the lateral ventricle is one of them, containing stem cells capable of slow division and able to produce progenitor cells. These progenitor cells can produce astrocytes, neurons or oligodendrocytes when stimulated from this state. For the induction of cell differentiation in these multipotent neural stem cells, accumulation in nucleus of FGFR1 (FGFreceptor type 1) is needed. This FGFR1 accumulation may be triggered by an stimuli, c AMP, or bone morphogenetic protein 7. These stem cells, have been proved to be evoked by inoculating with FGF2 protein or adenovirus expressing FGF2 in vitro.

Subsequently, whether in vivo DNA transfer into the neural stem cells of sub ventricular zone using organically modified silica nanoparticles (ORMOSIL) would moderate mechanisms and modulate their function, was studied which can, in turn be used for therapeutics. In this study, mouse brain was intraventricularly injected with ORMOSIL. This non viral gene delivery, successfully moderated the replication cycle of the neural progenitor cells, with EGFP (Enhanced green fluorescent protein) expression proving that thereupeutic manipulation is possible and the stem cells can be controlled by the nuclear receptor. This can be a base for more work, regarding an efficient non viral transfection vector (ORMOSIL nanoparticles) into the CNS for future gene therapies [55].

One of the common bone diseases, yet no plausible cure has been found for this disease of osteoporosis. Emphasis has been more on bone resorption inhibition than on bone regeneration. But gene therapy could hold the key for its treatment.

The following study aims at initiation of bone regeneration in treating osteoporosis. When controlled and continuous release of growth factors, PDGF-b and BMP-7 is provided, it triggers mesenchymal progenitor cells. This may be a turning point in treatment of osteoporotic patients with fractures. The study aimed at, a trial of mesoporous bioglass/silk scaffolds incorporated with adPDGF-b and adBMP-7 into osteoporotic femur defects of ovariectomised rats [56]. Follow up treatment period was 2 and 4 weeks.

In vivo bone forming ability was analysed by immunohistochemical study for BSP, osteopontin and type 1 collagen, Haemotoxylin and eosin staining and U–CT analysis. Scaffolds containing adenovirus for both, proved more osteogenic than with only BMP-7, and scaffolds alone. BMP-7 already known for its osteogenic potential, when combined with PDGF, a strong chemotactant aids osteblastic differentiation. These scaffolds on TRAP-positive staining showed biodegradability allowing the bone to remodel. As these scaffolds degrades, the viral vectors get released to initiate mesenchymal progenitor cells of the surrounding area. This promises a cost-effective delivery system for growth factors in treating osteoporosis. Degradation is also advantageous in this system of delivery.

Another area of notice, is that concentrations of growth factors need to be maintained by the delivery systems for optimizing of bone regeneration. At low concentrations the response of oteoblastic proliferation and differentiation to growth factors is minimal.

Traditionally, ex vivo cell transfection by use of adenovirus and subsequent in vivo re implantation was done. Direct delivery by way of injecting adenovirus into bone defects are being adopted to avoid complications and for easy methodology.

8 Drug Delivery, Ionic Release via Phosphate Glass Vehicles

8.1 Drug Delivery

Any good drug delivery system should have biological compatibility, good mechanical strength, inert nature, patient comfortability, no risk of accidental release, ability to carry heavy doses of the drug, easy administration, removal, fabrication and sterilization.

The three basic mechanisms of delivery are diffusion, solvent activation or swelling and degradation.

Bioglass has earned its place in controlled drug delivery, especially when the drug needs to be site-specific, when speed of release should be pre planned, where conventional methods do not fit in. It has been an excellent drug carrier, with teicoplanin and vancomycin in treating osteomyelitis [57, 58]. Indomethacin has been tried as a self setting bioactive cement. Mixture hardens and forms hydroxyapatite [59].

Nanofibers, which are electrospun [60] exhibits more advantages, due to the ease with which the variables during fabrication could be controlled. The fiber's size, surface area, topography and morphology can be altered by changing these parameters. The optimum use of this effective method, is on fabrication of polymeric nanofibers. Nanofibers range their application from gene delivery, tissue engineering, dressing of wounds, immobilizing enzymes and as filters and sensors. For drug delivery, medicated nanofibers find use in infection prevention and abdominal adhesions after surgery in addition to in implants, wound covering and transdermal methods. Single or multiple polymers, Hybrids, blend of polymers and composites can also be electrospun.

Metal ions, play a pivotal role in angiogenesis closely linked to osteogenesis. Zinc has been showed to be important, in osteogenesis because of its presence in proteins. Other important ions are calcium, strontium, magne/sium, boron, titanium, phosphate and copper. Choice of delivery systems also affects the kind of response elicited from tissues. Study of these ions effect has showed significant effect on osteogenesis, with importance to the range of doses with best efficacies. The bioactive glasses with their P_2O_5 concentration hiked to 50–55 mol% have shown best efficiency as carrier vehicles for metal ion release which in turn stimulates bone formation [51, 61].

Beneficial results of S53P4 [62] has been reported in multiple areas such as treating osteomyelitis, benign bone tumour graft, procedures in the craniofacial region like mastoid, orbital floor reconstruction and spondylodesis. Whether the present PMMA beads with antibiotics, would be able to get replaced with S53P4 bioactive glass has to be further investigated.

9 Neurite Regeneration by Phosphate Glass Fibres

Peripheral nerve regeneration is promoted by bioactive scaffolds. Phosphate glass fibre scaffolds improved rate of axonal regrowth, but physical guidance limited [63].

10 Toxicity

Microparticles and nanoparticles toxicity needs further evaluation. Studies have shown cytotoxicity in 15 nm and 45 nm SiO_2 particles. A thorough study with all variables significantly involved is essential, as only size consideration would be misleading.

Studies of Fenoglio [64], showed that pure quartz and iron deprived quartz dust produce hydroxyl free radicals, even when iron is not present.

As already mentioned, genes are also affected by ROS during transcription. More emphasis is needed for the study of signaling pathways of gene expression, when exposed to SiO_2 nanoparticles. Thus the mode of ROS production should be studied further.

When new materials are investigated and tried out, the application possibilities are as important as their interactions with the co-materials they act with. More so with, when their applications are in the medical field. Bioglass with polymers, are becoming a trend now. In medical applications, PCL and PLLA are finding to be used as drug delivery for long terms [65], temporary implants [66], PLCL copolymers [67, 68] are proposed to be complementing PLLA and PCL.

A new study has shown the effect of bioglass on degradation of these polymers [69]. Thermogravimetric analysis was carried out for the way thermal degradation occurred in poly(ε-caprolactone) (PCL), poly(lactide/ε-caprolactone) (PLCL) and poly(L-lactide) (PLLA). It showed PCL to be have the highest thermal degradation resistance. Polyester's ester group and SiO group of bioglass react, causing an activation energy decrease of 1.3–1.9 fold compared to polymers without bioglass. Random chain breakage and increased absorbance of carboxylate peak of infra red spectra at 210 C has proved the reaction. DSC (differential scanning calorimetry) showed a significant decrease in thermal transitions of the polymers.

Polymers can be made to have thermal stability by traditional processes of extrusion or injection moulding. But, addition of bioglass changes the characteristics of these polymers. So, careful assessment of the degradation by-products is essential, especially at high processing temperatures. At a high temperature of processing above 200 C PLCL and PLLA with 15 vol% bioglass underwent thermal changes in molecular weight and mass, compared to the increased stability of PCL. Thus, processing by the present methods, may limit their applications in medicine. Trials are necessary to overcome these pitfalls.

11 Conclusion

Critically analyzing the options, bioactive glasses are better performing than other bio ceramics. But, hurdles to match autografts in terms of toughness, vascularization, controlled release of ions, porosity creation without crystallizing of commercially available bioglass, are a few to mention.

Now, the understanding that porous inter connectivity is related to fabrication and sintering without crystallization, many new methods have evolved. To fabricate scaffolds with large pores, high compressive strength mimicking bone pores, solid free form, gel-cast foaming and sol–gel foaming techniques have evolved. But, still these can be used only in areas of less load or where there is only compressive load. The surgeons, need for the material to be able to be pressed into the defect, able to be cut into desired shapes, able to share load with host bone are yet to be addressed [70].

To overcome a few of the mechanical characteristic problems, degradation rates, the solution may be in inorganic-organic hybrids. Present Polymers are excellent for sutures, but degradation criterias must be improved for mechanical properties. New polymers must be synthesized optimizing the present characters and improvising load bearing. Material designing can be augmented by imaging, porosity in non destructive methods like uCT imaging and subsequent analysis. X-Ray, Neutron diffraction, NMR, Particle-induced X-Ray emission (PIXE) [71] help in detailed study of atomic structure of bioglass as well as the new hybrids. The detail allows for evoking better cellular response. Tissue engineering studies should adopt phase I–Iv clinical trials conforming to ATMP Regulation 1394/200/EC along with/or FDA regulations, local policy and clinical protocols [34]. Screening of cell culture and new standardizing methods, ideal test materials and animal models have to be worked out. Commercial production of bioglass and hybrids should be made possible with help of Regulatory Boards and medical device companies.

In concise, the other hurdles to be overcome are

- To analyse the basic mechanisms in the nucleus of cell, to make the gene activation a reality.
- To ensure the performance of bioactive materials, to longer term with adequate mechanical strength.
- To pinpoint the stem cell differentiation, to the phenotypes and achieve precision to a level of preventing tumor origin.
- To scrutinize, soft tissue reaction mechanisms with approvals for clinical trials to make them possible into clinical products
- Long term load bearing applications with permanent sustainability in normal physiological environment
- To achieve vascularity, either in vivo or in pre implant constructs [72].

Thus, till we find answers for these questions, this wonderful concept is going to be in a trial and error phase. The potential and results are to be reaped with large leaps in terms of more trials with novel clinical products, by way of better understanding at molecular levels. Required statutory approvals by regulatory boards to accelerate more clinical applications to produce them commercially.

References

1. Joughehdoust, S., et al.: Synthesis and in vitro investigation of sol–gel derived bioglass-58S nanopowders. Mater. Sci. Pol. **30**(1), 45–52 (2012)
2. Lutz-Christian, G., et al.: Bioactive glass and glass-ceramic scaffolds for bone tissue engineering. Materials **3**, 3867–3910 (2010)
3. Wei, L., et al.: Bioactive glasses; traditional and prospective applications in healthcare. Hot Top. Biomater. 56–68 (2014)
4. Werner, V., et al.: The development of bioglass for medical applications. Angew Wandte Chem. Int. Ed. **26**(6), 527(1987)
5. Gentleman, E., et al.: The effects of strontium-substituted bioactive glasses on osteoblasts and osteoclasts in vitro. Biomaterials **31**(14), 3949–3956 (2010)
6. Kim, H.W., et al.: Production and potential of bioactive glass nanofibers as a next-generation biomaterial. Adv. Funct. Mater. **16**, 1529–1535 (2006)
7. Ulrike, R., et al.: In vitro and in vivo biocompatibility of alginate dialdehyde/gelatin hydrogels with and without nanoscaled bioactive glass for bone tissue engineering applications. Materials **7**, 1957–1974 (2014)
8. Jell, G., et al.: Gene activation by bioactive glasses. J. Mater. Sci. Mater. Med. **17**, 997–1002 (2006)
9. Brahatheeswaran, D.: Polymeric scaffolds in tissue engineering application. Int. J. Polym. Sci. Article ID 290602 (2011)
10. Hafezi, F., et al.: Transplantation of nano-bioglass/gelatin scaffold in a non-autogenous setting for bone regeneration in a rabbit ulna. J. Mater. Sci. Mater. Med. **23**, 2783–2792 (2012)
11. Joao, C., et al.: Development and characterization of lanthanides doped hydroxyapatite composites for bone tissue application. Curr. Trends Glass Ceram. Mater. 87–115 (2012)
12. Day, R.M., et al.: In vitro and in vivo analysis of macroporous biodegradable poly(D,L-lactide-co-glycolide) scaffolds containing bioactive glass. J. Biomed. Mater. Res. Part A **75**, 778–787 (2005)

13. Gorustovich, A., et al.: Effect of bioactive glasses on angiogenesis: in-vitro and in-vivo evidence. A review. Tissue Eng. Part B Rev. **16**, 199–207 (2010)
14. Day, R.M., et al.: Bioactive glass stimulates the secretion of angiogenic growth factors and angiogenesis in vitr. Tissue Eng. **11**, 768–777 (2005)
15. Pity, I.S., et al.: Aniogenesis, p 53 and Bcl2 in colorectal carcinoma. Int. J. Adv. Res. Technol. **2**(3), p.i (2013)
16. Wren, A.W., et al.: Fabrication of CaO-NaO-SiO_2/TiO_2 scaffolds for surgical applications. J. Mater. Sci. Mater. Med. **23**(12), 2881 (2012)
17. Durgalakshmi, D., et al.: Nano-bioglass: a versatile antidote for bone tissue engineering problems. Proc. Eng. **92**, 2–8 (2014)
18. Nowakowska, D., et al.: Dynamic oxido reductive potential of astringent retraction agents. Folia Biol. (Praha) **56**(6), 263 (2010)
19. Labbaf, S., et al.: Spherical bioactive glass particles and their interaction with human mesenchymal stem cells in vitro. Biomaterials **32**, 1010–1018 (2011)
20. Conner S.D. et al: Regulated portals of entry into the cell. Nature **422**(6927), 37–44 (2003)
21. Hild W.A., et al.: Quantum dots-nano-sized probes for the exploration of cellular and intracellular targeting. Eur. J. Pharm. Biopharm. **68**(2), 153–168 (2008)
22. Foncea, et al.: Endothelial cell oxidative stress and signal transduction. Biol. Res. **33**, 89–96 (2000)
23. Kharasch et al.: Gene expression profiling of nephrotoxicity from the sevoflurane degradation product fluoromethyl-2,2-difluoro-1(trifluoromethyl)vinyl ether("compound a") in rats. Toxicol. Sci. **90**, 419–431 (2006)
24. Lin, W.S., et al.: In Vitro toxicity of silica nanoparticles in human lung cancer cells. Toxicol. Appl. Pharmacol. **217**(3), 252–259 (2006)
25. Yuan, Y., et al.: Size-mediated cytotoxicity and apoptosis of hydroxyapatite nanoparticles in human hepatoma HepG2 cells. Biomaterials **09**, 088 (2009)
26. Park, J.H., et al.: Magnetic iron oxide nanoworms for tumor targeting and imaging. Adv. Mater. **20**(9), 1630.5 (2008)
27. Park, J.H., et al.: Biodegradable luminescent porous silicon nanoparticles for in vivo applications. Nat. Mater. **8**(4), 331–336 (2009)
28. Tsai, C.P., et al.: High contrast paramagnetic fluorescent mesoporous silica nanorods as a multifunctional cell-imaging probe. Small **4**(2), 186–191 (2008)
29. Huang, X. et al: The effect of the shape of mesoporous silica nanoparticles on cellular uptake and cell function. Biomaterials **31**(3), 438–48 (2009)
30. Guang, D.L., et al.: Synthesis and characterization of magnetic bioactive glass-ceramics containing Mg ferrite for hyperthermia. Mater. Sci. Eng. C **30**(1), 148–153 (2010)
31. Shah, S.A., et al.: Magnetic and bioactivity evaluation of ferromagnetic $ZnFe_2O_4$ containing glass ceramics for the hyperthermia treatment of cancer. J. Magn. Magn. Mater. (Impact Factor 2) **322**(3), 375–381 (2010)
32. Jebahi, S., et al.: Therapeutic potential of curcumin encapsulated bioglass-chitosan: cytocompatibility, 1 anticoagulant, oxidative stress, mechanical properties and bone collagen cross-links 2 following exposure to ionizing radiation in a rat model. Turk. J. Biol. ISSN:1300-0152E-ISSN:1303 6092; online avlb;15/3/15
33. Hench, L.L., et al.: Interactions between bioactive glass and collagen: a review and new perspectives. J. Aust. Ceram. Soc. **49**(2), 1–40 (2013)
34. Farre-Guasch, E., et al.: Human maxillary sinus floor elevation as a model for bone regeneration enabling the application of one-step surgical procedures. Tissue Eng. Part B Rev., pp 1–14 (2012)
35. Hall, M.B., et al.: Early clinical trials of 45S5 bioglass for endosseous alveolar ridge maintainance implants. In: Excerpta medica proceedings international congress on tissue integration and maxillofacial reconstruction, Brussels, vol. 2, pp. 48–252. Elsevier Science Publishers BV, Amsterdam (1985)
36. Clark, A.E., et al.: Clinical trials of bioglass implants for alveolar ridge maintenance. J Dent Res **65**(spec issue), 304 (1986)

37. Stanley, H.R., et al.: The implantation of natural tooth from bioglass in baboons-long term results. Int. J. Oral Implant **2**, 26–36 (1980)
38. Stanley, H.R., Hall, M., et al.: Research protocol and consent form for project entitled: preservation of alveolar ridge with the intraosseous implantation of root shaped cones made of bio glass. Gainesville FL, University of Florida, J.H.Miller Health Center (1983)
39. Weinstein, A.M., et al.: Implant-bone characteristics of bioglass dental implants. J. Biomed. Mater. Res. **14**, 23–29 (1980)
40. Mistry, S., et al.: Indigenous hydroxyapatite coated and bioactive glass coated titanium dental implant system—fabrication and application in humans. J. Indian Soc. Periodontol. **15**(3), 215–220 (2011)
41. Gilam, D.G., Tang, J.Y., et al.: The effects of a novel bioglass dentrifice on dentine sensitivity: a scanning electron microscopy investigation. J. Oral Rahabil. **30**(4), 446 (2003)
42. Forsback, A.P., et al.: Mineralisation of dentin induced by treatment with bioactive glass s53p4 in vitro. Acta Odontol Scand. **62**(1), 14–20 (2004)
43. Curtis, et al.: Synthesis of nanobioglass and formation of apatite rods to occlude exposed dentine tubules and eliminate hypersensitivity. Acta Biomater. **6**(9), 3740–3746 (2010)
44. Prabhakar, A.R., et al.: Comparison of the remineralising effects of sodium fluoride and bioactive glass using bioerodible gel systems. Dent. Res. Dent. Clin. Dent. Prospect. **3**(4), 11–121 (2009)
45. Jennings, D., et al.: Quantitative analysis of tubule occlusion using NovaMin (sodium calcium phosphosilicate). J. Dent. Res. **83**, 2416 (2006)
46. Burwell, A., et al.: Quantitative tubule occlusion in an in vitro remineralization/demineralization model. J. Dent. Res. **85**, 568 (2006)
47. Litknowski L.J., et al.: A clinical study of the effect of calcium sodium phosphosilicate on dentin hypersensitivity—proof of principle. J. Clin. Dent. **21**, 77–81 (2010)
48. Du, M.Q., et al.: Clinical evaluation of a dentifrice containing calcium sodium phosphosilicate (NovaMin) for the treatment of dentin hypersensitivity. Am. J. Dent. **21**, 210–214 (2008)
49. Sharma, et al.: A clinical study comparing oral formulations containing 7.5 % calcium sodium phsophosilicate (NovaMin), 5 % potassium nitrate, and 0.4 % stannous fluoride for the management of dentin hypersensitivity. J. Clin. Dent. **21**(88–92), 178–180 (2010)
50. Zhang, D., et al.: Antibacterial effects and dissolution behavior of six bio active glasses. J. Control Release **139**(2), 118–26 (2009)
51. Han, P.P., et al.: The cementogenic differentiation of periodontal-ligament cells via the activation of Wnt/β-catenin signalling pathways by Li ions released from bioactive scaffolds. Biomaterials **33**, 6370–6379 (2012)
52. Kamitakahara, M., et al.: J. Ceram. Soc. Jpn. **108**(12), 1117–1118 (2000)
53. Diba, M., et al.: Magnesium-containing bioactive glasses for biomedical applications. Int. J. Appl. Glass Sci. **3**(3), 221–253 (2012)
54. Published Patent 3 July 2014. Pub no WO2014102538 A1 by inventors, Felora MIRVAKILY) Cheryl Miller, Paul V. HATTON
55. Bergey, D., et al.: Organically modified silica nanoparticles: a nonviral vector for in vivo gene delivery and expression in the brain. PNAS **102**(32), 11539–11544 (2005)
56. Zhang, Y., et al.: Delivery of PDGF-B and BMP-7 by mesoporous bioglass/silk fibrin scaffolds for the repair of osteoporotic defects. Biomaterials **33**, 6698e6708 (2012)
57. Zhang, X., et al.: Borate bioglass based drug delivery of teicoplanin for treating osteomyleitis. J. Inorg. Mater. **25**(3), 293–298 (2010)
58. Xie, Z., et al.: Treatment of osteomylelitis and repair of bone effect by degradable bioactive glass releasing vancomycin. J. Control. Release **39**(2), 8–26 (2009)
59. Makoto, O., et al.: A novel skeletal drug delivery system using self setting bioactive glass bone cement III: the invitro drug release from bone cement containing indomethacin and its physicochemical properties. J. Control. Release **31**(2), 118–126 (1994)
60. Pillay, V., et al.: A review of the effect of processing variables on the fabrication of electrospun nanofibers for drug delivery applications. J. Nanomater. Article ID 789289, (2013)

61. Lakhkar, N.J., et al.: Bone formation controlled by biologically relevant inorganic ions: Role and controlled delivery from phosphate-based glasses. Adv. Drug Deliv. Rev. **65**, 405–420 (2013)
62. Van Gestel, N.A.P., et al.: Clinical applications of S53P4 bioactive glass in bone healing and osteomyelitic treatment: a literature review. BioMed Res. Int. ArticleID 68482
63. Young-Phil, K., et al.: Phosphate glass fibres promote neurite outgrowth and early regeneration in a peripheral nerve injury model. J. Tissue Eng. Regen. Med. **9**, 236–246 (2015)
64. Fenoglio, I., et al.: Free radical generation in the toxicity of inhaled mineral particles: the role of iron speciation at the surface of asbestos and silica. Redox Rep. **6**, 235–241 (2001)
65. Prior, S., et al.: Int. J. Pharm. **196**(1), 115–125 (2000)
66. Andriano, K.P., et al.: J. Appl. Biomater. **5**(2), 133–140 (1994)
67. Cohn, D., et al.: Biomaterials **25**(27), 5875–5884 (2004)
68. Fernández, J., et al.: J. Mech. Behav. Biomed. Mater. **9**, 100–112 (2012)
69. Larranaga, A., et al.: Effect of bioactive glass particles on the thermal degradation behaviour of medical polyesters. Polym. Degrad. Stab. **98**, 751–758 (2013)
70. Jones, J.R., et al.: Review of bioactive glass: from Hench to hybrids. Acta Biomater. **9**, 4457–4486 (2013)
71. Martin, R.A. etal.: Characterizing the hierarchial structures of bioactive sol–gel silicate glass and hybrid scaffolds for bone regeneration. Philos. Trans. R. Soc. A 370, 1422–43 (2012)
72. Hench, L.H.: Opening paper 2015—some comments on bioglass: four eras of discovery and development. Biomed. Glasses **1**, 1–11 (2015); De Gruyter Open

MIX
Papier aus verantwortungsvollen Quellen
Paper from responsible sources
FSC® C105338

If you have any concerns about our products,
you can contact us on
ProductSafety@springernature.com

In case Publisher is established outside the EU,
the EU authorized representative is:
Springer Nature Customer Service Center GmbH
Europaplatz 3, 69115 Heidelberg, Germany

Printed by Libri Plureos GmbH
in Hamburg, Germany